GOOD HOUSEKEEPING

HIGH-PROTEIN MEDITERRANEAN COOKBOOK

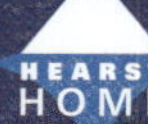

HEARST HOME

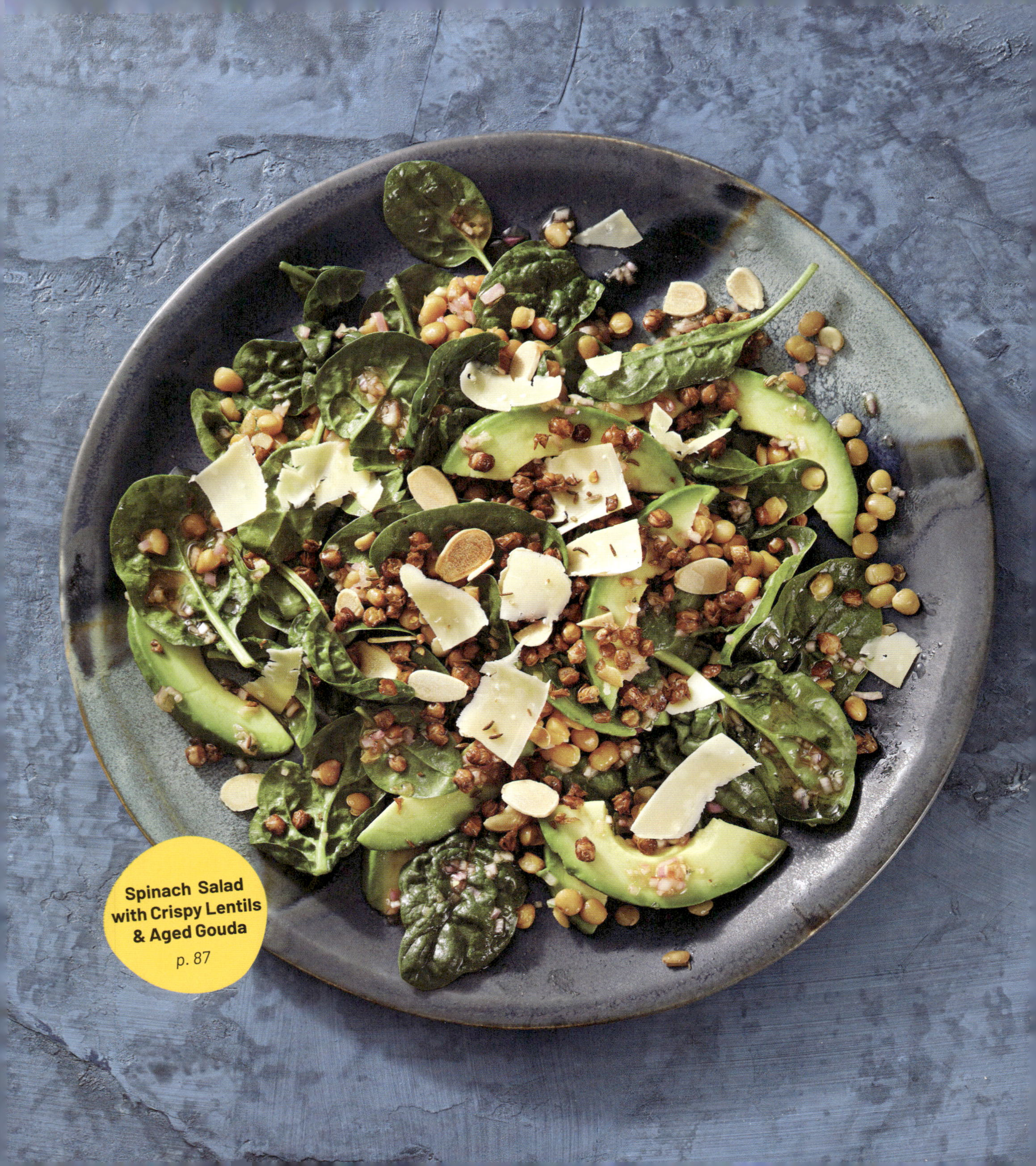
Spinach Salad
with Crispy Lentils
& Aged Gouda
p. 87

CONTENTS

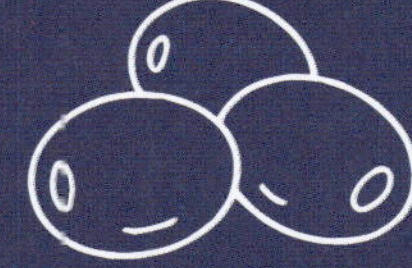

Meet the Editors

Behind every recipe is a team that tested, tasted, and fine-tuned the dish until it was just right. Here, our food and nutrition editors share their favorite dishes, protein hacks, and Mediterranean must-haves to inspire you.

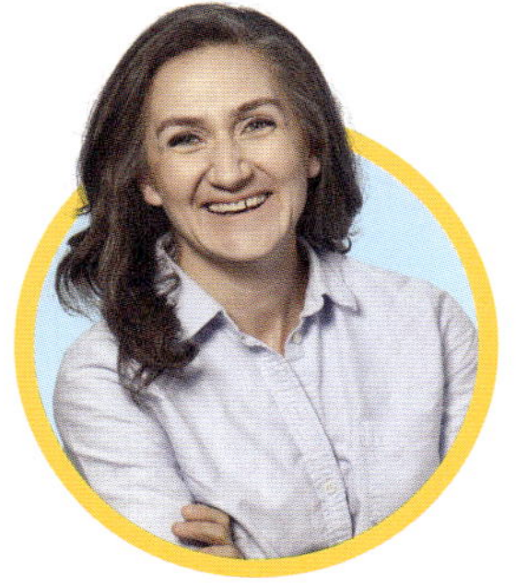

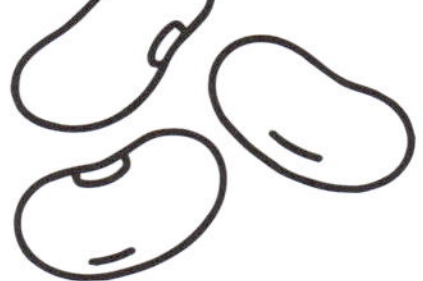

KATE MERKER

Chief Food Director

Q. What's the one ingredient you always keep stocked for quick protein meals?

A. Beans—always beans. They're endlessly versatile and packed with protein. I'll make them the star of a recipe (like in the **Saucy Beans & Farro** on page 106), toss them into salads, blend them into dips, or crisp them up for a crunchy snack. Simple, satisfying, and budget-friendly too.

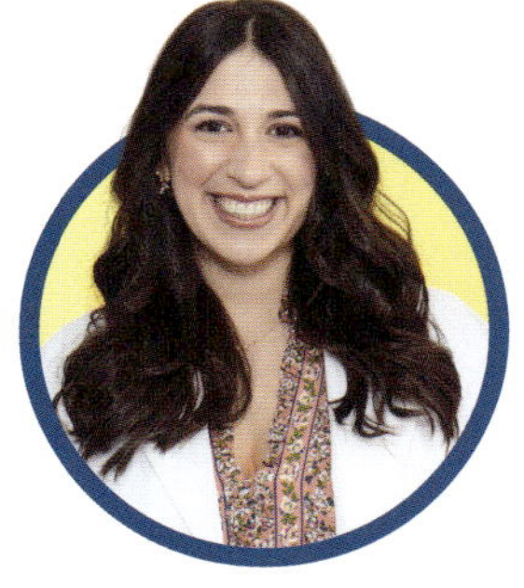

STEFANI SASSOS

MS, RD, CDN, NASM-CPT, Nutrition & Fitness Director

Q. What's your go-to way to hit your protein goals?

A. Definitely plain Greek yogurt! My Yiayia (grandmother) still makes it fresh, and there's truly nothing like it. It's rich, creamy, and packed with protein. I love topping it with walnuts, a drizzle of honey, and fresh berries for sweetness—it's simple, satisfying, and reminds me of home.

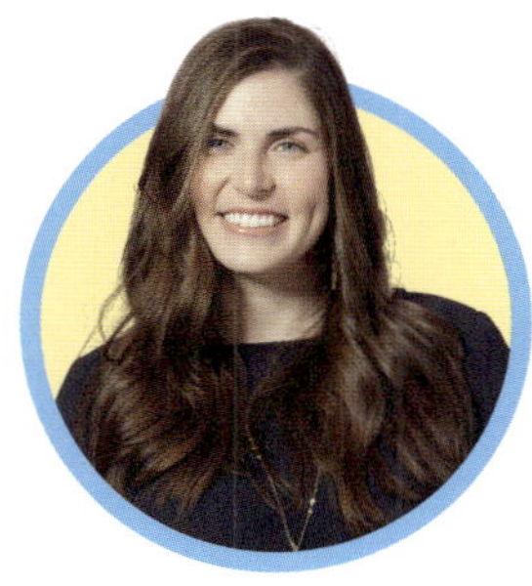

TRISH CLASEN MARSANICO

Deputy Food Editor

Q. What's your ultimate high-protein breakfast?

A. I'm not a big fan of eggs, so hitting my protein goals at breakfast used to be tricky. Then I discovered overnight oats, like the **Carrot Cake** version on page 51. With nut butter, chia seeds, flax, and a scoop of Greek yogurt, it's become my favorite make-ahead protein boost. Plus, it keeps me full all morning!

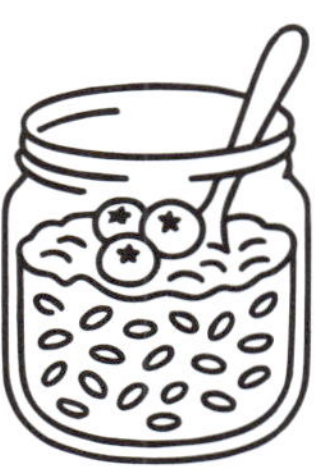

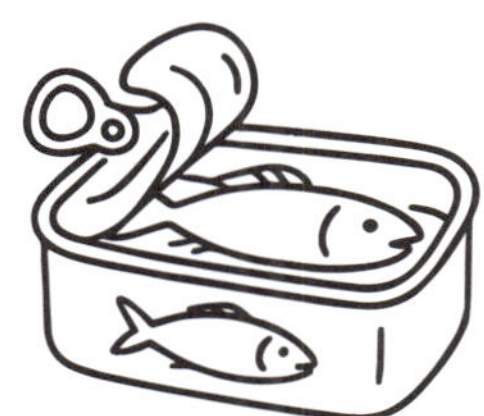

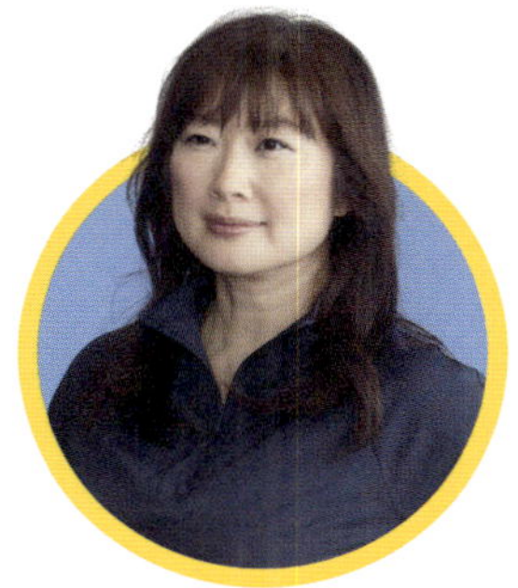

SUSAN CHOUNG

Recipe Editor

Q. What's your favorite high-protein Mediterranean snack?

A. I'm a tinned fish girlie, especially when it comes to canned sardines packed in good olive oil. I love making the **Sardine Toast with Quick-Pickled Spicy Shallots** on page 256. Or I pile these briny flavor bombs on crackers with a squeeze of lemon, crisp cucumber slices, and a dab of chili crisp. Quick, high in protein, and Mediterranean—with a kick.

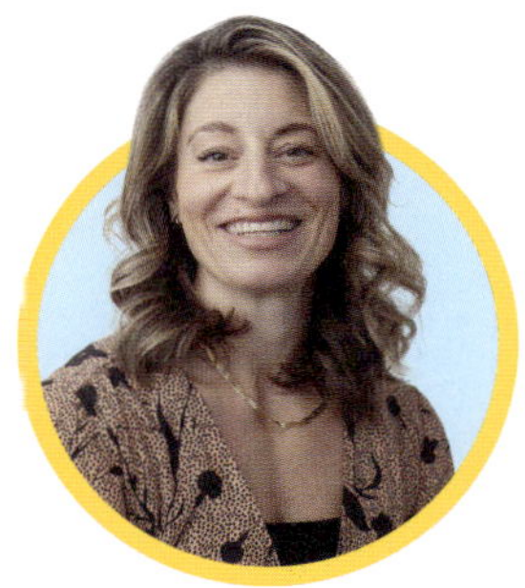

TINA MARTINEZ

Food Producer

Q. What's your go-to kitchen tip when cooking Mediterranean food?

A. When I think Mediterranean cooking, I think bright and fresh flavors. I always add plenty of herbs—parsley, mint, cilantro, or a mix—and finish with a squeeze of lemon and a drizzle of good olive oil. Those little touches make everything taste better.

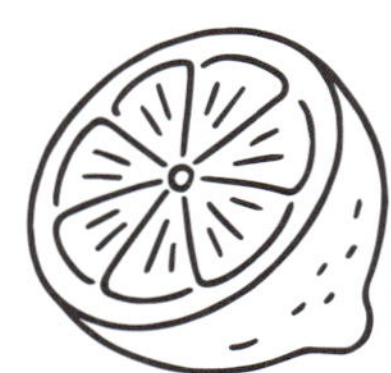

PART 1

GETTING STARTED

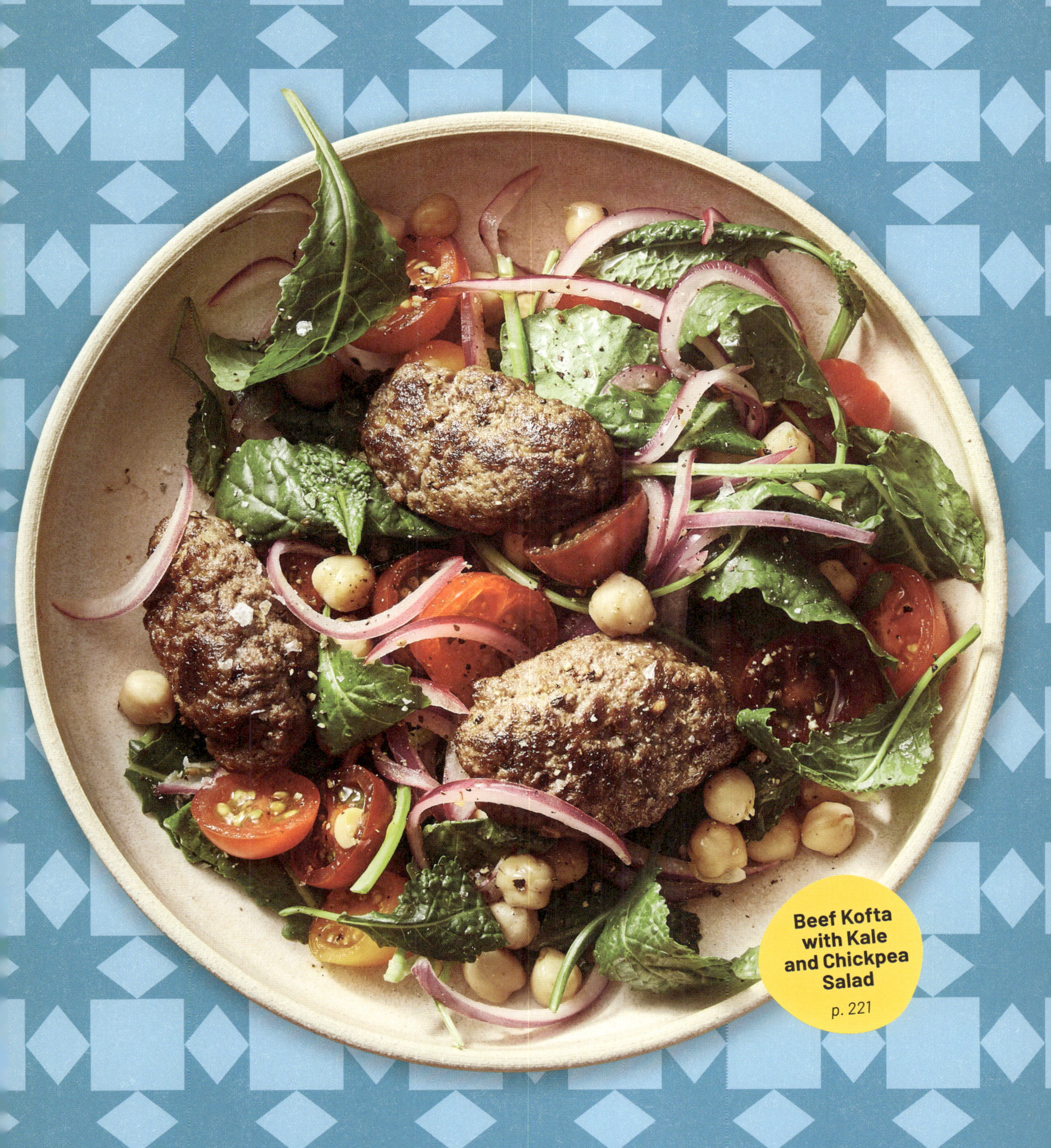

Beef Kofta with Kale and Chickpea Salad

p. 221

Eating the Mediterranean Way

Let's face it—these days, a lot of diets feel like a full-time job, with strict rules around macro-counting, meal timing, and, overall, too much stress. The good news is that a Mediterranean diet takes an entirely different approach. Inspired by the traditional cuisines of the countries bordering the Mediterranean Sea, this simple way of eating is actually more of a lifestyle than a strict plan, which makes it easier to stick with—and a whole lot more delicious.

Unlike fad diets, the Mediterranean style of eating doesn't require you to completely cut out any of your favorites. And how you eat is just as important as what you eat. Shared meals are a cornerstone of the lifestyle. Whether that involves cooking together or sitting down to eat together, community and connection is part of what makes this approach so special and successful.

For generations, people have been eating the Mediterranean way, with an emphasis on seasonal, local, and plant-based foods. But the Mediterranean diet as we know it today first came about in the United States in the 1950s when the Seven Countries Study analyzed the dietary patterns of people living in Italy, Greece, Japan, USA, Finland, the Netherlands, and Yugoslavia. The study found that people living in the Mediterranean had lower rates of heart disease compared to the other countries, due to their menus being rich in healthy fats, fruits and vegetables, lean proteins, legumes, nuts, and whole grains.

By the 1990s, the Mediterranean style of eating was widely promoted by organizations like the World Health Organization and Harvard School of Public Health. And the scientific evidence of the diet's effectiveness has piled up since then: A 2022 meta-analysis published in *Frontiers in Nutrition* found that elderly individuals can reduce their risk of mild cognitive impairment and Alzheimer's by adopting the Mediterranean diet. Evidence also suggests that this way of eating can fight inflammation as you age, which may play a role in protecting your brain and keeping your memory sharp. Plus, it may also prevent chronic diseases such as diabetes.

Today, we're combining this long-proven lifestyle with the power of protein for a fresh approach to the Mediterranean diet. An emphasis on protein is key for both long-term strength and weight health—helping you build muscle, burn fat, and feel fuller longer. The result? A delicious selection of wholesome foods, vibrant recipes, inventive meals, and a well-rounded emphasis on nutrition with long lasting benefits to your overall health—in the short term and in the years to come.

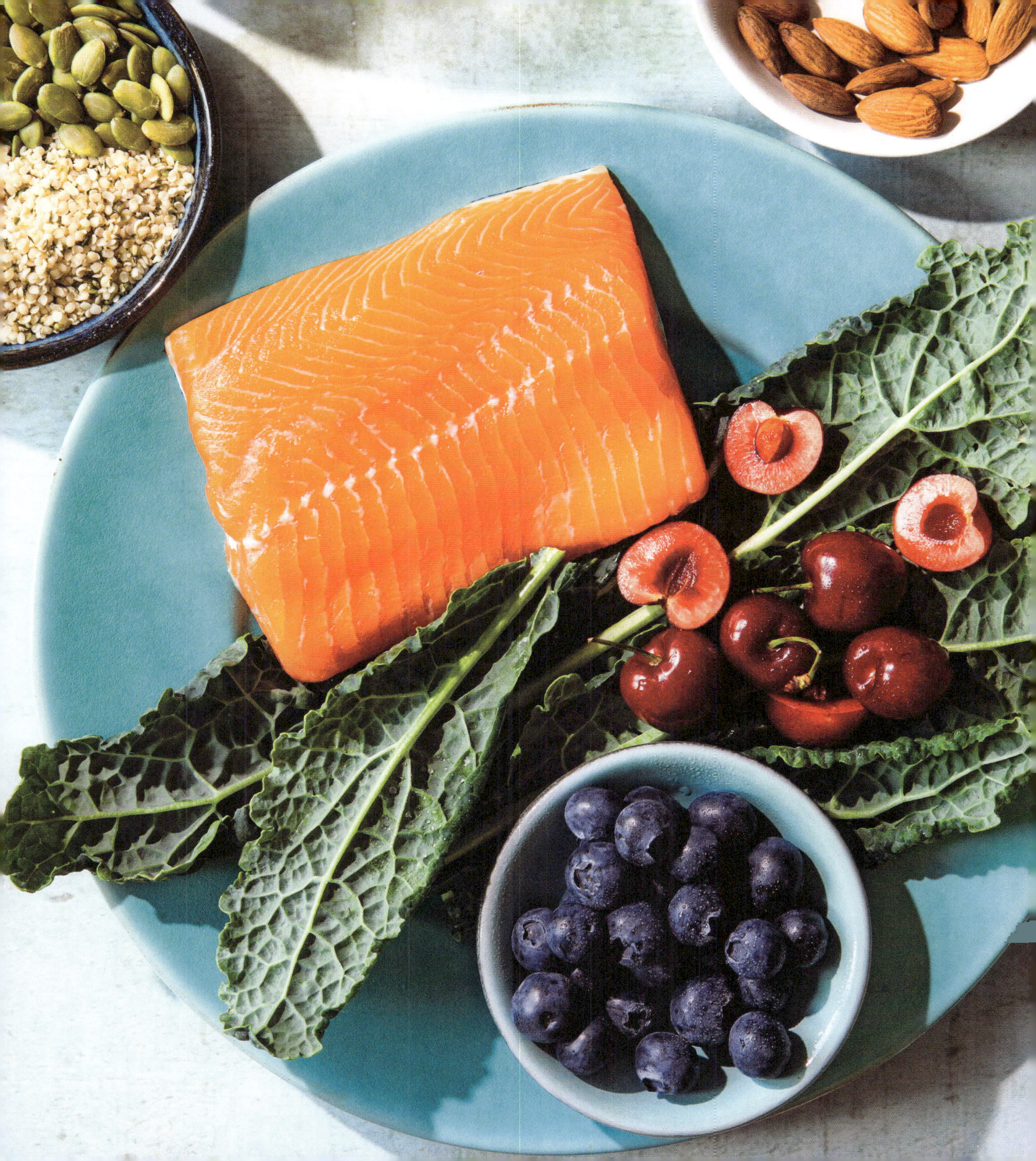

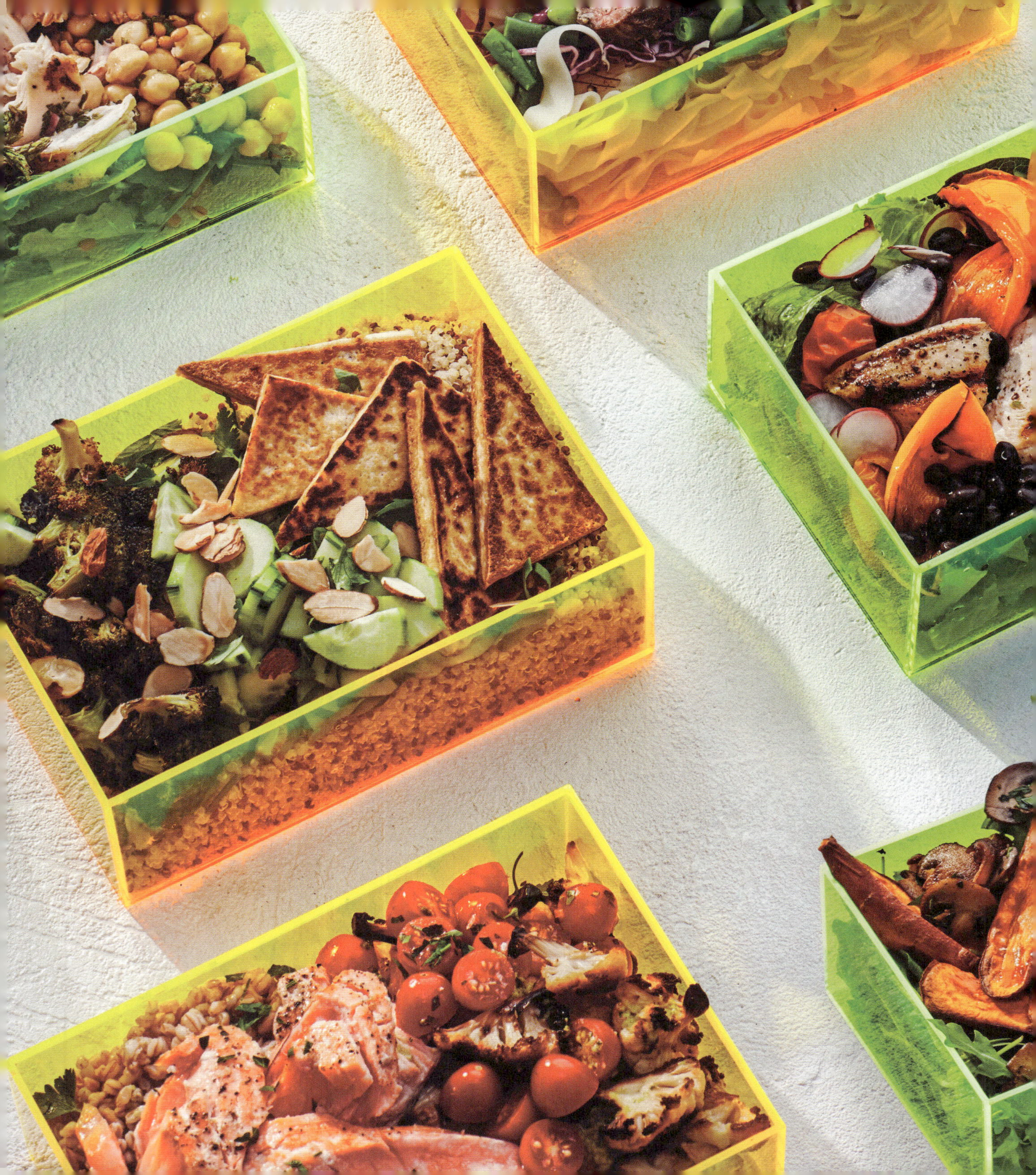

HOW THIS WAY OF EATING COULD CHANGE YOUR LIFE

Decades of research shows that a Mediterranean-style meal plan offers a wide range of health advantages that benefit both your body and mind.

1

SUPPORTS HEART HEALTH

Research has shown that the Mediterranean way of eating may provide heart-healthy benefits, likely thanks to the emphasis on healthy fats like olive oil, nuts, and fatty fish. In fact, women who followed the diet had 25% less risk of developing heart disease over the course of 12 years, according to a 2018 study in *JAMA Network Open*.

2

ASSISTS IN WEIGHT LOSS

A key part of managing weight is managing hunger. A classic Mediterranean-style plate features fiber- and nutrient-rich whole foods that help keep you fuller for longer—and fewer ultra-processed foods that can spike your hunger cravings. Bonus: with such an array of delicious foods to choose from, the Mediterranean style of eating isn't overly restrictive, making it easier to stick with in the long-term.

3

FIGHTS INFLAMMATION

Chronic inflammation is linked to the development of many diseases. But Mediterranean-style eating is packed with antioxidant-rich, anti-inflammatory foods, like dark leafy greens, avocados, and berries. The World Health Organization recommends it to help decrease the risk of dementia, which has been linked to diets high in inflammatory foods.

4

PROMOTES GUT HEALTH

According to a 2022 study published in the *BMJ journal*, people who followed the Mediterranean way of eating had a higher amount of "friendly" gut bacteria. Since all food is ultimately broken down in the gut, a healthy digestive system is crucial for processing and delivering nutrients throughout the body.

5

IMPROVES LONGEVITY

People who follow a Mediterranean way of living tend to live longer and have fewer chronic illnesses. And it's not just the food—it's the lifestyle, centered around slower meals, social connection, and daily movement. It's no wonder that Ikaria and Sardinia, both islands in Greece and Italy respectively, are two of the world's five Blue Zones, or regions where people live the longest.

WHY PROTEIN MATTERS MORE THAN EVER

For as popular as the Mediterranean way of eating is, recently protein has been taking the wellness world by storm—and for good reason. It turns out, the macronutrient isn't just for bodybuilders. Protein is essential for every cell in your body from your organs, muscles, skin, hair, and nails, to your bones. It's key for metabolism, hormone health, immunity, weight loss, and even healthy aging.

Unlike other fad diets, the science backs protein up: initial research from a 2005 Johns Hopkins University study found that a diet in which roughly a quarter of the calories come from lean protein sources reduced blood pressure, LDL ("bad") cholesterol levels, and triglycerides better than a traditional higher-carb diet. Other research finds that diets rich in protein can help prevent obesity, osteoporosis, and diabetes. It helps you feel energized and full for longer and also helps build and support your muscles so that your body can preserve lean body mass and muscle mass while prioritizing losing fat mass instead.

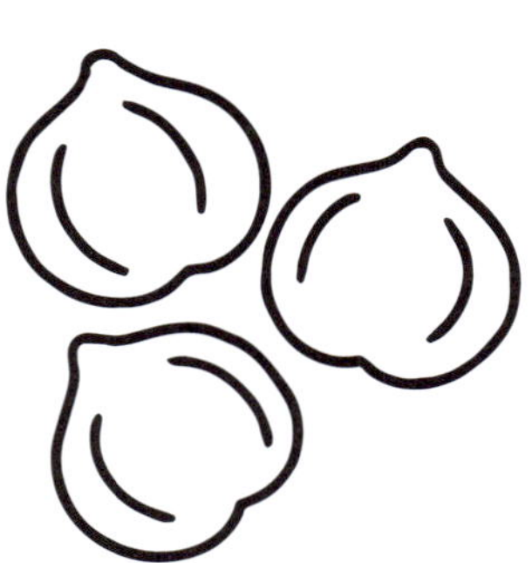

While the Mediterranean diet is best known for its focus on fruits, vegetables, whole grains, and healthy fats, protein also plays a key role. Getting enough protein is about making smart, balanced choices throughout your day. The best protein sources—like fatty fish, lean meats, dairy, beans, nuts, seeds, or soy products—can add delicious nutrition to your meals and snacks. With some simple tweaks and tasty options, hitting your protein goals can be easier than ever.

How Much Protein Do You Need?

Most of us don't have the time or energy to meticulously calculate our macros every meal of the day—particularly if you're following a Mediterranean lifestyle, which focuses on flexibility and sustainability instead of rigid rules. So instead of stressing, a good way to hit your protein goal is to aim for about 20 to 30 grams of protein per meal.

Luckily, that's actually easier to do than most people may think: A chicken breast or salmon fillet about the size of your palm (3-4 ounces), 1 cup Greek yogurt or cottage cheese, a little over half a block of tofu (5 ounces), 4 large eggs, 1.5 cups cooked lentils, a heaping cup of cooked quinoa—all can give you 20 to 30 grams of protein on their own.

Officially, the recommended daily allowance (RDA) from the Food and Nutrition Board of the National Academy of Sciences has long held that most adults need 0.8 grams of protein per kilogram of bodyweight (or 0.36 grams per pound). But other experts say that's simply

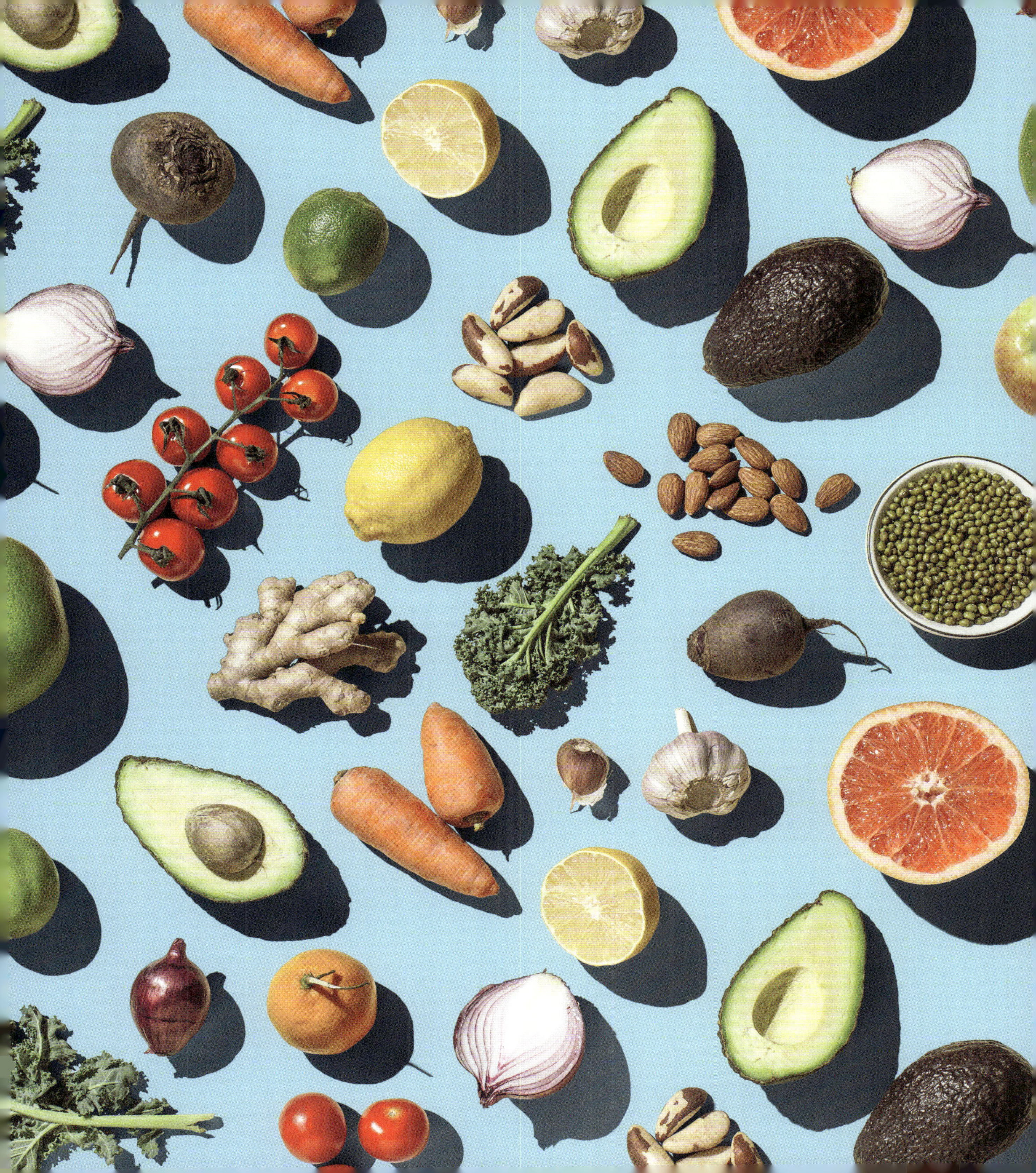

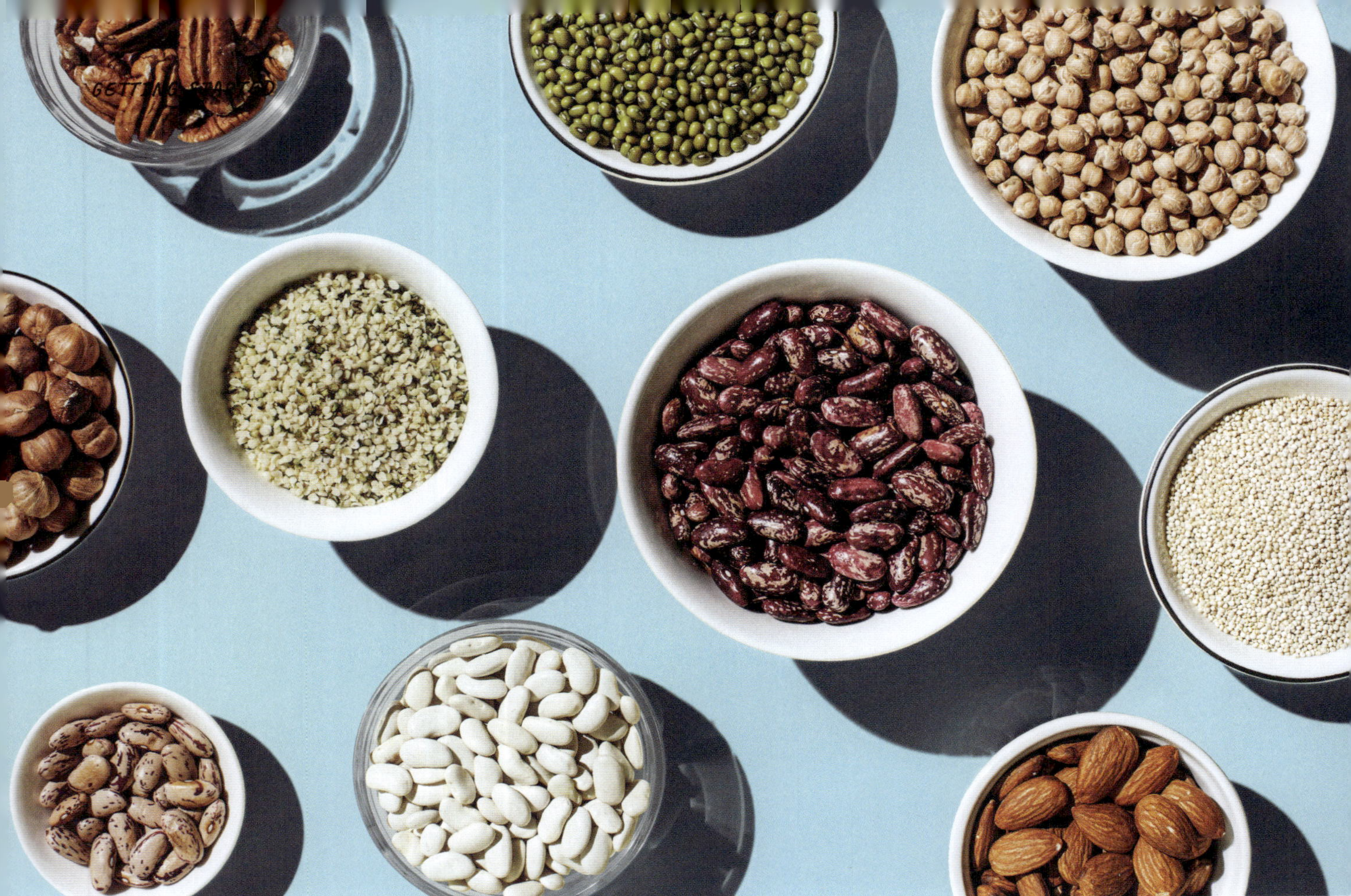

a baseline, or the minimum amount you need to eat daily to stay healthy—and that women, those over 60 years old, and those who are active, likely need much more than that, since those populations are even more prone to losing lean body mass.

Many researchers are now saying the recommendations should be closer to 1.2 to 1.5 grams of protein per kilogram of bodyweight (or 0.55 to 0.68 grams per pound). According to these recommendations, a 140-pound person should be eating at least 76 to 95 total grams of protein per day. If those numbers sound overwhelming, don't stress—start by aiming for the minimum RDA (0.36 grams of protein per pound) and slowly work your way up from there.

Timing Is Everything: When to Eat Protein

When we say to aim for 20 to 30 grams of protein per meal, we really do mean *per meal*. That's because the body doesn't store amino acids (which make up protein) the way it does carbs or fat. While extra carbohydrates are stored in the body as glycogen and surplus fat is stored as body fat, amino acids aren't stockpiled in the same way.

Rather, your body uses the protein you eat at that specific meal to support essential functions like metabolism, hormone production, bone maintenance, and muscle protein synthesis. Once your body takes what it needs, the excess amino acids are converted into fat or glucose. That's why it's crucial to include protein consistently throughout the day, from breakfast to lunch to dinner. This helps ensure a steady supply of amino acids to fuel your body's needs around the clock.

Now, if you're like most Americans, you're probably getting the bulk of your protein at dinner. Women between the ages of 20 and 49 were found, on average, to consume about 40% of their daily protein at dinner and just 18% at breakfast, according to a survey conducted by the U.S. Department of Agriculture's (USDA) Agriculture Research Service.

One of the biggest unsung benefits of spacing out your protein throughout the day instead of cramming it all in at dinner? You'll probably get less hungry.

Complete vs. Incomplete Proteins

COMPLETE PROTEINS

- Animal proteins *(chicken and turkey, fish and seafood, lean meat, eggs, etc.)*
- Dairy *(milk, cottage cheese, yogurt, etc.)*
- Whole soy *(tofu, tempeh, edamame, etc.)*
- Quinoa & buckwheat

INCOMPLETE PROTEINS

- Legumes/pulses *(beans, peas, lentils, chickpeas, etc.)*
- Nuts/seeds *(peanut butter, almonds, sunflower seeds, tahini, etc., apart from pistachios, which are a complete protein)*
- Whole grains *(steel-cut oats, brown rice, barley, farro, etc.)*

When you start to prioritize protein, particularly at breakfast, you'll feel more satiated throughout the day and your blood sugar will likely stay more stable as the day wears on, meaning more energy and fewer cravings. Even more reason to start your day with delicious Mediterranean protein-packed breakfasts like eggs with whole-grain bread or Greek yogurt with fruit and nuts.

The Proteins That Power a Healthier You

When it comes to protein, it's not just about how much you're eating. Quality plays a huge role too. Protein is made up of 20 amino acids—think of them as the building blocks for growing and repairing our body's tissues, as well as many other important functions. Only 11 of those amino acids are naturally produced by your body itself, which means that the remaining nine—called the "essential amino acids"—must come from the food you eat on a daily basis.

Luckily, some protein sources contain all nine essential amino acids—those are called complete proteins—and they're a great way to knock out all nine in one shot. Other incomplete proteins include some (but not all) of the essential amino acids, so eat a variety of those to ensure you're piecing together the daily puzzle of all the essential amino acids your body needs. When paired together, certain combos of incomplete proteins (like rice and beans, or peanut butter and whole-grain toast) can give your body all nine essential amino acids. (Don't worry—we've made this easy for you in our recipes and meal plan so you don't have to count amino acids all day long!)

So which is better: complete or incomplete proteins? While it's true that animal proteins are complete proteins and typically have higher protein counts, gram for gram, than their plant-based (and often incomplete) counterparts, incomplete sources also often come packed with fiber and antioxidants. So you need both types to keep your muscles strong and to support good collagen production. Don't worry about eating certain essential amino acids at every meal. Instead, focus on getting a variety of protein sources over the course of the entire day.

PAIRING PLANT PROTEINS

Some combos of incomplete proteins create a complete protein, giving your body all nine essential amino acids it needs.

PROTEIN COMBOS	COMPLETE PROTEIN MEALS
Legumes + Whole grains	Hummus + pita Beans + rice Lentil soup + whole-grain bread
Nuts or seeds + Legumes or whole grains	Peanut butter + chia + oatmeal Almonds + pumpkin seeds + lentil salad
Vegetables (leafy greens, broccoli) + legumes + whole grains	Broccoli + chickpea + barley bowl Spinach lentil stew + brown rice

Simple Strategies for Success

You don't need hours upon hours to make delicious and nourishing high-protein Mediterranean dishes. With the handy hints and shortcuts outlined here, you can spend less time in the kitchen and more time savoring every bite.

Prep Your Kitchen

You're more likely to make healthy choices when you have nutritious and delicious ingredients on hand. Use the list on page 18 to stock your fridge and pantry with high-protein Mediterranean staples to help you create flavorful dishes on the fly and stay consistent.

Find Your Favorite Ingredients

The key to mastering any new style of eating is planning ahead. After looking through the recipes in this book, select a handful of base ingredients you love and recipes you can quickly prepare, to save your future self time and effort on busy nights. Bonus: When you incorporate your favorite ingredients into your weekly menu, you'll look forward to every meal.

Batch Cook Base Ingredients

When you're short on time to cook, it's easy to turn to processed foods or your favorite takeout spot. Batch cooking is the easy answer. Grains, firm veggies, and certain proteins can be bulk-prepped at the beginning of the week, then added to lunches, dinners, and more. Many grocery stores also sell pre-prepped staples you can stock your fridge with as well, from steamed lentils to spiralized sweet potato and grilled chicken strips.

Get More Life From Leftovers

Save yourself the time and hassle of making a new dish for every meal by using leftovers. Most can be refrigerated in airtight containers for two to five days. Store meats, vegetables, and dressings separately to maintain optimal freshness and give yourself flexibility for future uses.

Freeze Now, Feast Later

Make a big-batch meal, then freeze some for when you're pressed for time. Nutrient-dense soups, stews, and chilis all freeze (and defrost) easily. Let your cooked food cool completely, then divide it into individual portions so you'll only defrost what you need. Label it with the name of the dish and the date, so you can follow the "first in, first out" rule.

PANTRY STAPLES

All the recipes in this book are packed with fresh produce, lean proteins, seafood, and healthy fats. Here are some delicious ingredients that you might find useful when stocking your fridge and pantry to add the power of protein plus Mediterranean flavor and flare to every meal.

HEARTY WHOLE GRAINS

- ☐ Barley
- ☐ Buckwheat
- ☐ Bulgur
- ☐ Couscous
- ☐ Farro
- ☐ Oats
- ☐ Quinoa
- ☐ Whole-grain bread & pasta

ANTIOXIDANT-RICH PRODUCE

- ☐ Apples
- ☐ Artichokes
- ☐ Berries
- ☐ Citrus (*oranges, lemons*)
- ☐ Cucumbers
- ☐ Dark leafy greens (*spinach, kale*)
- ☐ Dates & figs
- ☐ Eggplant
- ☐ Peppers
- ☐ Potatoes & root vegetables (*sweet potatoes, carrots*)
- ☐ Stone fruit (*apricots, cherries, peaches*)
- ☐ Tomatoes
- ☐ Zucchini

HEALTHY FATS

- ☐ Avocado
- ☐ Extra-virgin olive oil
- ☐ Nuts & seeds (*almonds, walnuts, pine nuts, pistachios, sunflower seeds*)
- ☐ Olives
- ☐ Tahini

POWERFUL PROTEINS

- ☐ Cheese (*feta, goat, Parmesan*)
- ☐ Eggs
- ☐ Fatty fish (*salmon, sardines, tuna, mackerel*)
- ☐ Greek-style yogurt
- ☐ Legumes (*lentils, chickpeas, beans*)
- ☐ Poultry (*chicken, turkey*)
- ☐ Red meat (*limited to a few times a month*)
- ☐ Shellfish (*shrimp, mussels, clams*)

HERBS & SPICES

- ☐ Fresh or dried herbs (*basil, dill, mint, oregano, rosemary, sage, thyme*)
- ☐ Spices (*black pepper, cinnamon, coriander, crushed red pepper flakes, cumin, garlic powder, onion powder, paprika, sumac, turmeric*)
- ☐ Spice blends (*za'atar*)

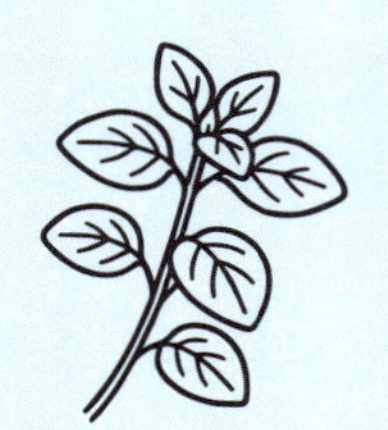

Spice Cabinet Smarts

Keep your seasonings in tip-top shape with these tricks.

- Replace dried herbs and spices at least every two years
- Buy spices you don't use often in smaller amounts—you'll have less waste
- Group spices together by type and usage on carousels, racks, or designated shelves

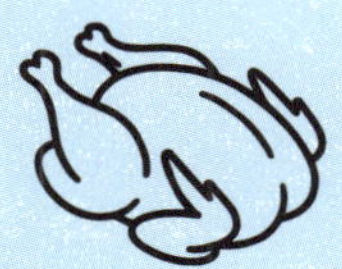

All-Star Ingredients

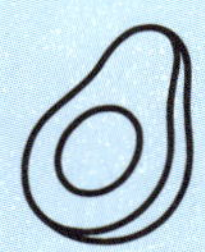

Ancient Grains

Grains like farro, quinoa, barley, buckwheat, and oats have great texture and rich flavor, and are also loaded with nutrients (particularly fiber). Whip up a batch for the week to use in pilafs, grain bowls, or salads. Quinoa is both gluten-free and a complete plant-based protein. Tip: Cook your grains in bone broth versus water for an added boost of protein and flavor.

Avocado

Avocados are rich in mono- and poly-unsaturated fats, the healthy kinds of fats that are abundant in Mediterranean-style meals and reduce your risk of heart disease and stroke. Slice and freeze leftover avocado to add to smoothies and more.

Beans & Lentils

Legumes are versatile staples in Mediterranean kitchens. They provide a shelf-stable protein source and a slew of vitamins and minerals. Use them to add a dose of filling fiber and plant-based protein to any meal. When choosing canned varieties, opt for low- or reduced-sodium. Dried beans require soaking, but offer a wider variety.

Eggs

Each egg provides a hefty dose of 6 grams of complete protein, plus choline, a nutrient that's essential for brain development, memory, and nerve function. Boiled eggs are popular in Mediterranean cuisine—plus, they make a great protein-rich snack

Extra-Virgin Olive Oil

The primary oil used in Mediterranean cooking, traditional uses include everything from salad dressings and roasted vegetables to seafood marinades and dips like hummus. Look for high-quality olive oils that ideally come from a single origin, like Greece, Italy, or Spain. When cooking at higher temps, opt for avocado oil, which has an even higher smoke point.

Greek Yogurt

This popular protein-rich food is incredibly versatile. It makes for a filling snack, a healthy substitute for sour cream or a creamy addition to salad dressings. Look for plain, unsweetened varieties and use fruit to naturally sweeten your yogurt parfait.

Herbs & Spices

Whether your spices and herbs come from the pantry or your garden, they offer tremendous health benefits and are a fantastic way to add depth, aroma, and flavor to food without the need for extra salt, which helps support heart health and lower blood pressure—both goals of the Mediterranean style of eating.

Leafy Greens

The Mediterranean way of eating relies heavily on vegetables, in particular vitamin- and antioxidant-rich leafy greens such as spinach, kale, arugula, or a mixed greens medley. Enjoy them in salads, sautéed dishes, or omelets.

Nuts & Seeds

A common snack in the Mediterranean, nutrient-packed nuts and seeds are powerhouses of protein, healthy fat, vitamins, minerals, and fiber. Regularly eating a moderate amount of nuts and seeds has been linked to a reduced risk of heart disease, improved brain function, and better weight management. Eat them raw or dry-roasted without added salt or sugar for the greatest health benefits.

Sumac

This unique spice comes from dried berries of the sumac bush. Typically sold in powder form, sumac has a beautiful red color and a tart, almost lemony flavor. Add some to hummus, stir into marinades, or sprinkle on kebabs.

PART 2

POWER PLATES

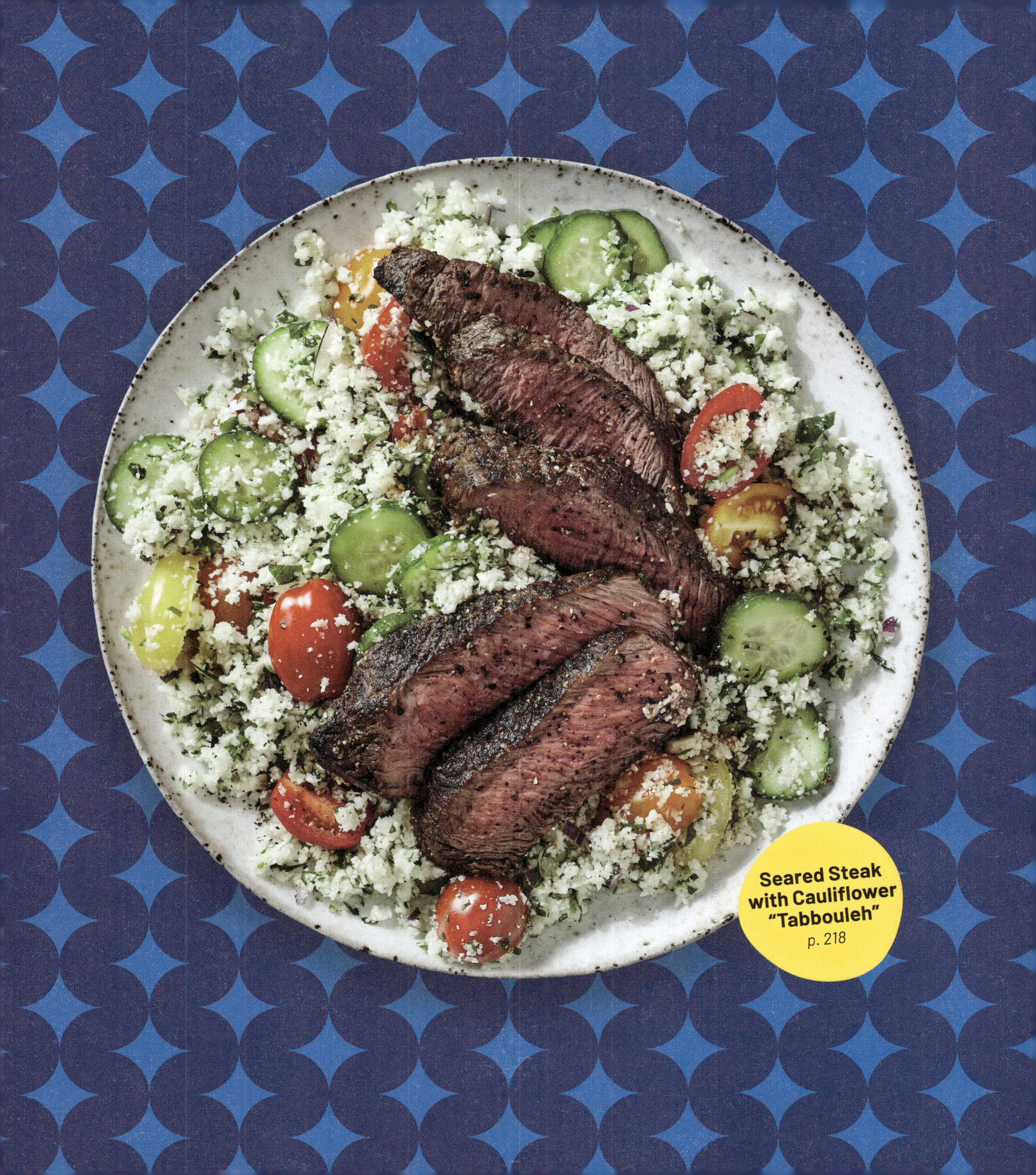
Seared Steak
with Cauliflower
"Tabbouleh"
p. 218

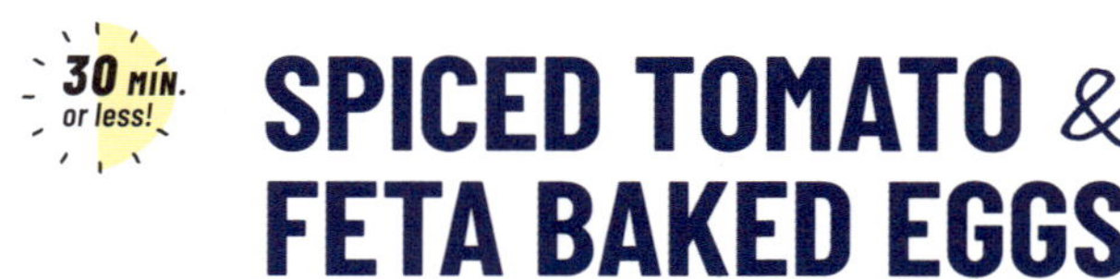

SPICED TOMATO & FETA BAKED EGGS

ACTIVE 20 min. **TOTAL** 25 min. **SERVES** 4

2 pints grape tomatoes, halved if large

2 Tbsp olive oil, divided

½ tsp smoked paprika

Kosher salt and pepper

¾ tsp coriander seeds

¾ tsp cumin seeds

6 oz feta cheese, crumbled

8 large eggs

⅓ cup basil leaves, roughly chopped

1 Tbsp fresh lemon juice

5-oz pkg. mixed greens

4 slices country bread, toasted

1. Heat the oven to 450°F. On a rimmed baking sheet, toss tomatoes with 1 tablespoon oil, smoked paprika, and ½ teaspoon each salt and pepper. Roast until tomatoes start to release liquid and break down, 8 minutes.
2. Meanwhile, using a mortar and pestle, crush coriander and cumin seeds until coarsely ground.
3. When tomatoes are ready, sprinkle evenly with feta. Using the back of a spoon, create 8 wells (1 for each egg) in tomatoes, then sprinkle with ground coriander and cumin seeds. Bake until cheese is slightly melted, 2 to 3 minutes. Crack 1 egg into each well and bake until egg whites are just set, 3 to 5 minutes more. Sprinkle with basil.
4. Meanwhile, in a large bowl, whisk lemon juice with remaining tablespoon oil. Add greens and ¼ teaspoon each salt and pepper and toss to coat. Serve alongside baked eggs with toast.

PER SERVING *About 452 cal, 27 g fat (10.5 g sat), 410 mg chol, 1,117 mg sodium, 38 g carb, 4 g fiber, 6 g sugar (1.5 g added sugar), 24 g pro*

KITCHEN TIP

A mortar and pestle is a traditional kitchen tool used to grind or mash herbs, spices, or seeds. Don't have one? Pop seeds into a zip-top bag, seal, then gently crush them with a rolling pin or a jar.

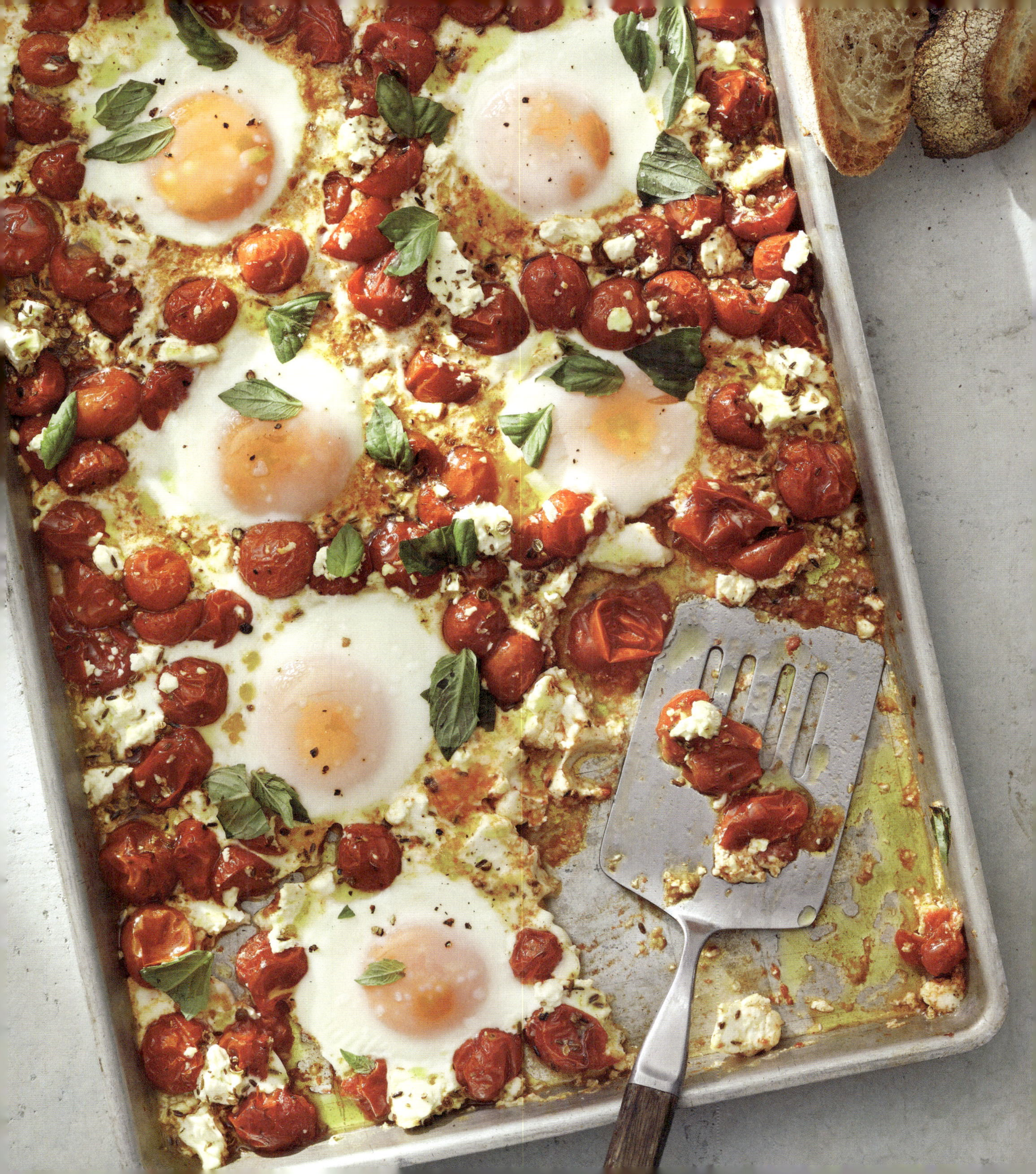

SMOKED TROUT, RED ONION & CRÈME FRAÎCHE

ACTIVE 15 min. **TOTAL** 15 min. **SERVES** 4

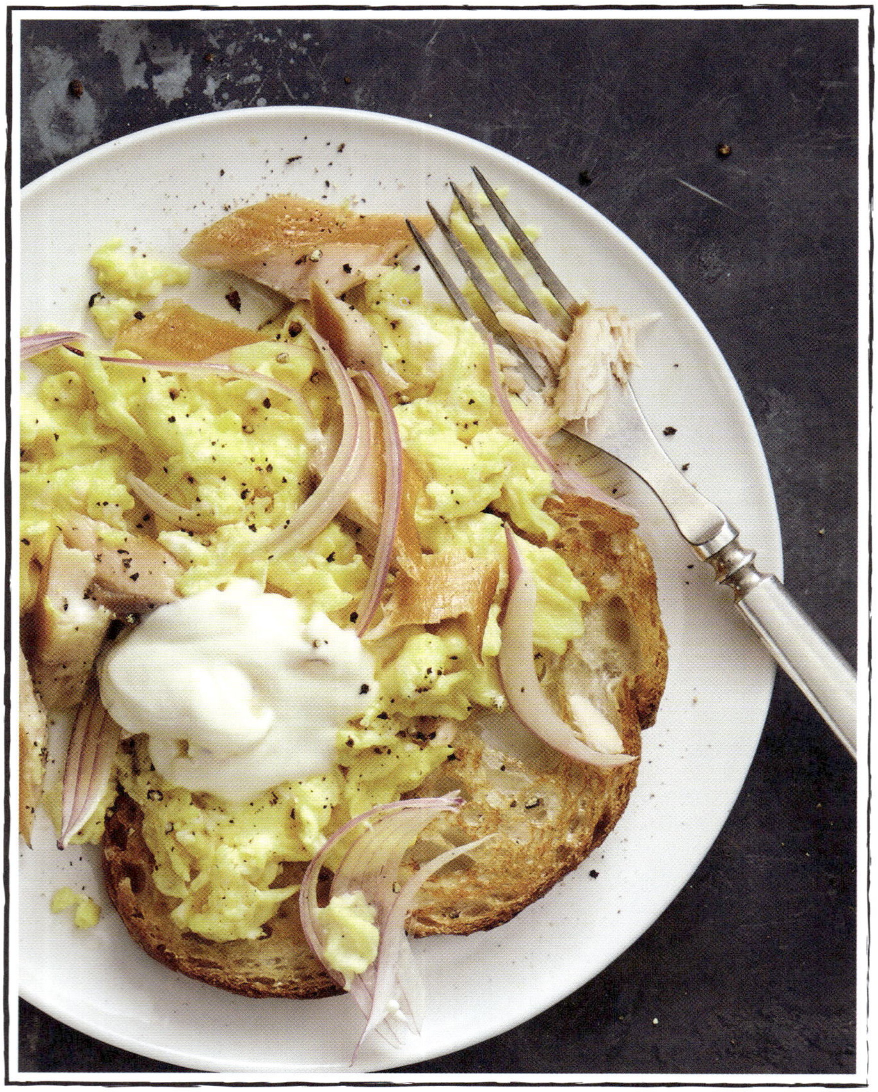

- 8 large eggs
- Kosher salt and pepper
- 1 Tbsp olive oil or unsalted butter
- ¼ cup crème fraîche, plus more for serving
- ½ cup flaked smoked trout
- ½ small red onion, thinly sliced
- 4 slices Ezekiel sprouted whole grain bread, toasted

1. In a large bowl, whisk together eggs, 1 tablespoon water, and ½ teaspoon each salt and pepper.

2. Heat oil or butter in a 10-inch nonstick skillet over medium heat. Add eggs and cook, stirring with a rubber spatula every few seconds, to desired doneness, 2 to 3 minutes for medium-soft eggs.

3. Fold crème fraîche, then trout and red onion into scrambled eggs. Dollop with additional crème fraîche and serve with toast.

PER SERVING *About 351 cal, 21 g fat (8 g sat), 417 mg chol, 464 mg sodium, 17 g carb, 3 g fiber, 1.5 g sugar (0 g added sugar), 21 g pro*

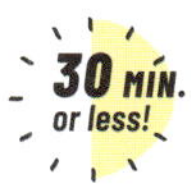

SMASHED AVOCADO TOAST *with* EGG

ACTIVE 25 min. **TOTAL** 25 min. **SERVES** 2

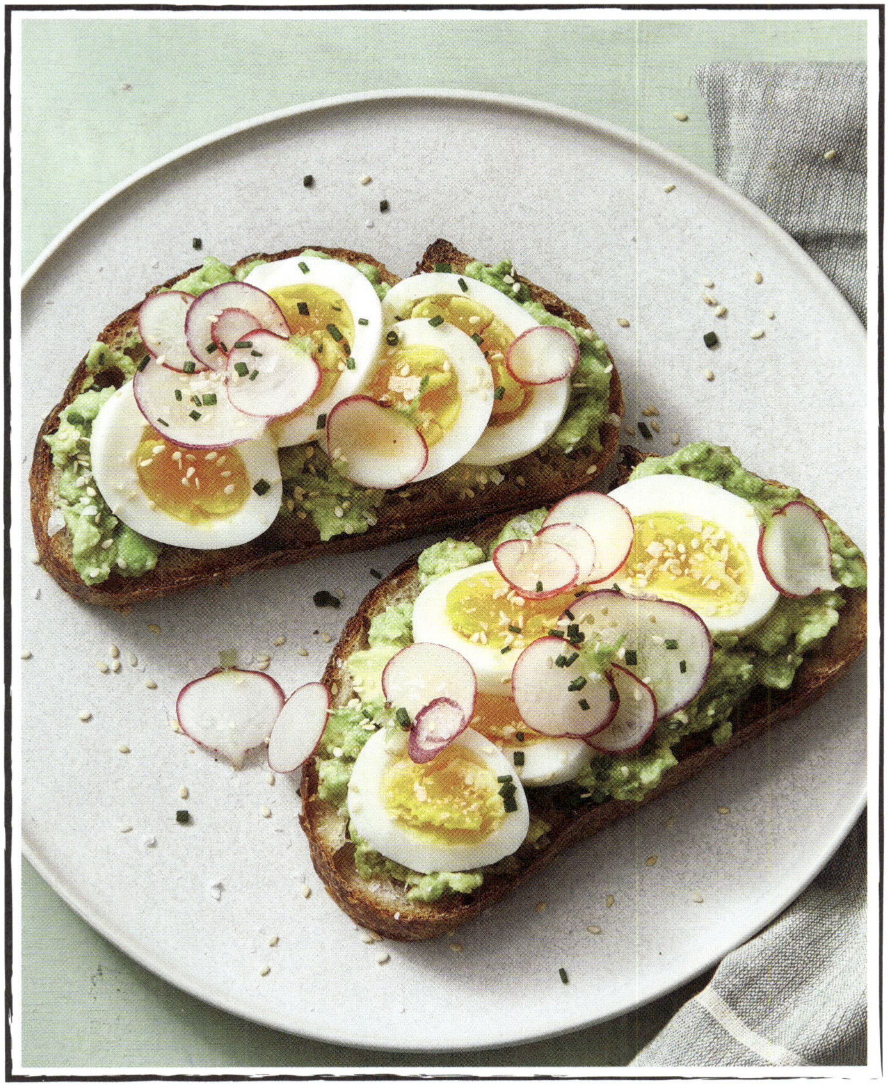

- 1 ripe avocado
- 1 Tbsp fresh lemon juice
- Kosher salt and pepper
- 4 slices Ezekiel sprouted whole grain bread, toasted
- 6 hard-boiled eggs, peeled and sliced
- 1 bunch small multicolored radishes, thinly sliced
- Chopped fresh chives and sesame seeds, for serving

1. In a medium bowl, smash avocado with lemon juice and ¼ teaspoon each salt and pepper.

2. Spread on toast and top with eggs and radishes and sprinkle with chives and sesame seeds.

PER SERVING *About 485 cal, 27 g fat (5.5 g sat), 373 mg chol, 527 mg sodium, 41 g carb, 13 g fiber, 2 g sugar (0 g added sugar), 23 g pro*

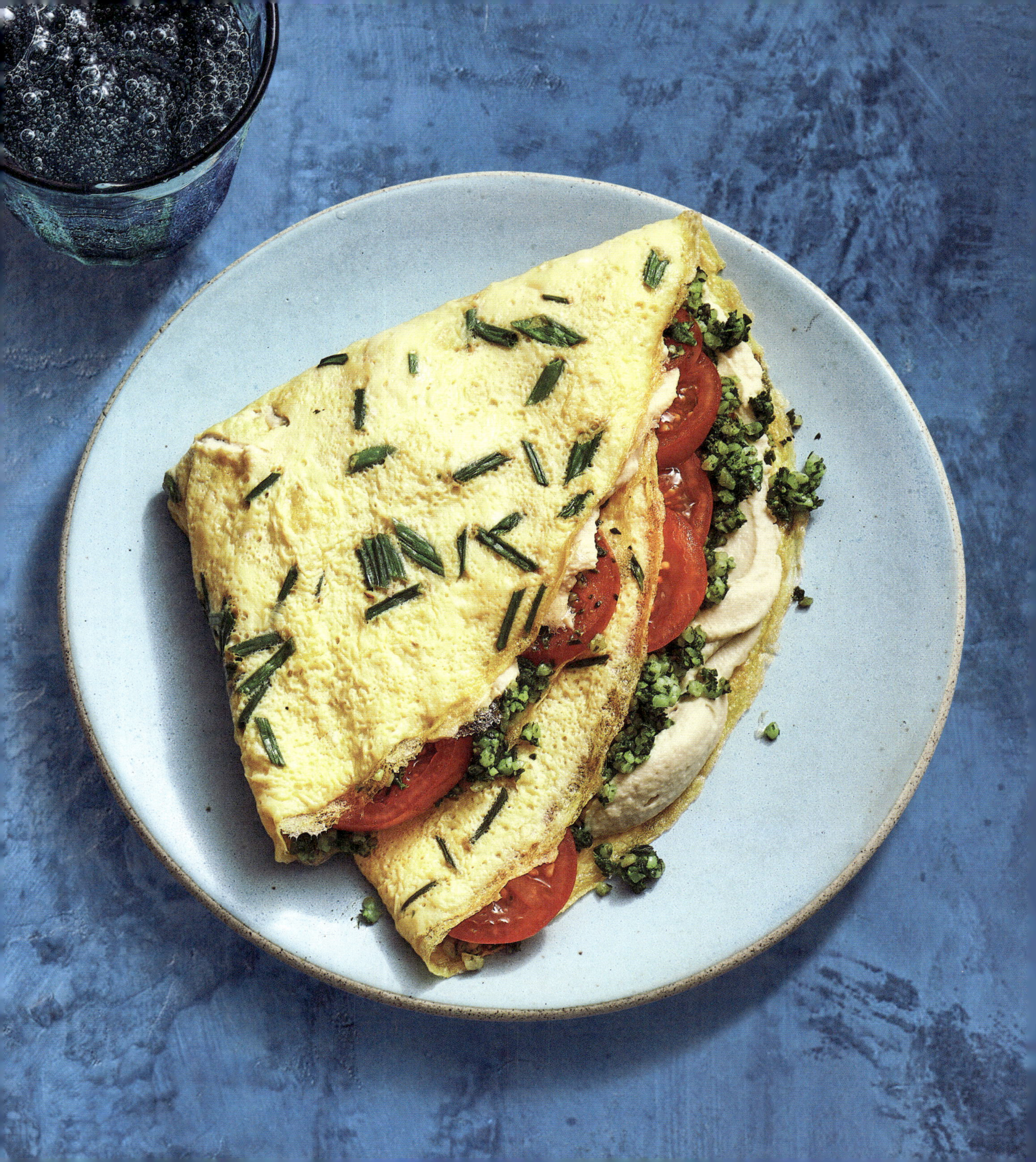

SPINACH & LEMON HUMMUS EGG WRAPS

ACTIVE 40 min. **TOTAL** 40 min. **SERVES** 4

½ cup bulgur

7 large eggs

Kosher salt

¼ cup bias-cut chives, plus ⅓ cup roughly chopped chives (from 1¼ bunches)

Nonstick cooking spray

2 cups baby spinach

1¼ cups flat-leaf parsley leaves

½ tsp ground cumin

1 cup roasted almonds

1 Tbsp olive oil

¾ cup lemon hummus

1 large heirloom tomato, very thinly sliced

1. Bring 1 cup water to a boil in a medium saucepan. Stir in bulgur and simmer, covered, until nearly tender, 9 minutes. Remove from heat and let sit, covered, 3 minutes, then fluff with a fork.
2. Meanwhile, in a food processor, pulse eggs, 3 tablespoons water, and ¼ teaspoon salt to combine. Stir in bias-cut chives. Transfer to bowl, then clean the food processor.
3. Heat a 10-inch nonstick pan over medium-low heat. Spray lightly with nonstick spray and add one-fourth of egg mixture, swirling to coat surface. Cook, undisturbed, until bottom just barely turns golden brown and top is set, 3 to 4 minutes. Release edges with a spatula; then, using fingers, carefully grab edges and flip wrap. Cook 10 seconds. Transfer to a wire rack and repeat with remaining egg mixture to make 3 more wraps.
4. In a food processor, pulse spinach, parsley, cumin, and remaining ⅓ cup chives to finely chop. Add almonds, oil, and ½ teaspoon salt and pulse to finely chop nuts. Fold into bulgur.
5. Lay egg wraps on work surface, pretty side down, and spread each bottom half with hummus. Top with bulgur (about ½ cup per wrap; you will have some left over), pressing to adhere, and then with tomato. Fold over top half of wrap. Fold once more to create a quarter-fold, then serve.

PER SERVING *About 426 cal, 27.5 g fat (4.5 g sat), 326 mg chol, 903 mg sodium, 27 g carb, 8 g fiber, 4 g sugar (0 g added sugar), 20 g pro*

OPEN-FACE FRITTATA SANDWICHES

ACTIVE 25 min. **TOTAL** 55 min. (plus cooling) **SERVES** 8

- 2 pints grape tomatoes
- 1 Tbsp olive oil, plus more for greasing
- ½ tsp red pepper flakes
- 14 large eggs
- Kosher salt and pepper
- 1 lb broccoli crowns, finely chopped
- 4 scallions, chopped
- 11-oz pkg. fully cooked Italian chicken sausage, halved lengthwise and sliced
- 4 oz sharp white Cheddar, coarsely grated (about 1¼ cups), divided
- 8 slices Ezekiel 4:9 bread, toasted

1. Arrange the racks in upper and lower thirds of oven. On a small rimmed baking sheet, toss tomatoes with oil and red pepper flakes, place in oven on lower rack and then heat oven to 450°F (this may take 15 to 30 minutes). Continue roasting until tomatoes begin to burst and are golden brown on top, 6 to 15 minutes, depending on initial preheat time. Let cool 5 minutes, then gently mash to create a thick spread.
2. Meanwhile, line a large rimmed baking sheet (11½- by 17-in.) with parchment paper; coat parchment and sides of pan with oil.
3. In large bowl, whisk eggs with ½ teaspoon each salt and pepper; fold in broccoli and scallions, then sausage and all but ½ cup cheese. Spread mixture on the prepared baking sheet.
4. Sprinkle with remaining cheese and bake until frittata is set, slightly puffed, and starting to turn golden brown, 17 to 20 minutes. Cut into 16 portions.
5. To serve, spread each toast with 2½ to 3 tablespoons tomato jam and top with 2 slices frittata.

PER SERVING *About 376 cal, 19.5 g fat (7 g sat), 370 mg chol, 666 mg sodium, 27 g carb, 6 g fiber, 2.5 g sugar (0 g added sugar), 28 g pro*

MAKE IT AHEAD

The tomatoes and frittata can be refrigerated separately for up to four days. When ready to serve, gently warm frittata slices in a 325°F oven for 10-15 minutes to keep them fluffy and avoid drying out. Toast the bread, then top with the tomato jam just before serving. You can also wrap frittata slices individually in plastic and freeze for up to two months. Thaw in the refrigerator overnight.

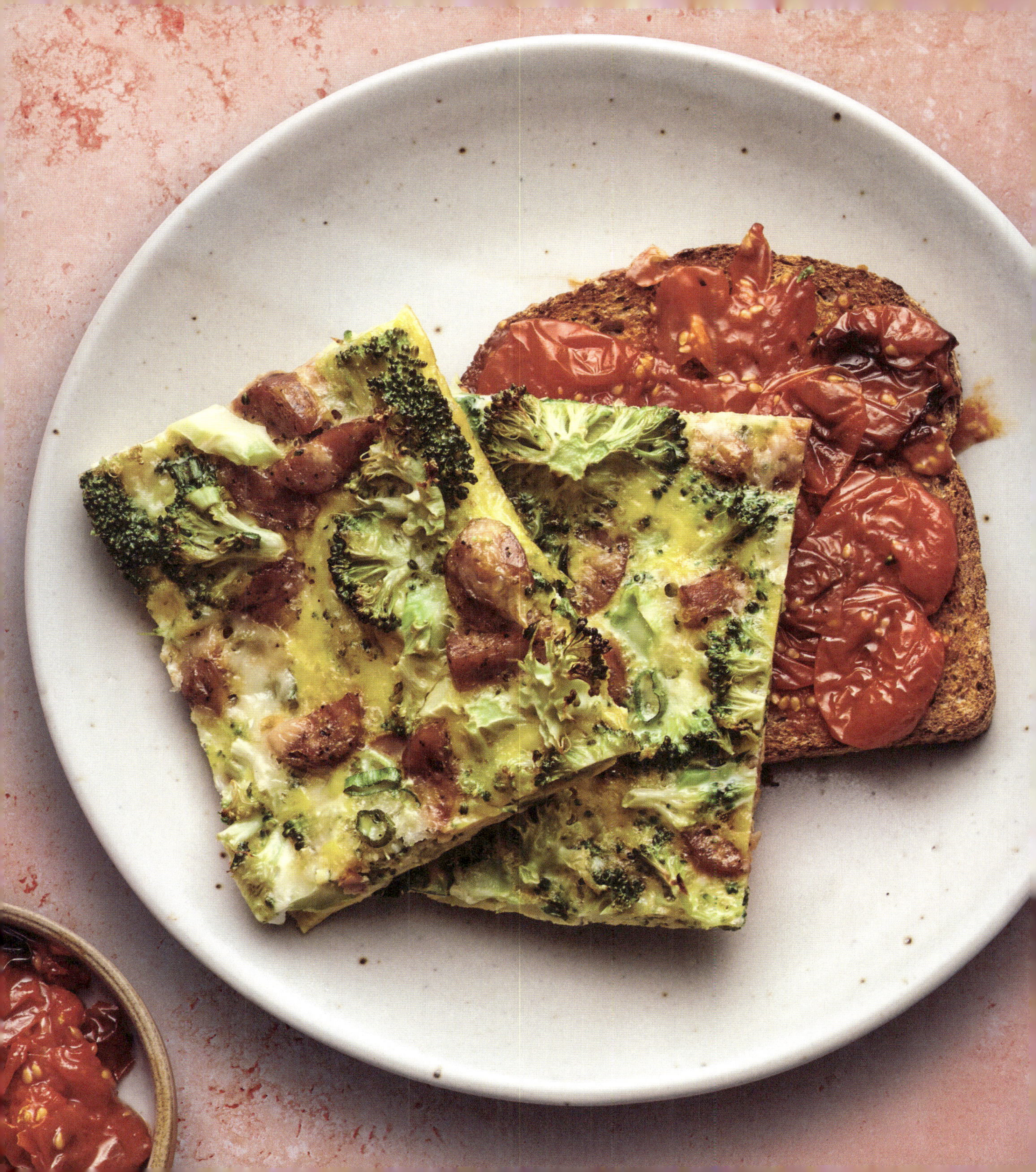

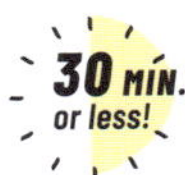

CLASSIC OMELET & GREENS

ACTIVE 20 min. **TOTAL** 20 min. **SERVES** 2

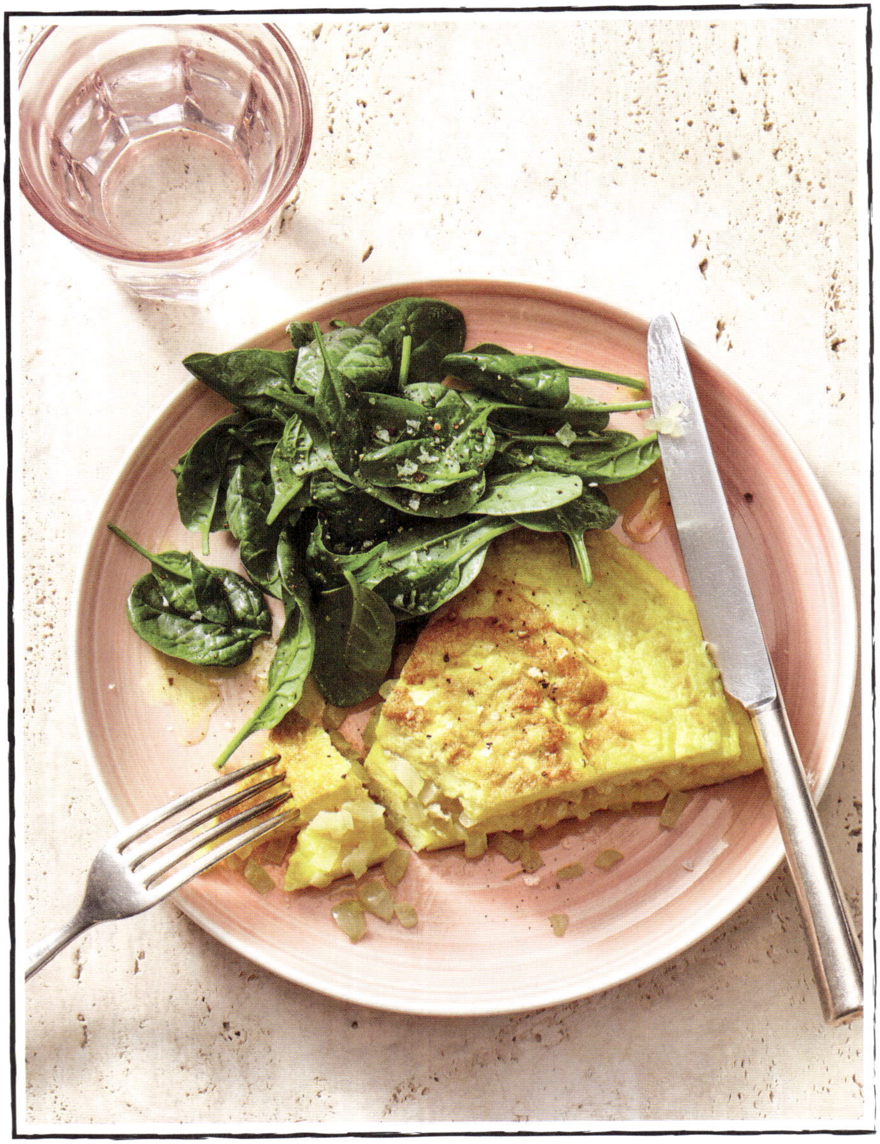

2 Tbsp olive oil, divided
1 small yellow onion, finely chopped
5 large eggs
Kosher salt and pepper
1 Tbsp unsalted butter
½ oz Parmesan, finely grated (about ¼ cup)
1 Tbsp fresh lemon juice
4 cups baby spinach

1. Heat 1 tablespoon oil in a medium nonstick skillet over medium heat. Add onion and sauté until tender, about 6 minutes. Transfer to a bowl.

2. In a large bowl, whisk eggs, 1 tablespoon water, and ½ teaspoon salt. Return the skillet to medium and add butter. Add eggs and cook, stirring constantly with rubber spatula, until partially set. Turn heat to low and cover the pan tightly until eggs are just set, 2 to 4 minutes. Top with onion and Parmesean; fold in half.

3. In a bowl, whisk lemon juice, remaining tablespoon oil and pinch each salt and pepper. Toss with spinach and serve with omelet.

PER SERVING *About 415 cal, 33.5 g fat (10.5 g sat), 486 mg chol, 948 mg sodium, 9 g carb, 3 g fiber, 2.5 g sugar (0 g added sugar), 21 g pro*

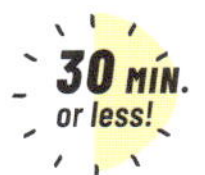

GRAIN BOWL *with* SAUTÉED SPINACH

ACTIVE 10 min. **TOTAL** 10 min. **SERVES** 2

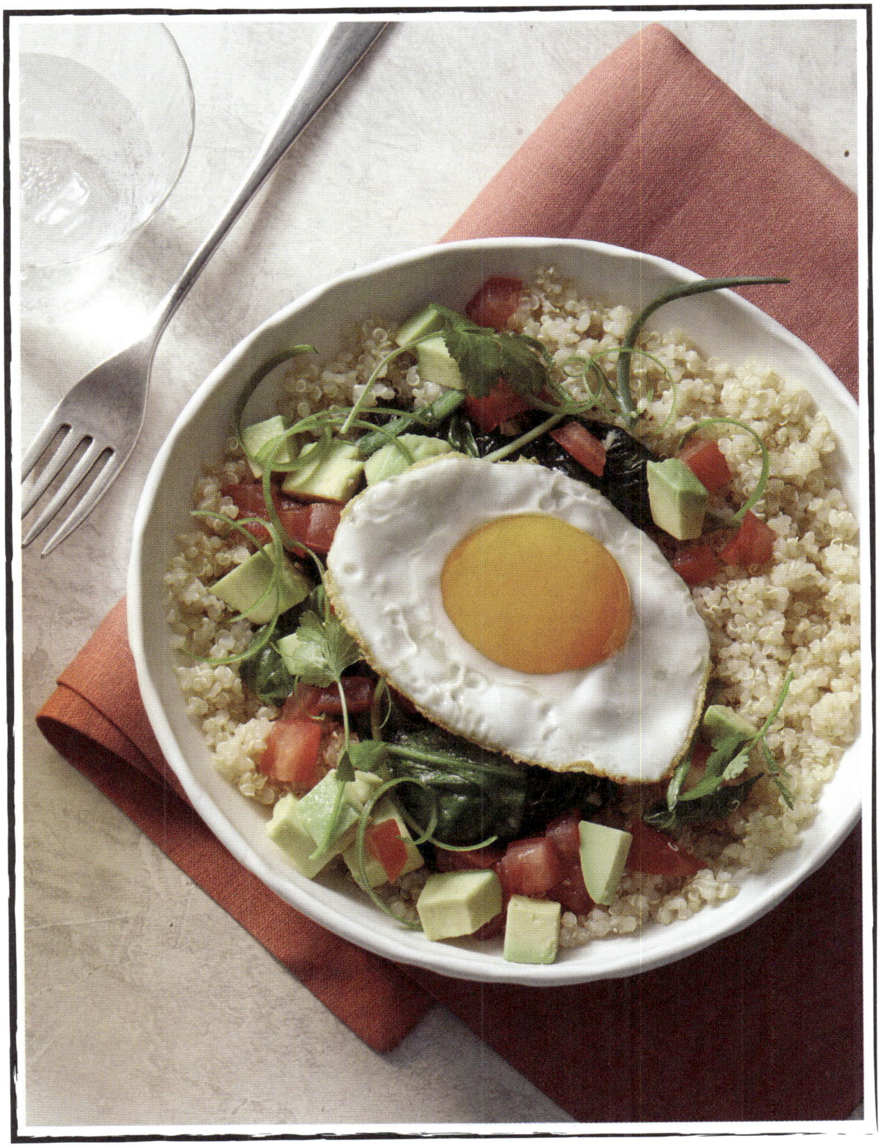

- 2 cups cooked grains (such as farro, brown rice, quinoa), warmed
- 1 Tbsp olive oil
- 1 clove garlic, finely chopped
- 1 bunch spinach, thick stems discarded, leaves roughly chopped (about 4 cups)
- Kosher salt and pepper
- 1 medium tomato, cut into 1-in. pieces
- ½ avocado, diced
- 4 large eggs

1. Divide grains between 2 bowls. In a large nonstick skillet over medium heat, heat oil and garlic until garlic starts to turn golden brown, 1 minute. Add spinach, and ¼ teaspoon each salt, and pepper and cook, tossing, until leaves begin to wilt, 1 to 2 minutes. Spoon on top of grains along with tomato and avocado.

2. Return the skillet to medium heat and cook eggs to desired doneness, 2 to 3 minutes for runny yolks. Serve on top of grain bowls.

PER SERVING *About 534 cal, 27.5 g fat (5.5 g sat), 372 mg chol, 450 mg sodium, 50 g carb, 11 g fiber, 4 g sugar (0 g added sugar), 24 g pro*

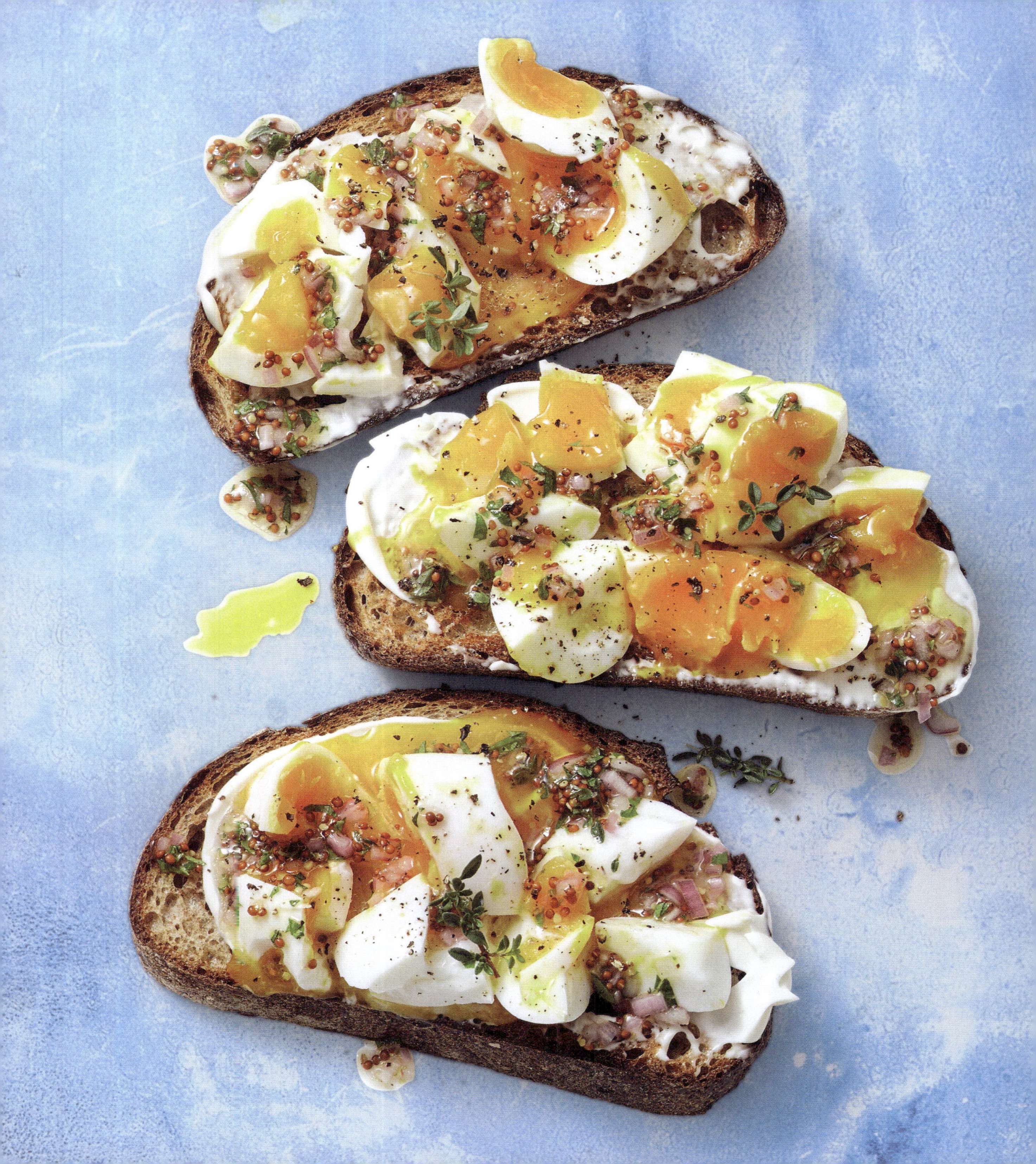

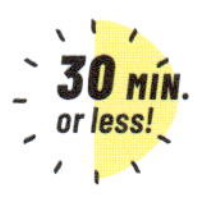

JAMMY EGG TOASTS *with* SHALLOT VINAIGRETTE

ACTIVE 10 min. **TOTAL** 15 min. **SERVES** 2

- 2 Tbsp white wine vinegar
- 1 small shallot, finely chopped
- ½ tsp fresh thyme, plus more for sprinkling
- Kosher salt and pepper
- 4 large eggs
- 1 Tbsp olive oil
- 2 tsp whole-grain mustard
- 1 Tbsp chopped flat-leaf parsley, plus more for sprinkling
- 2 Tbsp small curd cottage cheese
- 1 Tbsp mayonnaise
- 4 thick slices country bread, toasted

1. In a small bowl, combine vinegar, shallot, thyme, and ¼ teaspoon each salt and pepper. Let sit, tossing occasionally, 10 minutes.
2. Meanwhile, bring a medium saucepan of water to a boil and fill a medium bowl with ice water. Reduce heat so water is at rapid simmer, gently add eggs and simmer 6 minutes. Immediately transfer eggs to ice water to stop cooking. Drain and peel eggs.
3. Stir oil, mustard, and parsley into shallot mixture. Combine cottage cheese and mayo and spread on bread, then coarsely chop eggs and arrange on top of bread. Spoon shallot vinaigrette over top and sprinkle with more thyme, parsley, and cracked pepper if desired.

PER SERVING *About 505 cal, 24.5 g fat (5 g sat), 377 mg chol, 1083 mg sodium, 48 g carb, 3 g fiber, 4 g sugar (0.5 g added sugar), 21 g pro*

KITCHEN TIP

Letting shallots sit in vinegar softens their sharp bite and mellows their flavor, turning them tangy, sweet, and deliciously pickled—perfect for adding a zesty kick to salads, sandwiches, or grains.

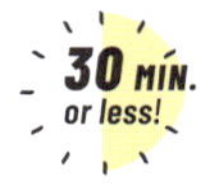

TURKISH EGGS *with* GREEK YOGURT

ACTIVE 15 min. **TOTAL** 15 min. **SERVES** 2

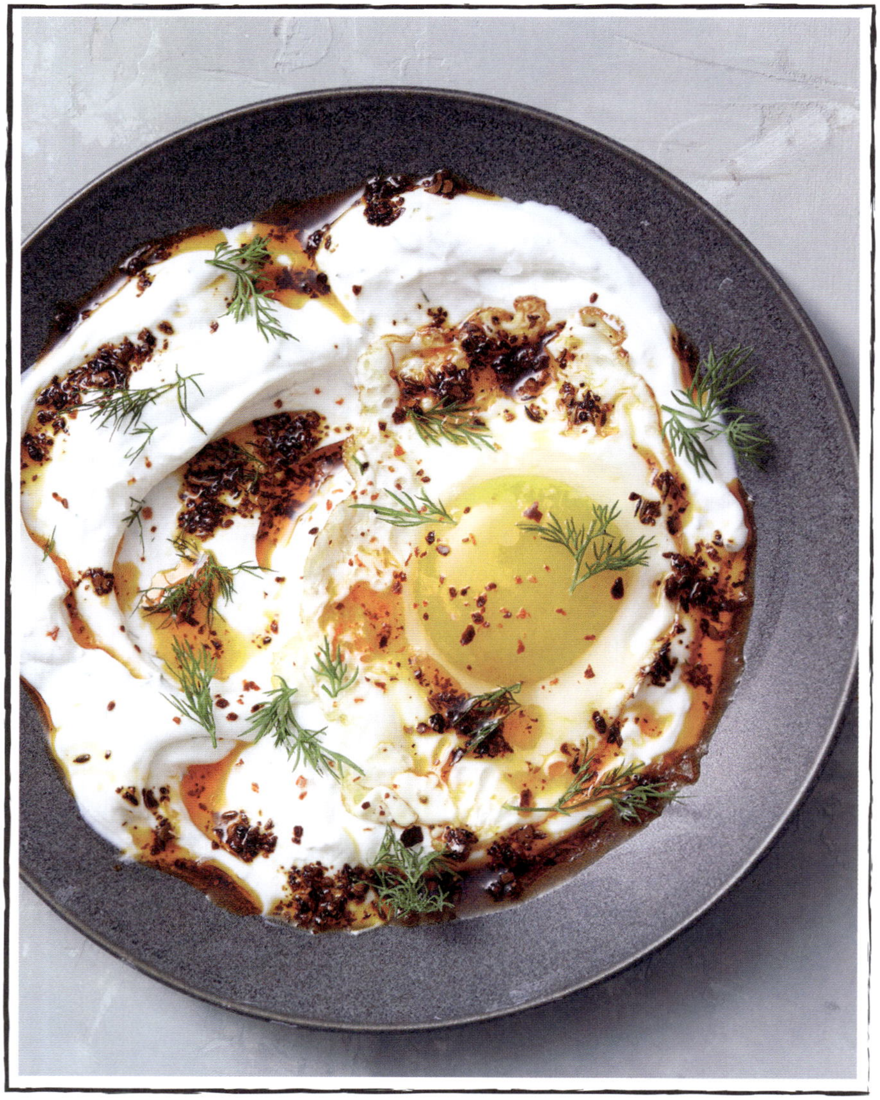

1. In a bowl, combine ¾ cup plain **Greek yogurt** (at room temp), ¼ cup **dill** (chopped), ½ teaspoon grated **garlic**, and ¼ teaspoon **kosher salt**. Heat 1 tablespoon **olive oil** in a medium nonstick skillet over medium heat until warm. Remove from heat, stir in 1¼ teaspoon **Aleppo pepper** and ¼ teaspoon **cumin seeds**, and let sit 4 minutes. Spoon half of oil into small bowl and reserve.

2. Return skillet with remaining oil to medium heat and cook 2 **large eggs** to desired doneness, about 2 minutes for runny yolks.

3. Spoon yogurt onto 2 plates, spreading out. Top with eggs, reserved oil, and dill. Sprinkle with additional Aleppo pepper and **flaked salt** if desired and serve with toasted **Ezekiel sprouted whole grain bread**.

PER SERVING *About 230 cal, 16.5 g fat (5 g sat), 198 mg chol, 346 mg sodium, 5 g carb, 1 g fiber, 4 g sugar (0 g added sugar), 20 g pro*

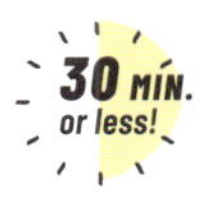

SCRAMBLED EGG TOAST *with* TOMATO AND PARMESAN

ACTIVE 10 min. **TOTAL** 10 min. **SERVES** 4

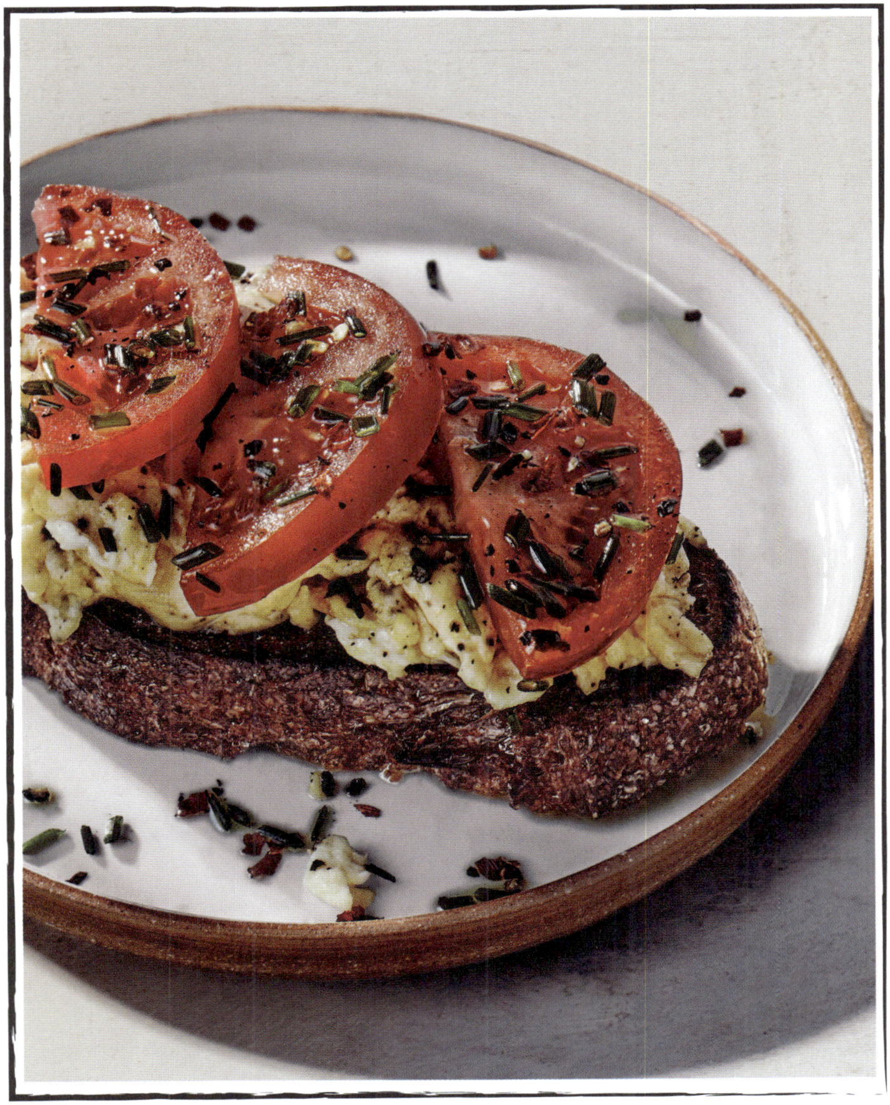

1. Heat 1 tablespoon **olive oil** in a medium nonstick skillet over medium-low heat. In a large bowl, whisk together 3 large **eggs** and ½ teaspoon each **kosher salt** and **pepper**. Add eggs to a skillet and cook, stirring often, until eggs are beginning to set.

2. Once eggs are nearly set, stir in 2 tablespoons chopped fresh **chives** and 2 tablespoons freshly grated **Parmesan**, then spoon over 4 slices **Ezekiel sprouted whole grain bread**, toasted. Top with 1 large **tomato**, halved and sliced, and a drizzle of oil if desired. Sprinkle with chives and cracked pepper.

PER SERVING *About 303 cal, 14.5 g fat (4 g sat), 374 mg chol, 580 mg sodium, 23 g carb, 4 g fiber, 5.5 g sugar (3 g added sugar), 24 g pro*

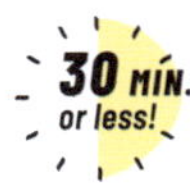

SMOKED SALMON OMELET

ACTIVE 10 min. **TOTAL** 10 min. **SERVES** 1

½ small red onion, thinly sliced

1½ cup watercress (tender leaves and stems)

1 tsp fresh lemon juice

1¼ tsp avocado oil, divided

Kosher salt and pepper

2 large eggs

1 Tbsp Greek yogurt

1½ oz smoked salmon, torn into pieces

1. In a medium bowl, gently toss together red onion, watercress, lemon juice, ¼ teaspoon oil, and a pinch each of salt and pepper.
2. Heat remaining teaspoon oil in a small to medium nonstick skillet over medium heat. In a bowl, whisk eggs and a pinch of salt until no visible strands of egg white remain. Add eggs to the pan and cook, shaking the pan and stirring constantly with silicone spatula, pulling in more-cooked eggs at perimeter of the pan to mingle with less-cooked interior. When eggs look like wet scrambled eggs, in 30 to 45 seconds, remove from heat and spread to cover surface of the pan, letting residual heat cook and set eggs. Run spatula around the pan's perimeter and shake the pan to loosen omelet.
3. Spread yogurt over half of omelet and top with watercress mixture and smoked salmon. Season with pepper. Fold other half of omelet over filling. Serve immediately.

PER SERVING *About 268 cal, 18 g fat (4.5 g sat), 384 mg chol, 681 mg sodium, 3 g carb, 1 g fiber, 1.5 g sugar (0 g added sugar), 22 g pro*

PROTEIN POWER

Smoked salmon is brunch-worthy fancy and a protein-packed delight with about 18 grams of protein per 3-ounce serving. Perfect for boosting your meals with flavor and fuel.

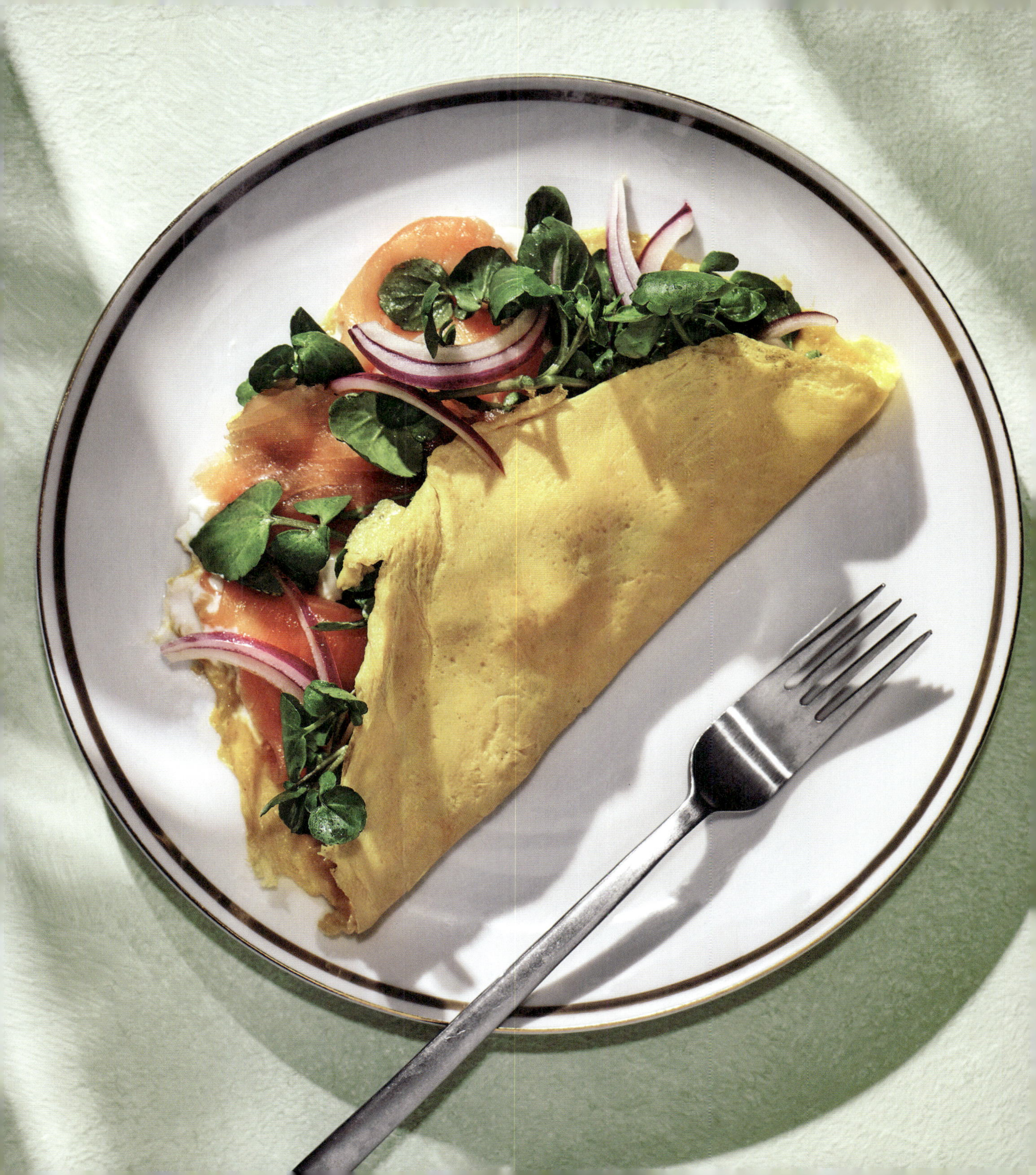

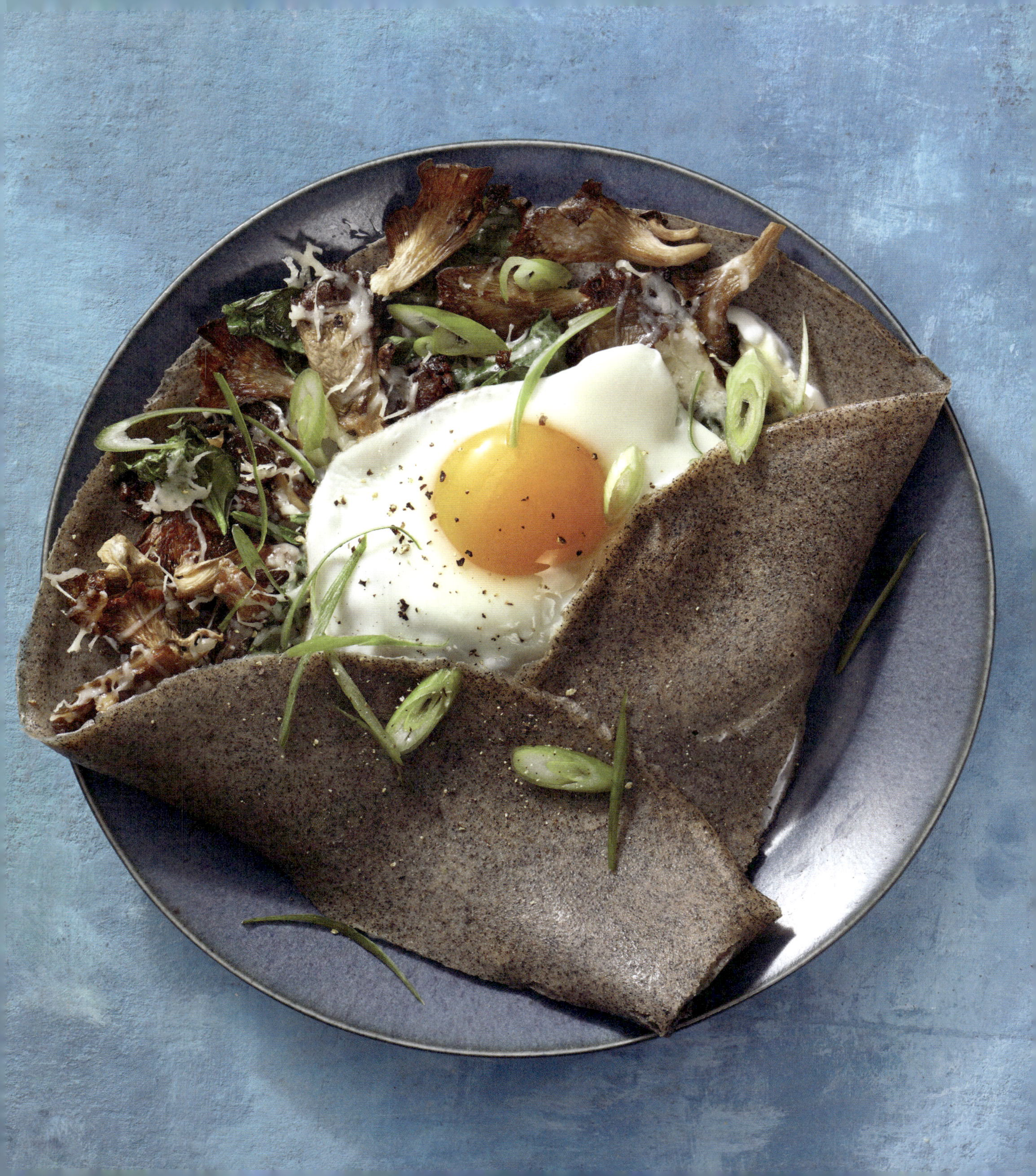

GRUYÈRE VEGGIE CREPES *with* FRIED EGGS

ACTIVE 50 min. **TOTAL** 50 min. (plus resting) **SERVES** 4 (with 2 crepes left over)

- 1 cup whole milk
- 6 large eggs, divided
- Kosher salt and pepper
- ¾ cup buckwheat flour
- ½ cup all-purpose flour
- 1 lb oyster mushrooms, torn into pieces
- 2 Tbsp olive oil, plus more for greasing
- 5-oz pkg. baby spinach
- 1½ oz Gruyère cheese, finely grated (about ½ cup)
- 4 Tbsp low-fat Greek yogurt
- 2 scallions, thinly sliced
- Grated Parmesan cheese, for serving

1. In a blender, purée milk, 2 eggs, ⅔ cup water, and ¼ teaspoon salt until smooth. Add both flours and process until smooth, 10 to 15 seconds. Let sit at room temp 1 hour.
2. Heat oven to 425°F. On a rimmed baking sheet, toss mushrooms with oil and ¼ teaspoon each salt and pepper. Roast, tossing halfway through, until starting to brown, 20 to 22 minutes. Scatter spinach on top and return to oven until starting to wilt, 1 to 2 minutes. Toss spinach with mushrooms and sprinkle with Gruyère. Return to oven until cheese melts, 1 minute.
3. Meanwhile, heat a large nonstick skillet over medium heat and lightly brush with oil. Stir batter until smooth, then add one-sixth of batter (scant ½ cup) to the skillet, swirling to coat. Cook, adjusting heat as necessary, until lightly browned, 2 to 3 minutes. Flip and cook 1 minute more. Transfer to a plate. Repeat with remaining batter, brushing with additional oil for each crepe.
4. Brush oil onto the same skillet, add remaining eggs, and cook on medium to desired doneness, 3 to 4 minutes for runny yolks.
5. Spread 1 tablespoon yogurt on each of 4 crepes (you will have 2 left over), then top with mushroom mixture and fried eggs. Sprinkle with scallions and Parmesan if desired, then fold crepes.

PER SERVING *About 405 cal, 20.5 g fat (6.5 g sat), 264 mg chol, 445 mg sodium, 34 g carb, 4 g fiber, 4.5 g sugar (0 g added sugar), 22 g pro*

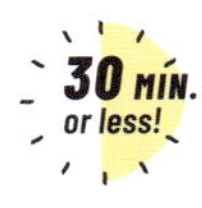

SUNRISE BUCKWHEAT SALAD *with* GOUDA & EGGS

ACTIVE 25 min. **TOTAL** 30 min. (plus cooling) **SERVES** 4

- 1 cup buckwheat groats, divided
- ¼ tsp smoked paprika
- 3 Tbsp olive oil, divided
- Kosher salt and pepper
- 1 Tbsp sherry vinegar
- 1 tsp country-style Dijon mustard
- ½ tsp honey
- 4 small heads oak leaf lettuce (8 oz total), leaves separated
- 1 small head frisée (4 oz), torn into pieces
- 8 large jammy eggs, halved lengthwise
- 2 oz aged Gouda, shaved with vegetable peeler
- Flaky sea salt
- Cracked pepper

1. Heat oven to 300°F. On a small rimmed baking sheet, toss ½ cup groats with smoked paprika, 1 tablespoon oil, and ⅛ teaspoon each kosher salt and pepper. Spread in even layer and bake, stirring halfway through, until golden brown, 25 to 30 minutes. Let cool.
2. Meanwhile, cook remaining ½ cup groats per package directions; set aside.
3. In a large bowl, whisk together vinegar, mustard, honey, and ¼ teaspoon each salt and pepper, then whisk in remaining 2 tablespoons oil.
4. Toss with greens to coat. Divide among bowls and top with cooked buckwheat, eggs, Gouda, toasted buckwheat, and flaky salt and cracked pepper if desired.

PER SERVING *About 460 cal, 27 g fat (8 g sat), 429 mg chol, 499 mg sodium, 35 g carb, 6 g fiber, 1.5 g sugar (0.5 g added sugar), 22 g pro*

PROTEIN POWER

Despite its name, buckwheat isn't actually wheat—it's a gluten-free seed and one of a few plant-based complete proteins, meaning it packs all nine essential amino acids your body needs.

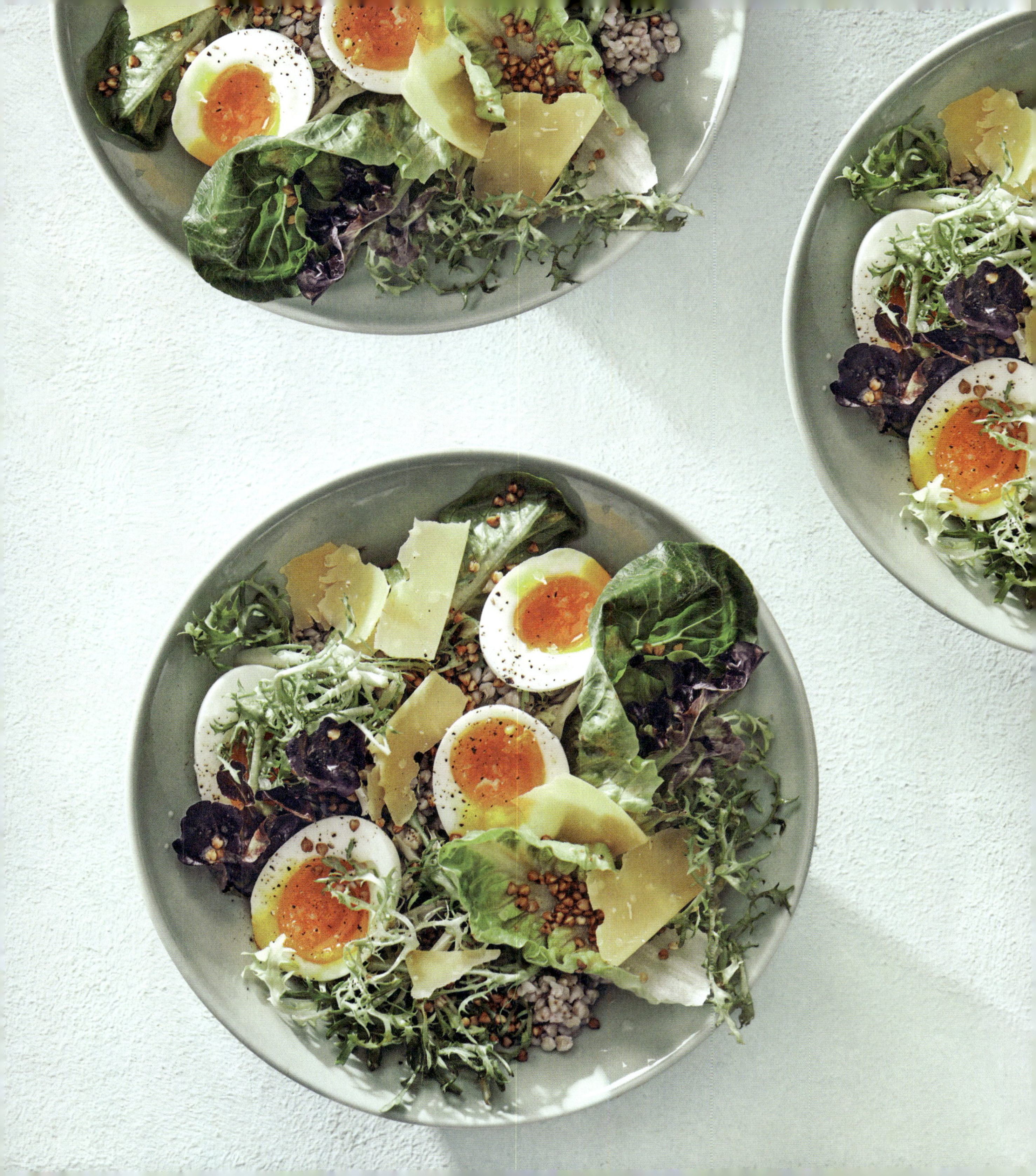

SHAKSHUKA

ACTIVE 15 min. **TOTAL** 35 min. **SERVES** 4

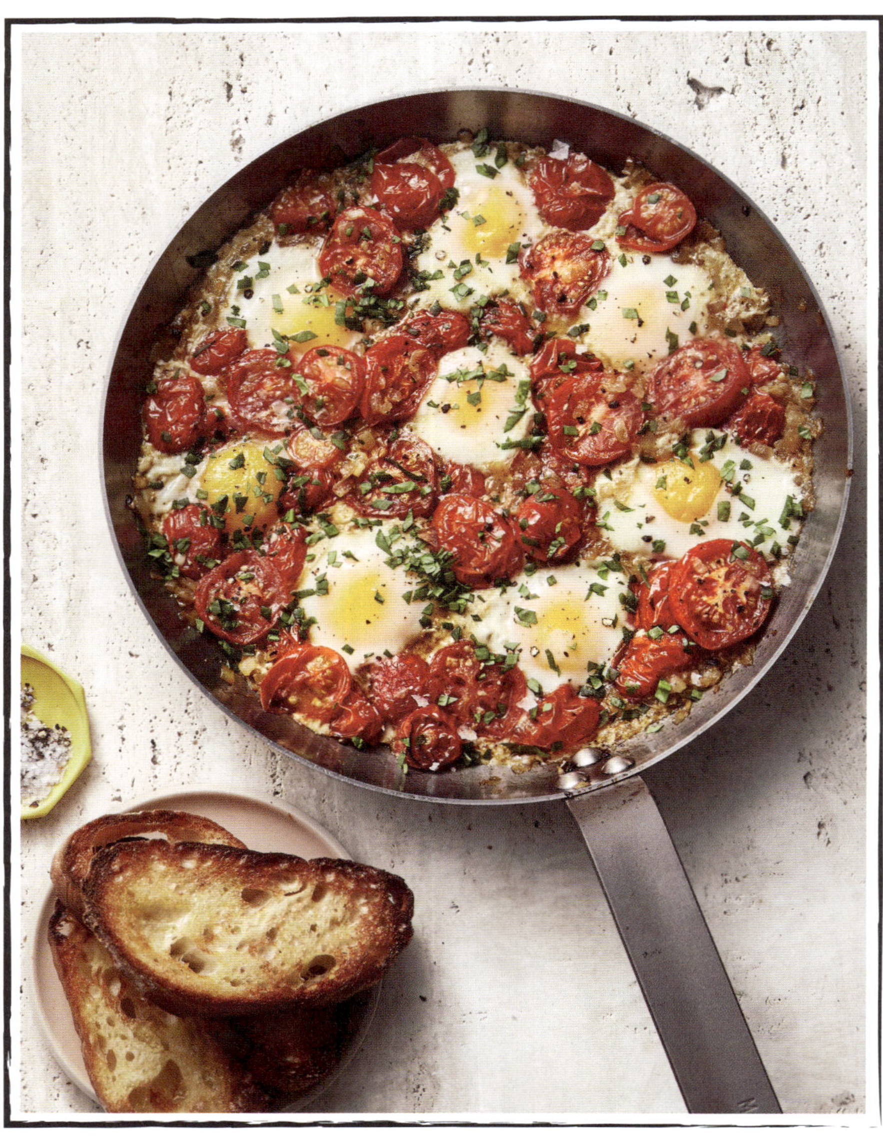

1. Heat oven to 400°F. Heat 2 tablespoons **olive oil** in a large oven-safe skillet over medium heat. Add 1 **onion** (finely chopped) and sauté until golden brown and tender, 8 minutes. Stir in 1 clove **garlic** (finely chopped), 1 teaspoon **ground cumin**, and ½ teaspoon each salt and pepper and cook 1 minute. Stir in 1¼ lb **Campari tomatoes** (halved), transfer to oven and roast 10 minutes.

2. Remove the pan from oven, stir, then make 8 small wells in vegetable mixture and carefully crack 1 large **egg** into each (8 eggs total). Bake eggs to desired doneness, 7 to 8 minutes for slightly runny yolks.

3. Sprinkle with ⅓ cup **baby spinach** (finely chopped). Serve dolloped with one 7-oz container plain **Greek yogurt** and 4 slices **Ezekiel sprouted whole grain bread** (toasted).

PER SERVING *About 359 cal, 19 g fat (5.5 g sat), 378 mg chol, 483 mg sodium, 26 g carb, 6 g fiber, 6.5 g sugar (0 g added sugar), 22 g pro*

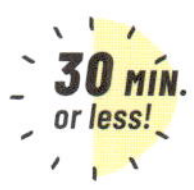

GREEK CHICKPEA WAFFLES

ACTIVE 30 min. **TOTAL** 30 min. **SERVES** 4

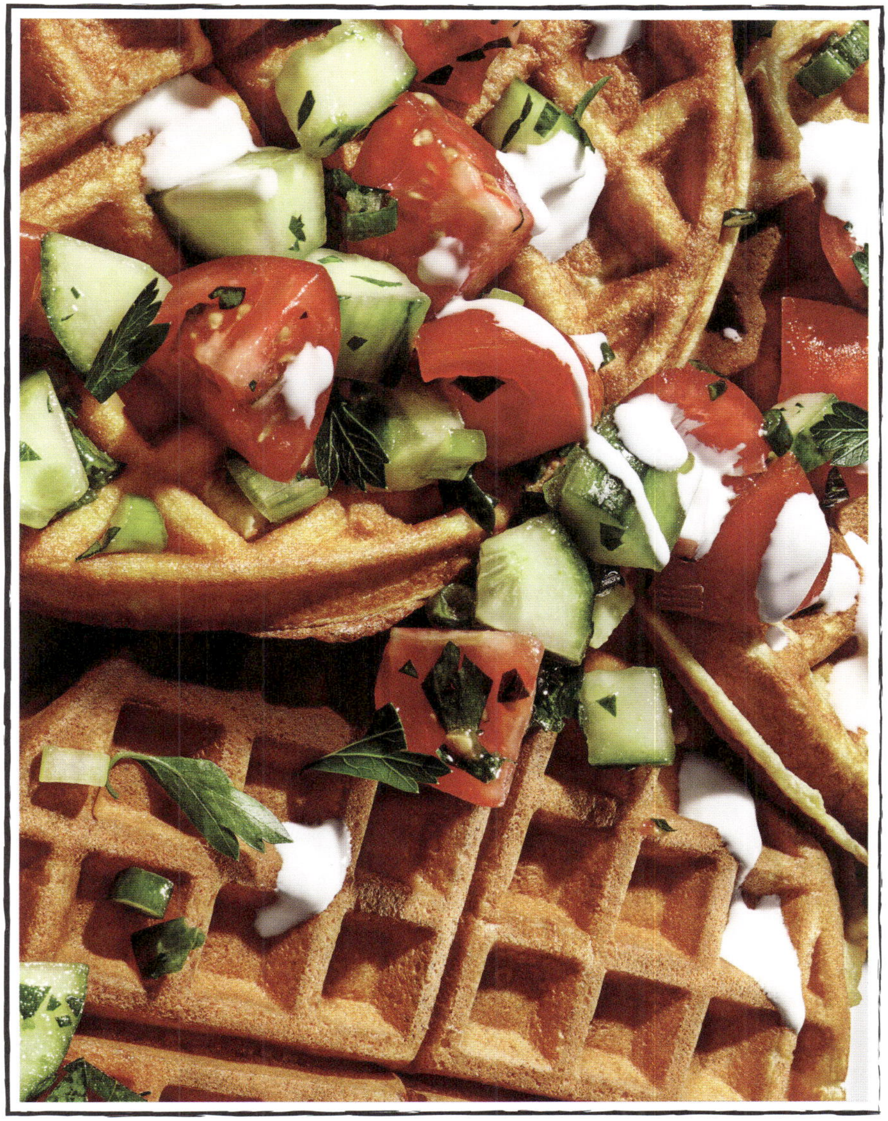

1. Heat oven to 200°F. Set a wire rack over a rimmed baking sheet and place in oven. Heat waffle iron per directions.

2. In a large bowl, whisk together ¾ cup **chickpea flour**, and ½ teaspoon each **baking soda** and **salt**. In a small bowl, whisk together ¾ cup **2% plain Greek yogurt** and 6 large **eggs**. Stir wet ingredients into dry ingredients.

3. Lightly coat a waffle iron with nonstick cooking spray and, in batches, drop ¼ to ½ cup batter into each section of iron and cook until golden brown, 4 to 5 minutes. Transfer to oven and keep warm. Repeat with remaining batter.

4. Serve topped with **tomatoes**, **cucumbers**, and **scallion** tossed with **olive oil**, **salt**, **pepper**, and **flat-leaf parsley**. Drizzle with **yogurt** mixed with **lemon juice**.

PER SERVING *About 272 cal, 12.5 g fat (4 g sat), 376 mg chol, 573 mg sodium, 16 g carb, 2 g fiber, 5 g sugar (0 g added sugar), 22 g pro*

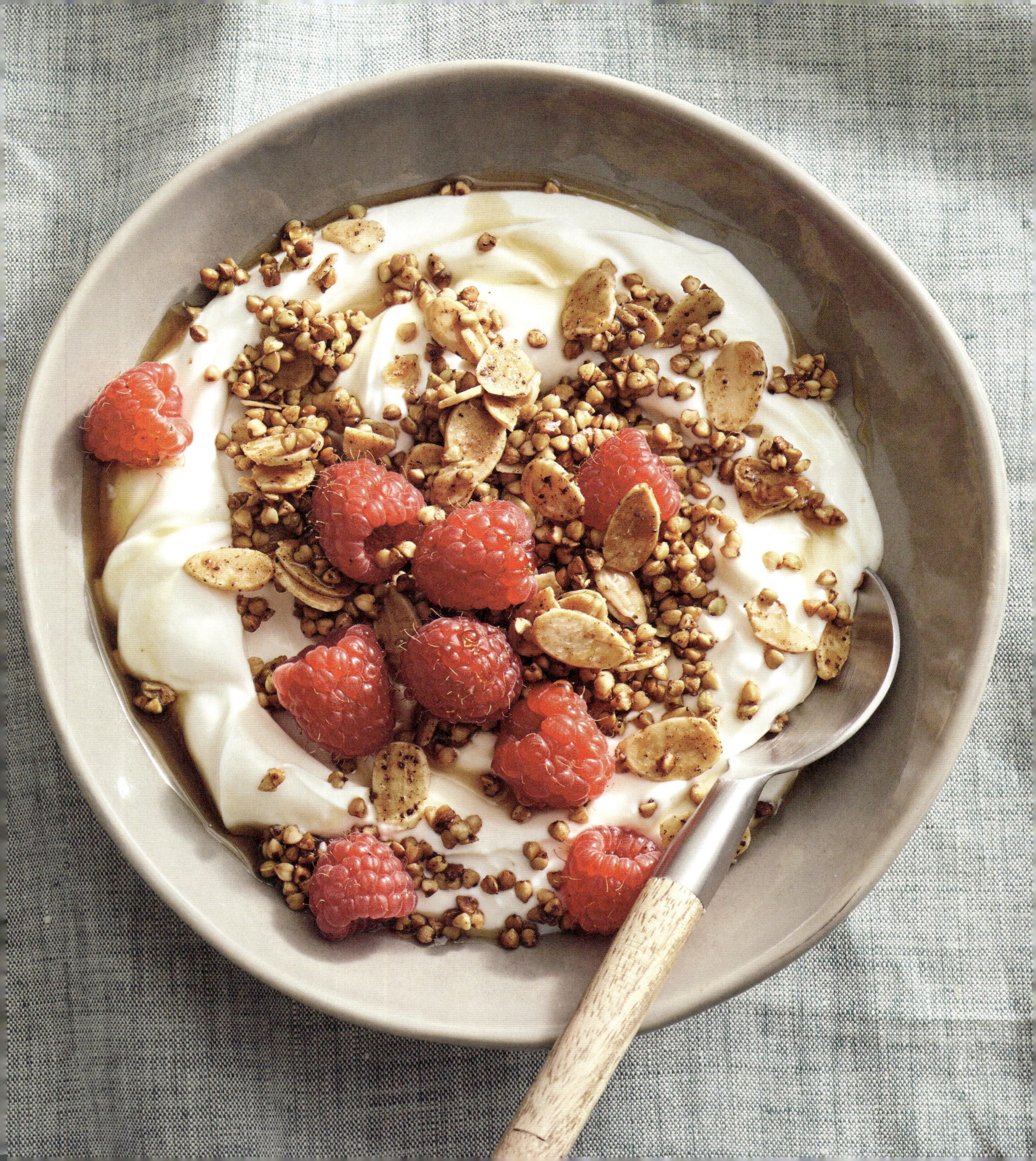

ALMOND-BUCKWHEAT GRANOLA *with* YOGURT & BERRIES

ACTIVE 30 min. **TOTAL** 40 min. **SERVES** 4

- 1 Tbsp olive oil
- 1½ Tbsp pure maple syrup, divided
- Kosher salt
- ½ cup buckwheat groats
- ¼ tsp ground cinnamon
- ⅓ cup sliced almonds
- 2 cups mixed berries
- 3 cups plain Greek yogurt

1. Heat oven to 300°F. Line a rimmed baking sheet with parchment paper. In a medium bowl, whisk together oil, 1 tablespoon maple syrup, and ¼ teaspoon salt.
2. Heat a medium cast-iron skillet over medium-high heat. Add groats and toast, shaking and tossing often and adjusting heat as needed, until crisp and light golden brown, 2 to 4 minutes. Transfer to a bowl with maple syrup mixture and toss to coat (it will sizzle), then stir in cinnamon and almonds.
3. Spread mixture onto a prepared baking sheet and bake, stirring halfway through, until golden brown, 15 to 20 minutes. Let cool.
4. In a bowl, toss berries with remaining ½ tablespoon maple syrup and pinch of salt; let sit 5 minutes. Spoon berries and juices over yogurt and top with granola.

PER SERVING *About 332 cal, 17 g fat (5.5 g sat), 25 mg chol, 250 mg sodium, 27 g carb, 4 g fiber, 18 g sugar (4.5 g added sugar), 20 g pro*

MAKE IT AHEAD
Double the granola and store in an airtight container at room temperature for up to 10 days. Serve on yogurt or try sprinkled over salads.

SAVORY SEEDY GRANOLA *with* GREEK YOGURT & CUCUMBER

ACTIVE 5 min. **TOTAL** 35 min. **SERVES** 4

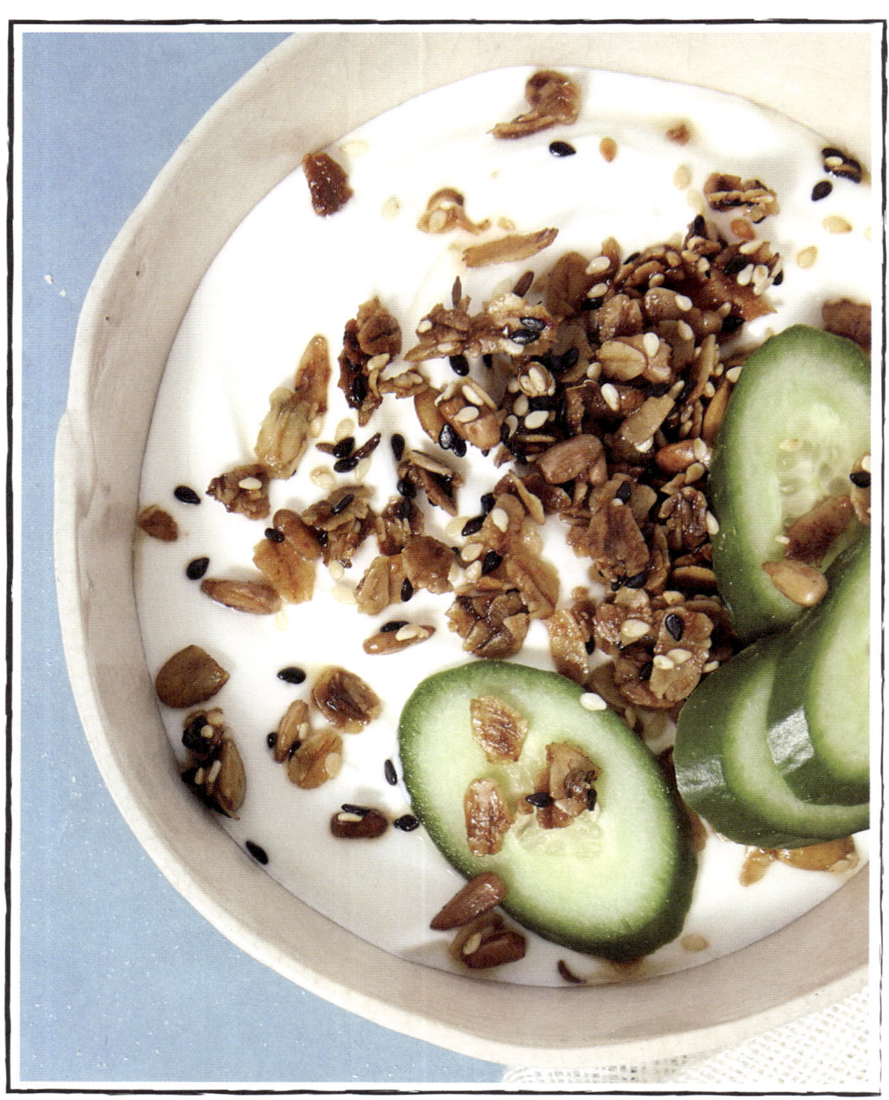

1. Heat oven to 300°F. In a large bowl, whisk together ¼ cup each **olive oil** and **pure maple syrup**, 2 tablespoons whole **coriander** (lightly crushed), 1 tablespoon **cumin seeds**, and ¼ teaspoon each **smoked paprika** and **kosher salt**. Fold in 1½ cups **old-fashioned rolled oats**, ½ cup each **raw pumpkin seeds** and **sunflower seeds**, and ¼ cup **sesame seeds** (both black and white).

2. Spread mixture on a parchment-lined rimmed baking sheet and bake, stirring every 10 minutes, until granola is lightly golden brown, 30 to 35 minutes; let cool, then store in airtight container up to 2 weeks.

3. For each serving, top ¾ cup plain **Greek yogurt** with ⅓ cup granola and ½ **Persian cucumber** (sliced).

PER SERVING *About 430 cal, 26.5 g fat (6.5 g sat), 25 mg chol, 125 mg sodium, 28 g carb, 4 g fiber, 14 g sugar (5.5 g added sugar), 24 g pro*

BLUEBERRY-and-MIXED-NUT PARFAIT

ACTIVE 25 min. **TOTAL** 35 min. **MAKES** 4 parfaits

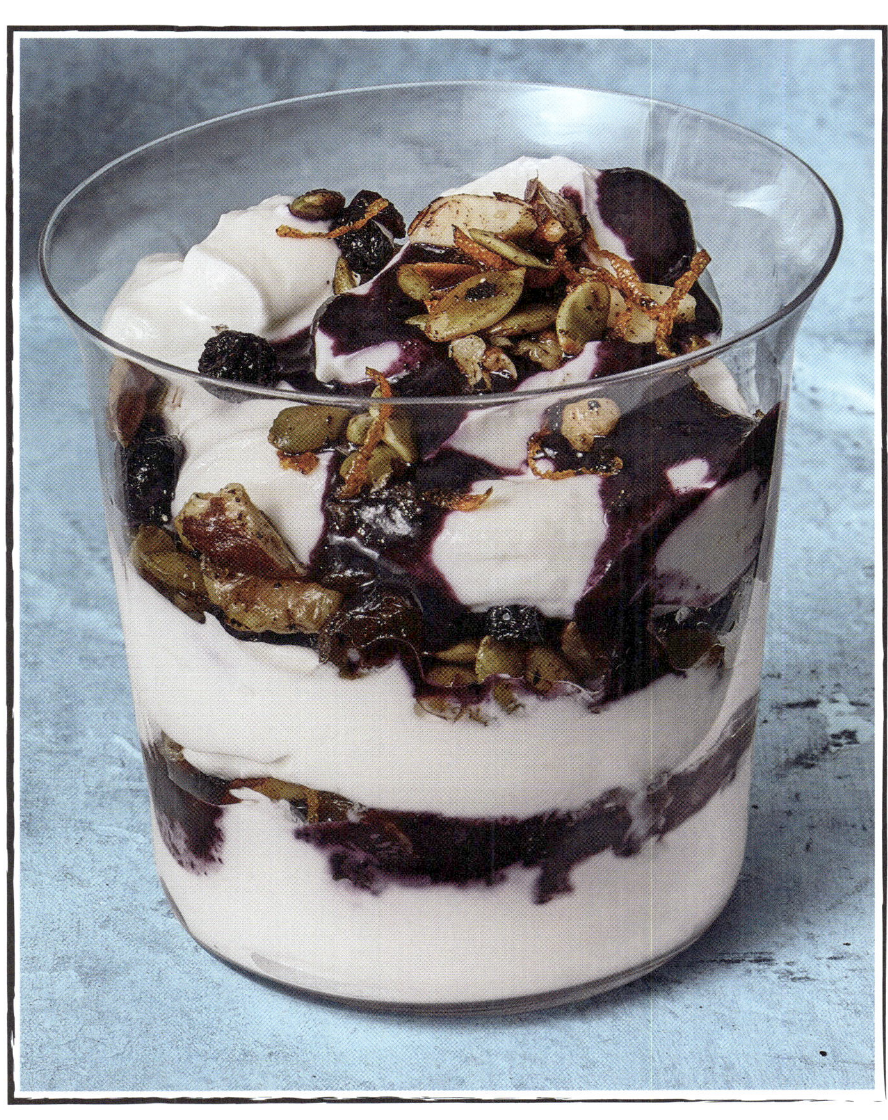

1. In a food processor, pulse ½ cup **freeze-dried blueberries** to form a powder; transfer to a small saucepan. Whisk in 1 cup **water** and simmer until sauce is thickened, about 15 minutes. Stir in pinch **salt**; let cool.

2. Meanwhile, on a rimmed baking sheet toss 3 tablespoons each **walnuts**, **almonds**, **pecans**, and **pepitas** with 1 tablespoon **olive oil**, 1 teaspoon **cinnamon**, ⅛ teaspoon **cardamom**, and ½ teaspoon **flaky sea salt**. Roast at 400°F until toasted, about 6 minutes, then toss with 1 tablespoon **orange zest**, ½ cup additional **freeze-dried blueberries**, and ¼ cup **golden raisins**.

3. Make 4 parfaits, layering plain **Greek yogurt** (about ¾ cup each), blueberry sauce (about 1 heaping tablespoon), and nut mixture (heaping ¼ cup).

PER SERVING *About 413 cal, 25.5 g fat (6.5 g sat), 25 mg chol, 388 mg sodium, 28 g carb, 4 g fiber, 21.5 g sugar (0 g added sugar), 22 g pro*

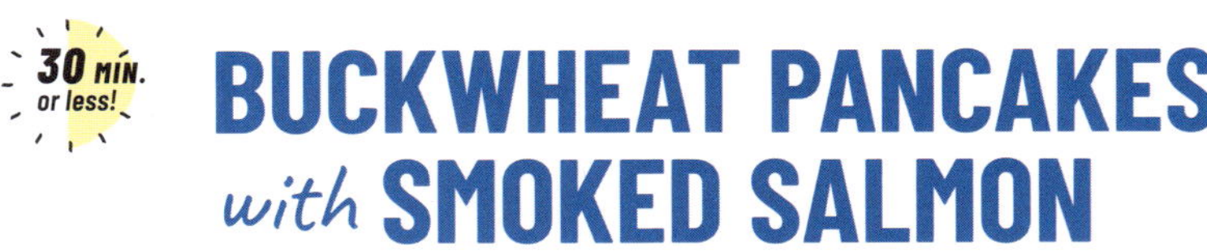

BUCKWHEAT PANCAKES *with* SMOKED SALMON

ACTIVE 25 min. **TOTAL** 25 min. **SERVES** 4

- 1 large egg, separated
- ⅔ cup cashew milk or milk of choice
- ½ cup buckwheat flour
- Kosher salt and pepper
- 3 Tbsp roasted sunflower seeds
- 3 Tbsp toasted sesame seeds
- 2 tsp avocado oil, divided
- ½ cup plain Greek yogurt
- ½ small red onion, thinly sliced
- 8 oz smoked salmon
- ¼ cup dill
- Lemon wedges, for serving

1. In a bowl, whisk together egg yolk and milk. Stir in flour and a pinch each of salt and pepper until just combined.
2. In second bowl, beat egg white until soft peaks form. Fold into buckwheat mixture, along with sunflower and sesame seeds, until just combined.
3. Rub 1 teaspoon oil in large nonstick skillet, then heat over medium heat. In batches, cook ¼-cupfuls of batter, coating pan with more oil as needed, until nearly set and bottoms are golden brown, about 3 minutes. Flip and cook until just cooked through, 1 minute. Transfer to a plate and cover to keep warm.
4. Top with yogurt, onion, salmon, dill, and pepper. Serve with lemon wedges.

PER SERVING *About 278 cal, 15 g fat (2.5 g sat), 64 mg chol, 477 mg sodium, 16 g carb, 3 g fiber, 2.5 g sugar (0 g added sugar), 20 g pro*

MAKE IT AHEAD

Let the pancakes cool completely, then stack with parchment paper in between and pop them in an airtight container or freezer bag. To reheat, pop in the toaster or warm in a skillet for a few minutes, then top as directed.

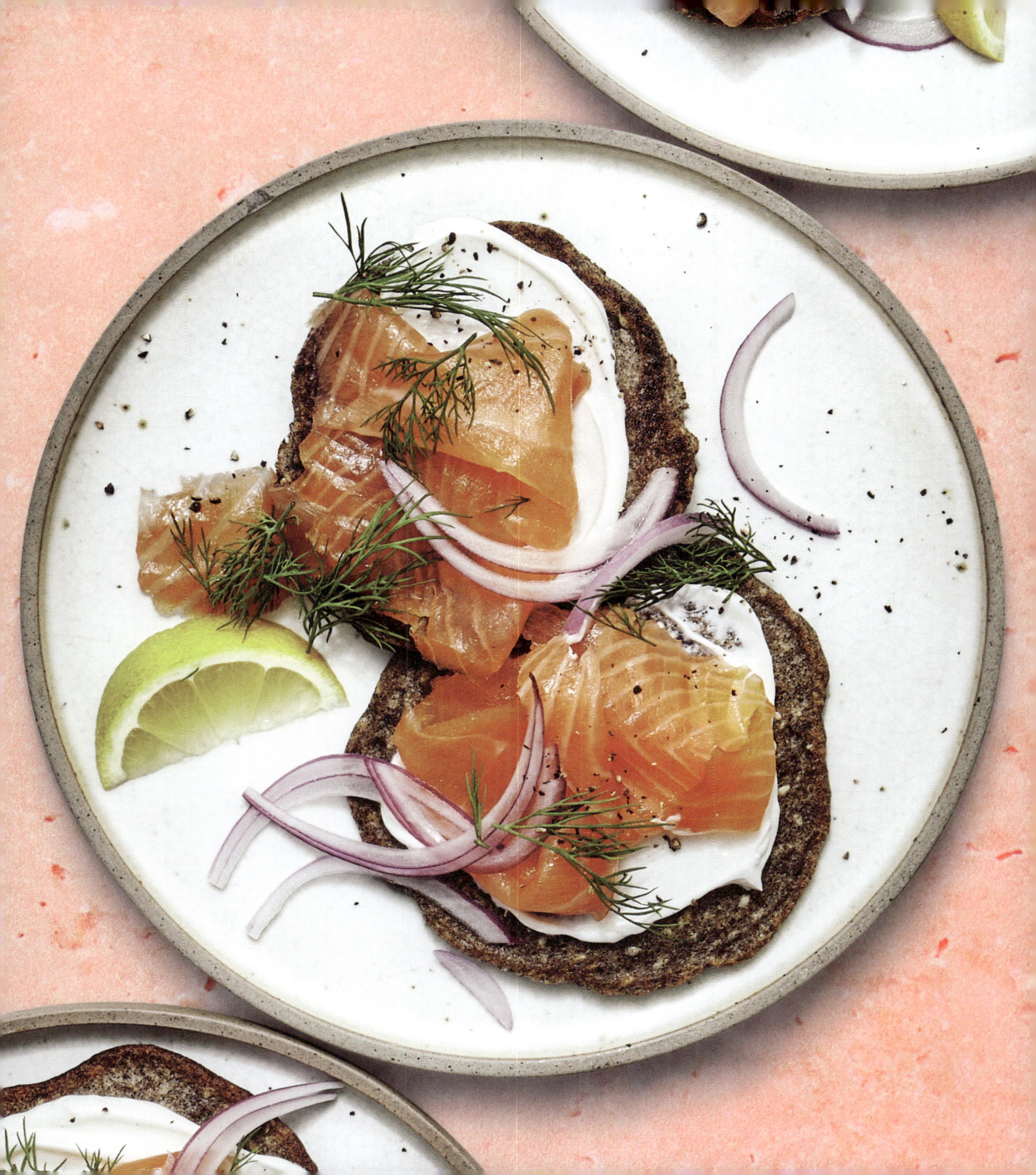

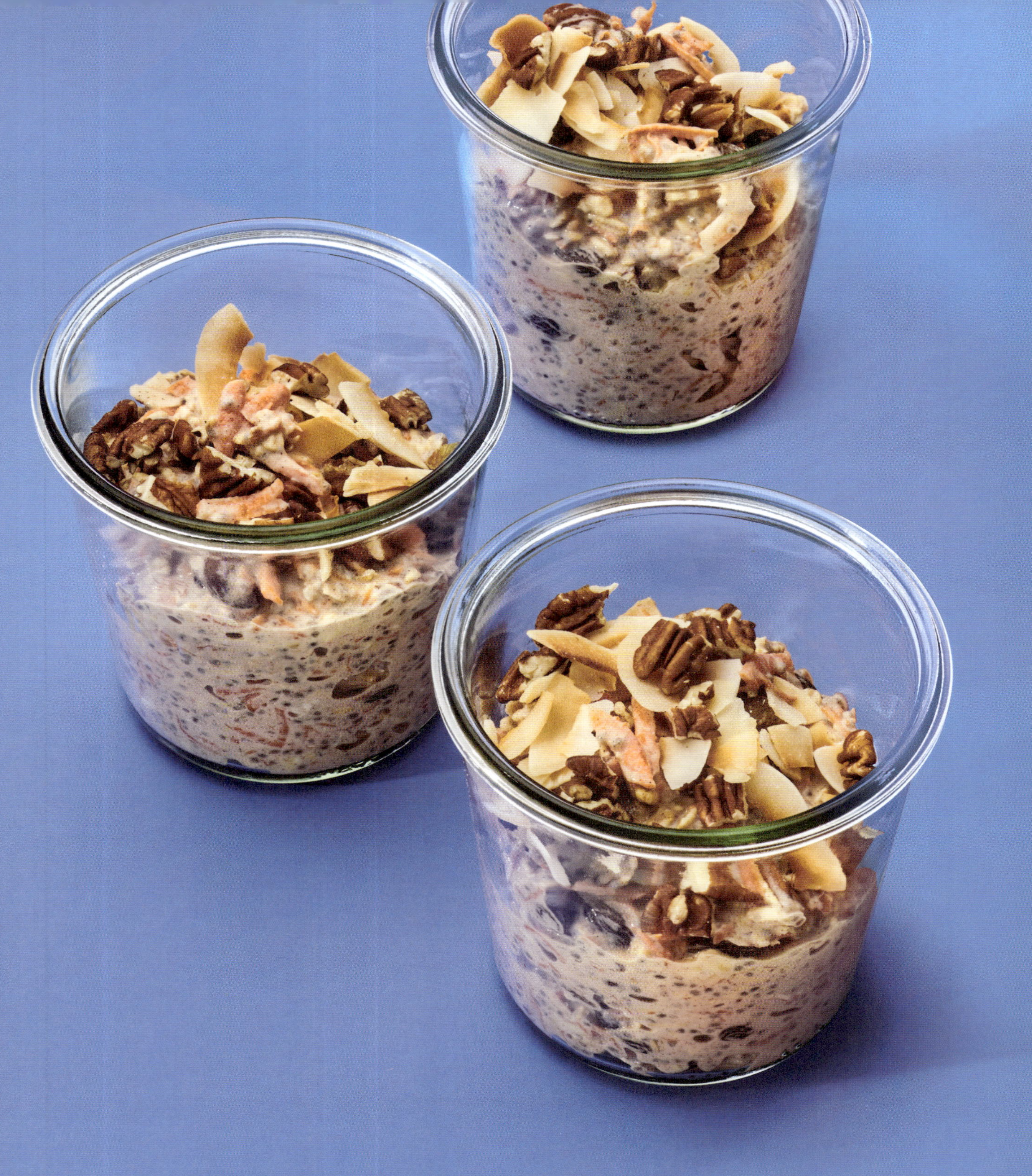

OVERNIGHT "CARROT CAKE" OATS

ACTIVE 20 min. **TOTAL** 10 min. (plus overnight chilling) **SERVES** 4

2 cups unsweetened soy milk, plus more for thinning

1½ cups whole milk plain Greek yogurt

3 tsp pure maple syrup

2 tsp ground cinnamon

1½ tsp pure vanilla extract

Kosher salt

1¼ cups rolled oats

1 large carrot (8 oz), scrubbed and coarsely grated (2½ cups)

⅔ cup toasted pecans, chopped, plus more for topping

½ cup raisins, roughly chopped, plus more for topping

¼ cup toasted unsweetened coconut chips, lightly crushed

¼ cup chia seeds

1. In large bowl, whisk together soy milk, yogurt, maple syrup, cinnamon, vanilla, and ½ teaspoon salt.
2. Stir in oats, carrot, pecans, raisins, coconut, and chia seeds until well combined. Divide among 4 jars, cover, and refrigerate overnight.
3. Serve, adjusting consistency with additional soy milk as needed.

PER SERVING *About 541 cal, 27 g fat (6 g sat), 9 mg chol, 348 mg sodium, 60 g carb, 13 g fiber, 26.5 g sugar (3 g added sugar), 21 g pro*

PROTEIN POWER

One cup of Greek yogurt delivers around 15-20 grams of protein, making it a simple and satisfying way to add high-quality protein to your day.

SPINACH & COTTAGE CHEESE SPOONBREAD MUFFINS

ACTIVE 20 min. **TOTAL** 40 min. (plus cooling) **SERVES** 6

Canola oil spray, for greasing

6 Tbsp finely ground yellow cornmeal

¾ tsp baking powder

Kosher salt and pepper

½ tsp freshly grated nutmeg (optional)

6 large eggs

1½ cups lowfat cottage cheese

4 oz Gruyère, coarsely grated (1¼ cups), divided

4 scallions, thinly sliced

16-oz bag frozen chopped spinach, thawed and squeezed very well

1. Heat oven to 475°F. Line a 12-cup muffin pan with foil liners and coat with canola oil spray.
2. In a small bowl, whisk together cornmeal, baking powder, ½ tsp each salt and pepper, and nutmeg (if using).
3. In large bowl, whisk eggs, then stir in cottage cheese and 1¼ cups Gruyère. Stir in scallions, spinach, then dry ingredients. Divide among prepared liners (about ⅓ cup each), then sprinkle with remaining Gruyère.
4. Bake until golden brown and puffy, 16 to 18 minutes Let cool 5 minutes before serving.

PER SERVING *About 250 cal, 13 g fat (6 g sat), 214 mg chol, 676 mg sodium, 13 g carb, 4 g fiber, 3.5 g sugar (0 g added sugar), 22 g pro*

MAKE IT AHEAD

These quiche-like muffins are gluten-free and delicious both warm and at room temperature. Refrigerate in an airtight container for up to five days. Gently reheat in the microwave or toaster oven.

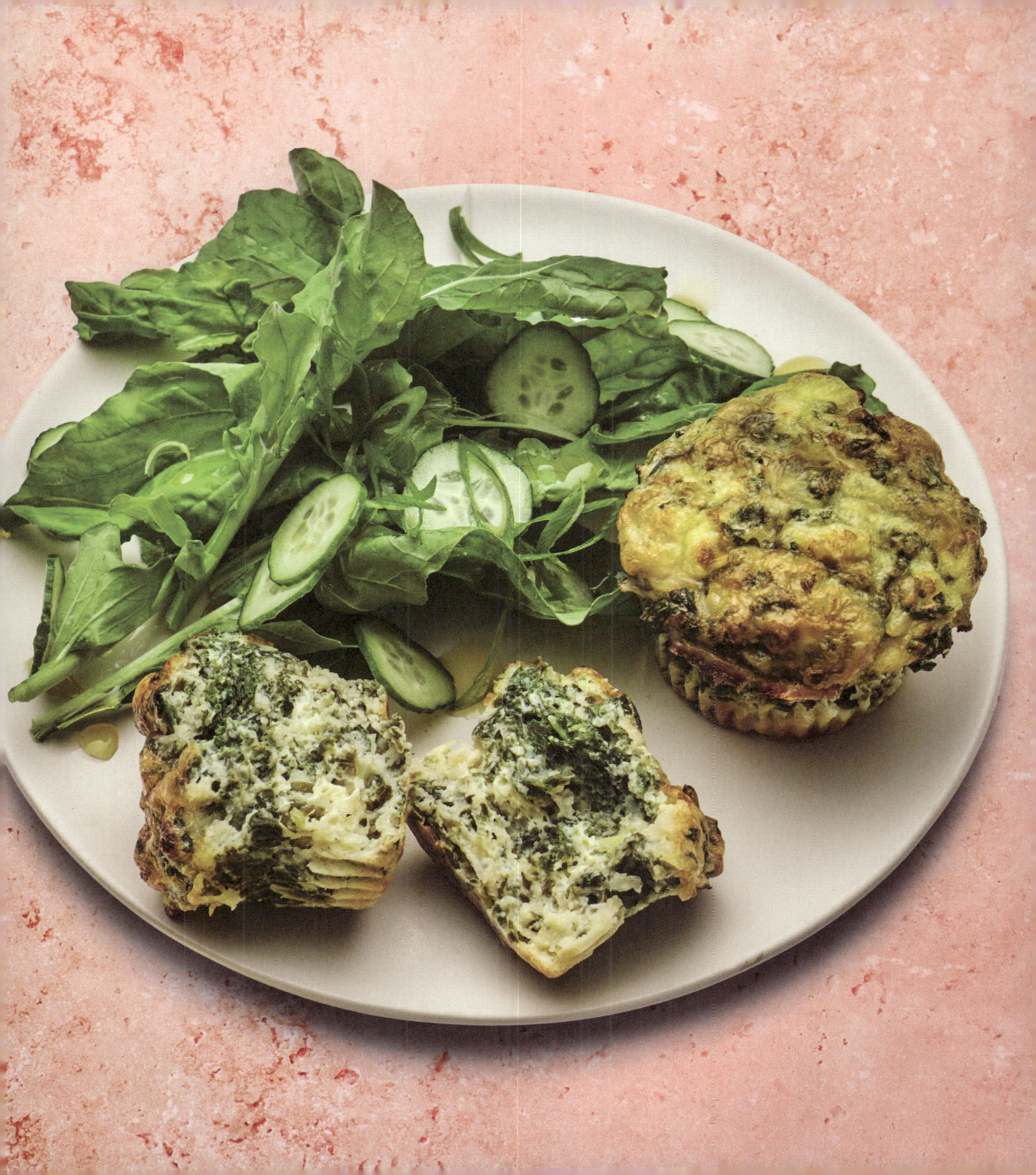

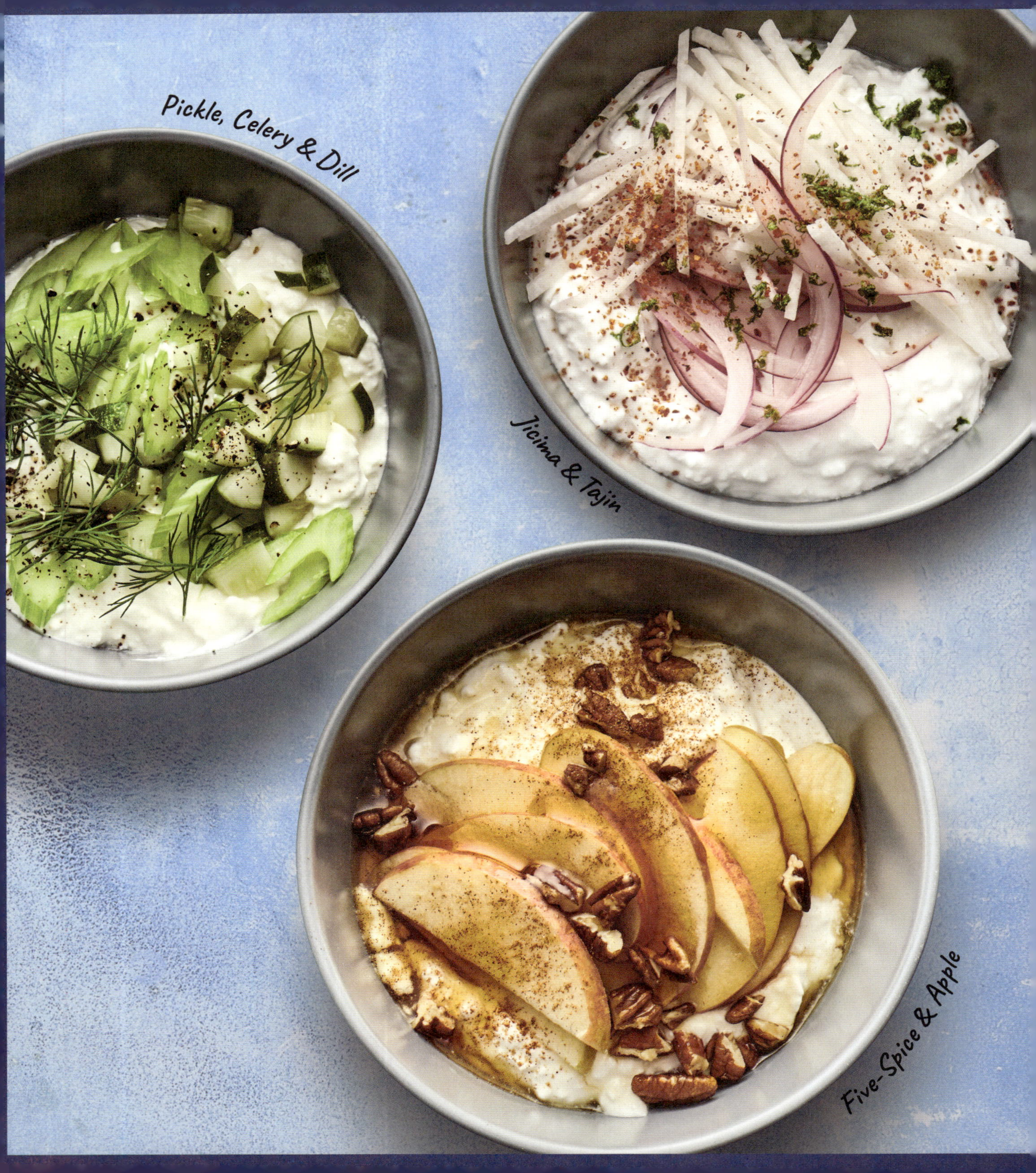

Pickle, Celery & Dill

Jicima & Tajin

Five-Spice & Apple

Cottage Cheese Bowls

Creamy cottage cheese is a sneaky source of protein that makes the perfect base for any flavor.

PICKLE, CELERY, AND DILL

ACTIVE 5 min.
TOTAL 5 min.
SERVES 1

1. In a small bowl, stir together ½ cup each **lowfat cottage cheese** and plain **2% Greek yogurt**.

2. Top with 1 rib **celery** (thinly sliced), ¼ **dill pickle spear** (chopped), and 1 teaspoon chopped **fresh dill**.

PER SERVING *About 190 cal, 5 g fat (3 g sat), 26 mg chol, 508 mg sodium, 11 g carb, 1 g fiber, 9.5 g sugar (0 g added sugar), 25 g pro*

JICAMA AND TAJIN

ACTIVE 5 min.
TOTAL 5 min.
SERVES 1

1. In a small bowl, combine ¼ small **red onion** (thinly sliced) and 1 tablespoon **lime juice**, let sit 5 minutes.

2. In another small bowl, stir together ½ cup each **lowfat cottage cheese** and plain **2% Greek yogurt**.

3. Top with ½ small **jicama** (cut into matchsticks, about ¼ cup), **onion**, and ½ teaspoon **lime zest**. Sprinkle with **Tajín**.

PER SERVING *About 206 cal, 5 g fat (3 g sat), 26 mg chol, 481 mg sodium, 16 g carb, 2 g fiber, 10.5 g sugar (0 g added sugar), 25 g pro*

FIVE-SPICE AND APPLE

ACTIVE 5 min.
TOTAL 5 min.
SERVES 1

1. In a small bowl, stir together ½ cup each **lowfat cottage cheese** and plain **2% Greek yogurt**.

2. Top with ½ crisp **pink apple** (cored and sliced) and 1 tablespoon chopped **pecans**.

3. Drizzle with 1 teaspoon pure **maple syrup** and sprinkle with pinch **five spice powder**.

PER SERVING *About 287 cal, 9.5 g fat (3.5 g sat), 26 mg chol, 405 mg sodium, 26 g carb, 3 g fiber, 21.5 g sugar (4 g added sugar), 25 g pro*

PROTEIN POWER
If you're not a fan of regular cottage cheese's taste or texture, try small-curd cottage cheese—it's creamier and milder, making it easier to love (and sneak into meals).

PORTOBELLOS *with* CANNELLINI *and* CHIMICHURRI

ACTIVE 30 min. **TOTAL** 50 min. **SERVES** 4

4 cloves garlic, divided

1 cup flat-leaf parsley leaves

½ cup cilantro

2 Tbsp oregano leaves

2 Tbsp red wine vinegar

9 Tbsp olive oil, divided

Kosher salt

¼ tsp red pepper flakes

2 15.5-oz can cannellini beans, rinsed

1 Tbsp smoked paprika

6 large portobello mushrooms (1¾ lb), stemmed and gilled

5-oz pkg. baby arugula

4 oz fresh goat cheese, crumbled

1. Heat oven to 475°F. In a food processor, pulse 2 cloves garlic to finely chop. Scrape the bowl, then add herbs, vinegar, 6 tablespoons oil, and ½ teaspoon salt; pulse to chop finely, scraping the bowl as needed. Transfer to a small bowl and stir in red pepper flakes; transfer ¼ cup to a large bowl and toss with beans (reserve rest for topping).

2. Grate remaining 2 cloves garlic into a small bowl. Add paprika, ½ teaspoon salt, and remaining 3 tablespoons oil; stir to combine. Brush onto both sides of portobellos and place portobellos, gill sides down, on a rimmed baking sheet; roast 11 minutes. Flip and roast until deep brown and cooked through, 6 to 9 minutes. When cool enough to handle, transfer to a cutting board and slice.

3. Add arugula to beans and toss to coat; divide among plates, then top with sliced mushrooms, goat cheese, and reserved chimichurri.

PER SERVING *About 664 cal, 38.5 g fat (8.5 g sat), 13 mg chol, 986 mg sodium, 58 g carb, 15 g fiber, 9 g sugar (0 g added sugar), 27 g pro*

KITCHEN TIP

Roasting portobellos gill sides down first helps them release moisture and brown nicely, keeping them juicy without getting soggy.

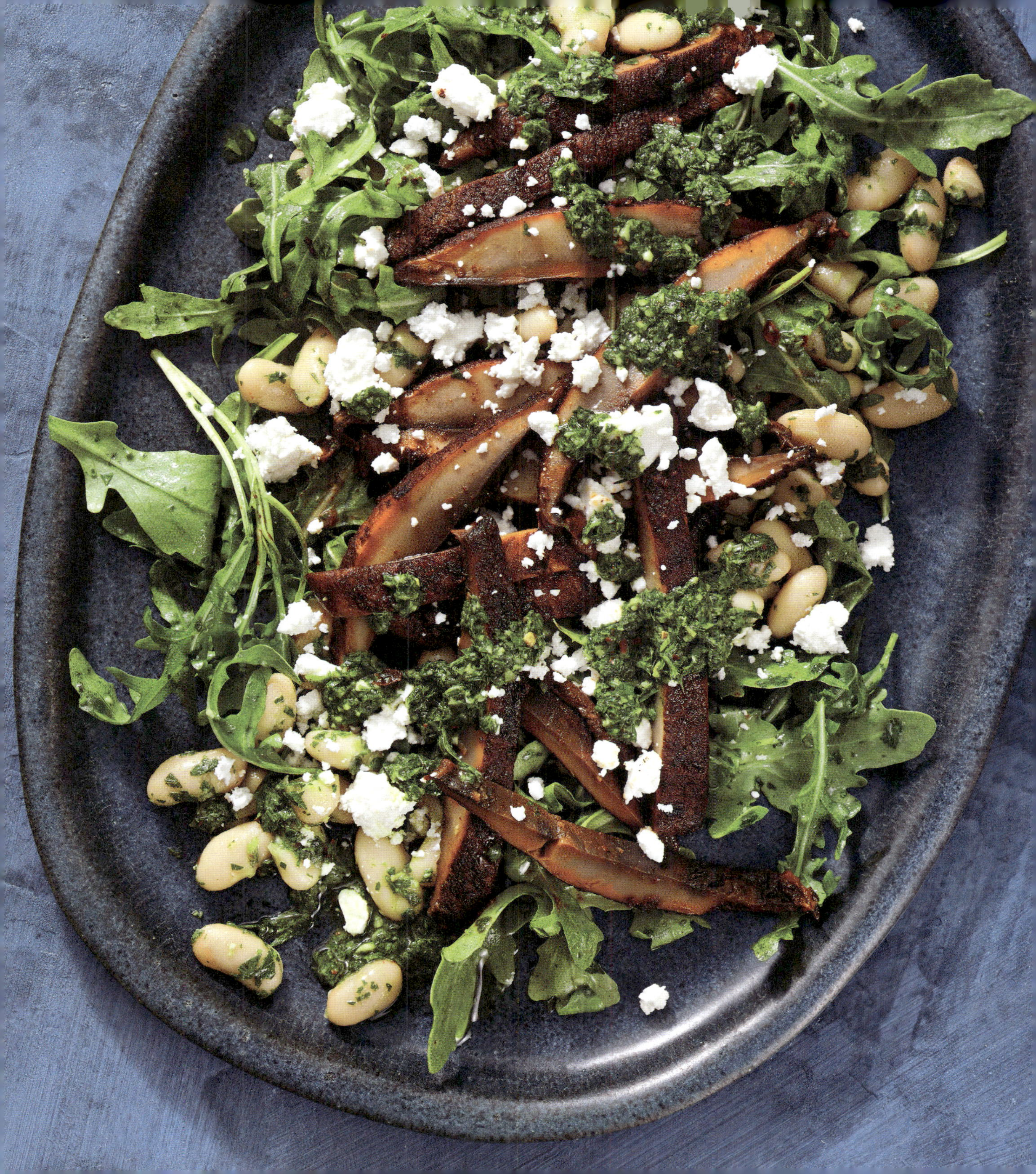

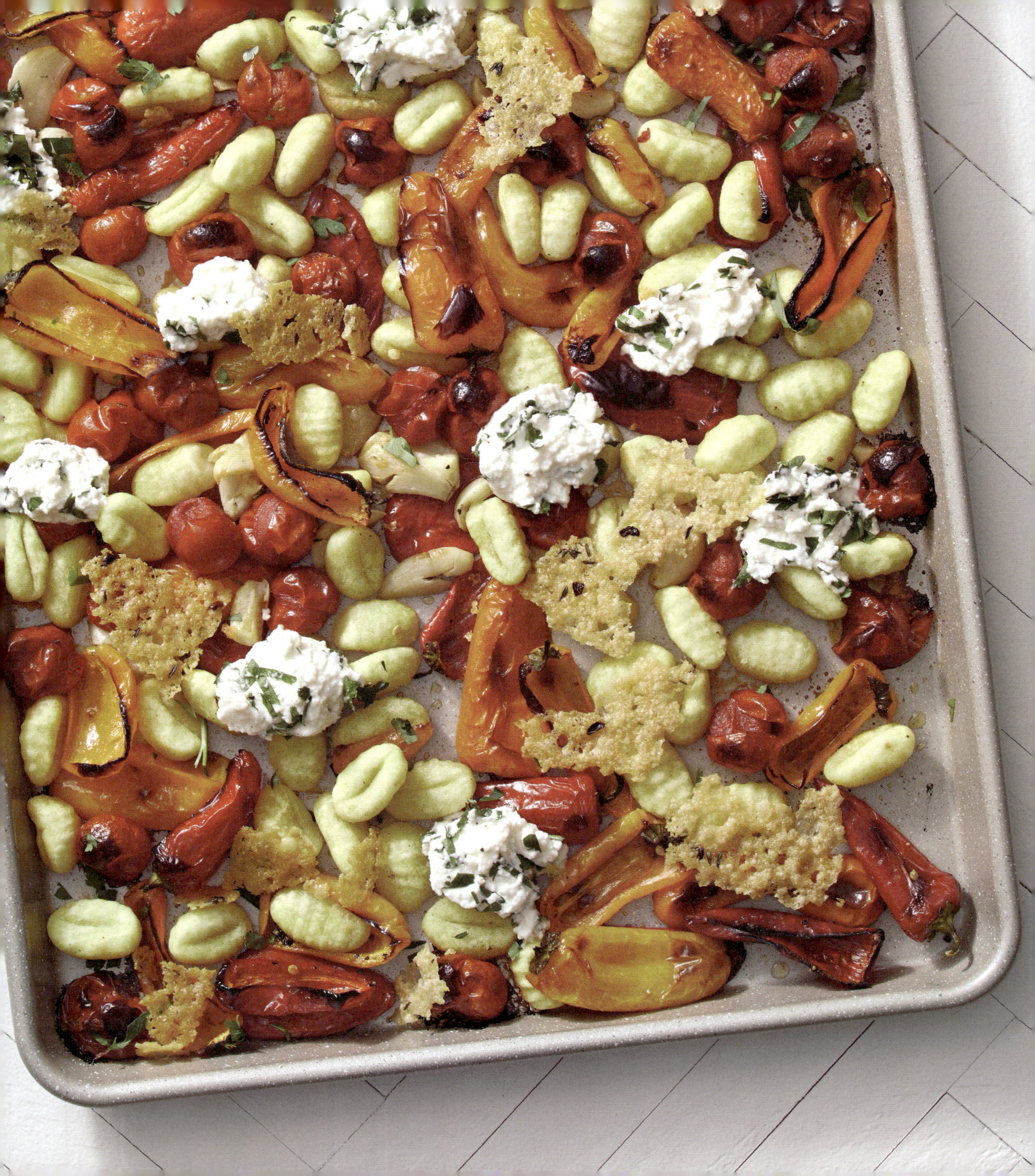

ROASTED GNOCCHI & PEPPERS *with* THYME FRICO

ACTIVE 25 min. **TOTAL** 40 min. **SERVES** 4

1 lb baby peppers, halved lengthwise and seeded

2 Tbsp olive oil, divided

Kosher salt and pepper

17.5-oz pkg. shelf-stable gnocchi

1 cup cherry or grape tomatoes

6 cloves garlic, smashed

2 Tbsp nutritional yeast

1 cup grated Parmesan cheese

2 tsp thyme leaves

Pinch of red pepper flakes

¾ cup ricotta cheese

¼ cup flat-leaf parsley leaves, chopped, plus more for serving

1. Heat oven to 425°F. In a large bowl, toss peppers with 1 tablespoon oil and ¼ teaspoon each salt and black pepper. Transfer to a large rimmed baking sheet. Roast until slightly brown on edges, 10 minutes.
2. Meanwhile, in the same large bowl, toss gnocchi, tomatoes, and garlic with remaining tablespoon oil and ¼ teaspoon each salt and black pepper. Add to peppers on same baking sheet and roast until gnocchi and peppers are golden brown and tender, 20 to 22 minutes more.
3. Meanwhile, make Frico: In a small bowl, combine nutritional yeast and ¾ cup Parmesan, then sprinkle on parchment-lined baking sheet in an even layer. Sprinkle with half of thyme and red pepper flakes. Roast until Parmesan is golden brown and crisp, 4 to 5 minutes. Let cool until ready to use.
4. In a small bowl, combine ricotta, remaining ¼ cup Parmesan, parsley, and a pinch each of salt and black pepper. Dollop over gnocchi and vegetables. Break frico into pieces and scatter over gnocchi and vegetables. Serve sprinkled with additional parsley if desired.

PER SERVING *About 589 cal, 22 g fat (8.5 g sat), 39 mg chol, 1,246 mg sodium, 70 g carb, 10 g fiber, 9.5 g sugar (0 g added sugar), 20 g pro*

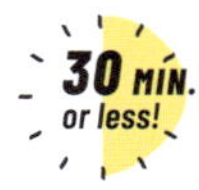

QUINOA ROMESCO and TEMPEH

ACTIVE 25 min. **TOTAL** 25 min. **SERVES** 4

- 1⅓ cups quinoa
- 2 Tbsp sherry vinegar
- 1 large clove garlic, grated (1 tsp)
- 2 tsp smoked paprika
- 5 Tbsp olive oil, divided
- Kosher salt
- 2 8-oz pkg. tempeh, cut into ½-in. cubes
- 12-oz jar roasted piquillo or red peppers, drained and chopped
- 1 cup raw almonds, well toasted and chopped, plus more for serving
- ¾ cup flat-leaf parsley leaves, chopped
- 2 oz Manchego, grated, plus more for serving

1. In a medium saucepan, combine quinoa with 2½ cups water and simmer, covered, until just tender, about 12 minutes. Remove from heat, keep covered 3 minutes, then fluff with fork.
2. In a large bowl, whisk together vinegar, garlic, smoked paprika, 4 tablespoons oil, and ½ teaspoon salt.
3. Heat remaining 1 tablespoon oil in a large nonstick skillet over medium heat. Add tempeh and cook, flipping occasionally until warmed through and golden brown, 5 to 6 minutes. Transfer to dressing and toss to coat.
4. Fluff quinoa, then add to tempeh and toss to combine. Add peppers, almonds, parsley, and Manchego and toss well. Top with additional almonds and cheese, if desired.

PER SERVING *About 706 cal, 34 g fat (5.5 g sat), 15 mg chol, 399 mg sodium, 53 g carb, 7 g fiber, 4.5 g sugar (0 g added sugar), 37 g pro*

PROTEIN POWER

Tempeh is made from a mix of fermented soybeans and other seeds and grains. Just 3 ounces packs 11 grams of complete plant-based protein, plus fiber, iron, potassium, and calcium.

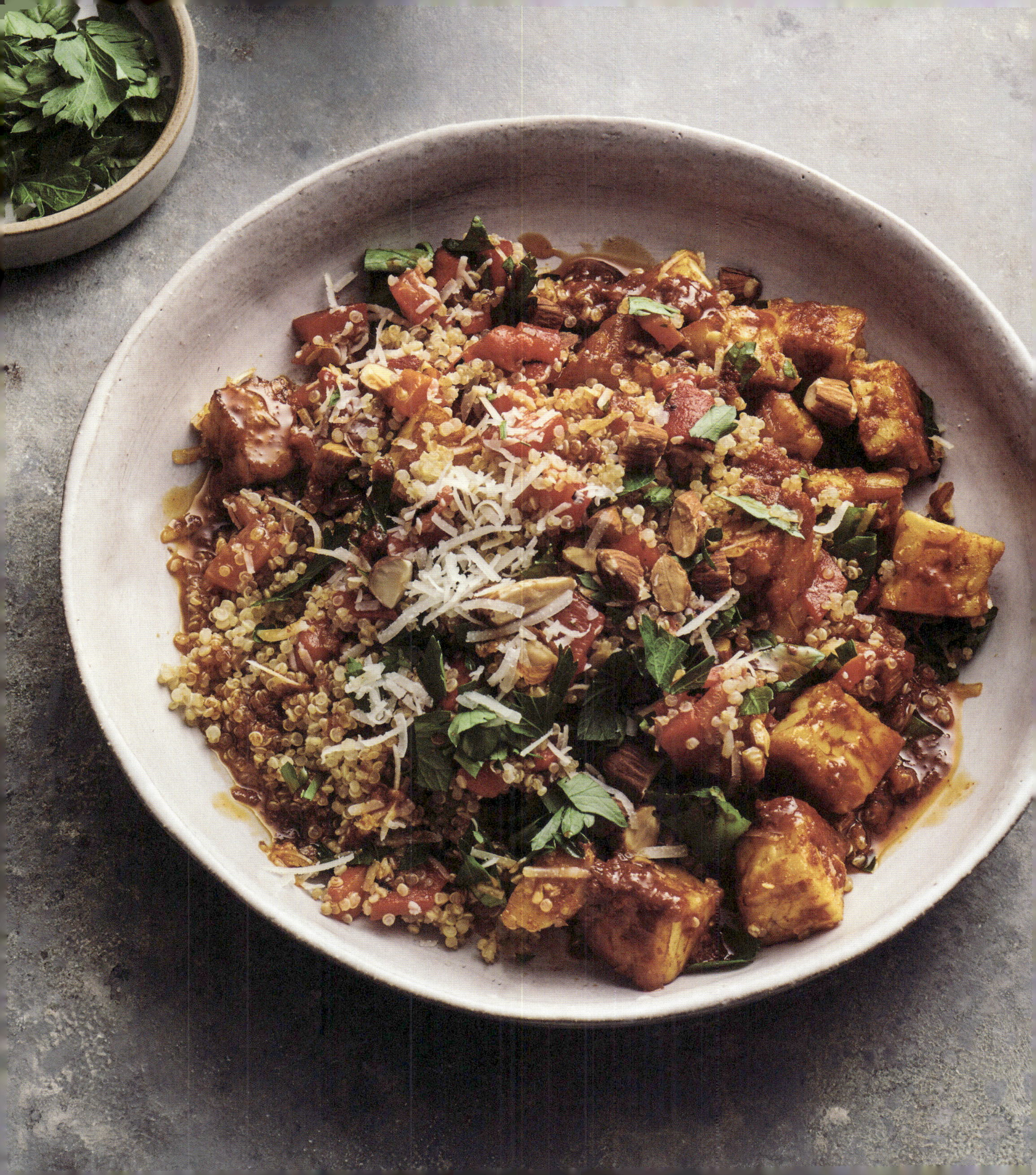

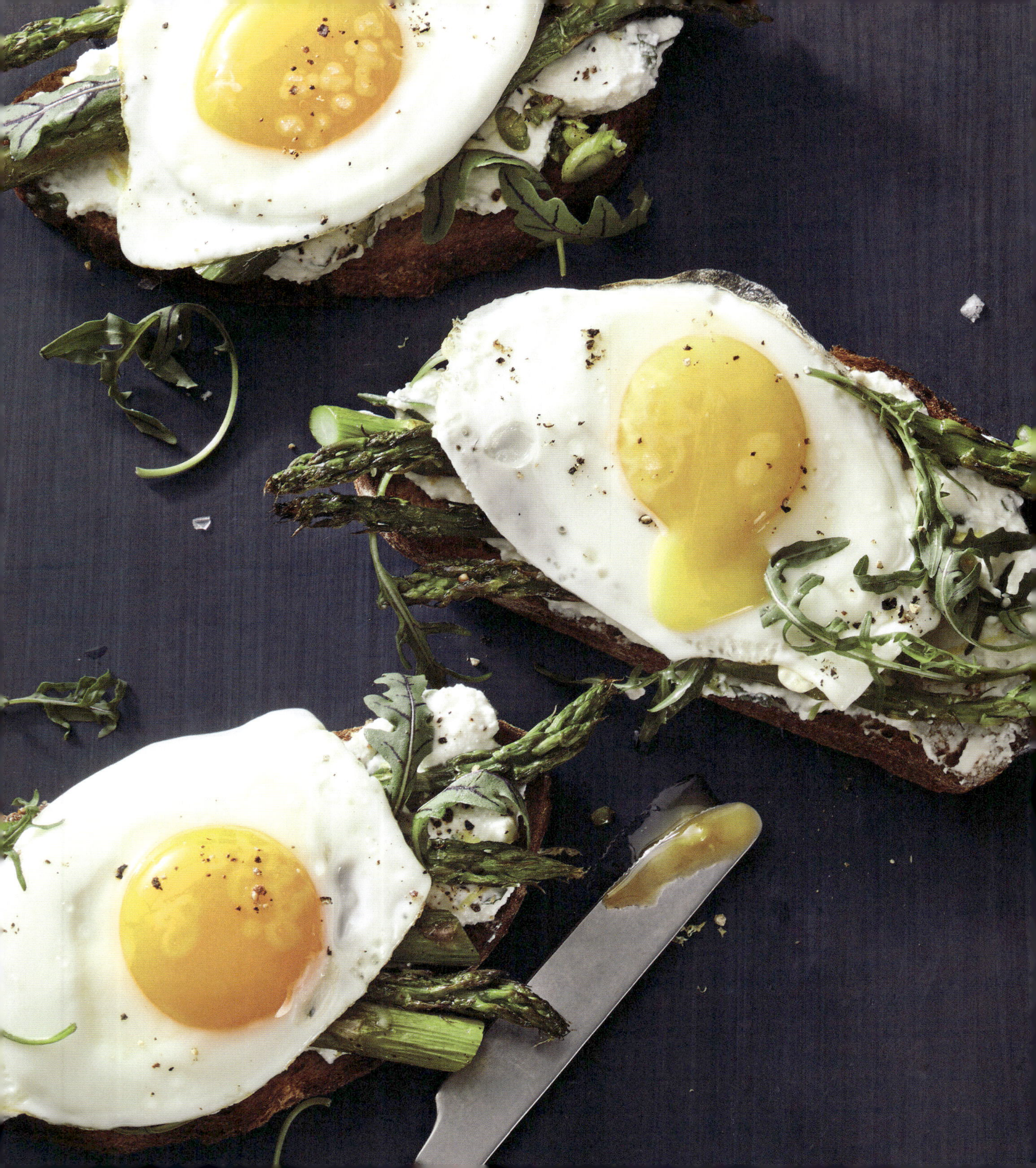

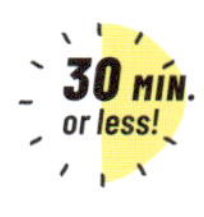

ASPARAGUS TARTINES *with* HERBED RICOTTA AND EGGS

ACTIVE 30 min. **TOTAL** 30 min. **SERVES** 4

4 slices multigrain sourdough bread

1 lb asparagus, ends trimmed

1½ Tbsp olive oil, divided

Kosher salt and pepper

½ tsp lemon zest plus ½ Tbsp lemon juice

3 scallions, thinly sliced, whites and greens separated

1 cup part-skim ricotta cheese

¼ cup grated Pecorino Romano cheese

1 Tbsp milk, plus more if needed

¼ cup mint leaves, chopped and divided

8 large eggs

Flaky sea salt (optional)

Mixed greens, for serving

1. Arrange oven rack 6 inches from broiler and another rack a few inches below and heat to broil.
2. On a large rimmed baking sheet, arrange bread. On a separate rimmed baking sheet, toss asparagus with 1 tablespoon oil and ¼ teaspoon each salt and pepper. Broil bread on top rack and asparagus on lower rack until bread is crisp, 1 to 3 minutes per side (depending on broiler). Remove bread, transfer asparagus to upper rack, and broil until just tender, 3 to 6 minutes more (depending on thickness).
3. Drizzle ½ tablespoon lemon juice over asparagus, toss with scallion whites, then transfer to a plate. Adjust oven temperature to 450°F.
4. In a medium bowl, stir together ricotta, Pecorino Romano, 1 tablespoon milk, reserved lemon zest, half each of mint and scallion greens, and ¼ teaspoon each salt and pepper. If ricotta seems dry, fold in a teaspoon or more of milk at a time as needed. Set aside.
5. Brush the baking sheet used for asparagus with remaining ½ tablespoon oil. Crack eggs on top (eggs will spread) and bake on lower rack until just set, 6 to 7 minutes.
6. Spread herbed ricotta on toast and top with asparagus and eggs. Sprinkle with remaining scallion greens and mint. Sprinkle with flaky sea salt if desired and serve with mixed greens.

PER SERVING *About 451 cal, 24 g fat (8.5 g sat), 397 mg chol, 765 mg sodium, 33 g carb, 8 g fiber, 2 g sugar (0 g added sugar), 28 g pro*

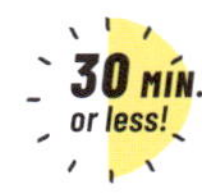

LINGUINE with ARUGULA PESTO

ACTIVE 25 min. **TOTAL** 30 min. **SERVES** 4

1 small head cauliflower (1½ lbs), cored and cut into small florets

5 Tbsp olive oil, divided, plus more for drizzling

Kosher salt and pepper

12 oz linguine

2 scallions, roughly chopped

Grated lemon zest for serving plus 1 Tbsp juice

5-oz. pkg. baby arugula, divided

2 basil leaves

⅓ cup grated Parmesan, plus more for serving

⅓ cup cottage cheese

Red pepper flakes, for sprinkling

1. Heat oven to 450°F. On a large rimmed baking sheet, toss cauliflower with 3 tablespoons oil and ½ teaspoon each salt and pepper; roast, tossing halfway through, until golden brown and tender, 20 to 25 minutes.
2. Meanwhile, cook linguine per package directions. Reserve ½ cup pasta cooking water, drain, and return to the pot.
3. While pasta cooks, in a food processor, pulse scallions, lemon juice, and 3 cups arugula to chop finely. Add basil, Parmesan, cottage cheese and ½ teaspoon each salt and pepper and pulse to chop basil. Scrape down sides; then, with the machine running, gradually add remaining 2 tablespoons oil and purée until smooth.
4. Toss pasta with pesto to coat, then toss with remaining arugula, adding a couple of tablespoons of reserved pasta water as needed to wilt arugula slightly. Fold in cauliflower and serve topped with more grated Parmesan, lemon zest, red pepper flakes, and a drizzle of oil if desired.

PER SERVING *About 568 cal, 22.5 g fat (4.5 g sat), 11 mg chol, 734 mg sodium, 72 g carb, 6 g fiber, 4 g sugar (0 g added sugar), 20 g pro*

KITCHEN TIP

Use your blender to finely grate fresh Parmesan. Cut a few big hunks away from the rind and blend them on high speed until they're a fine powder, 10 to 20 seconds.

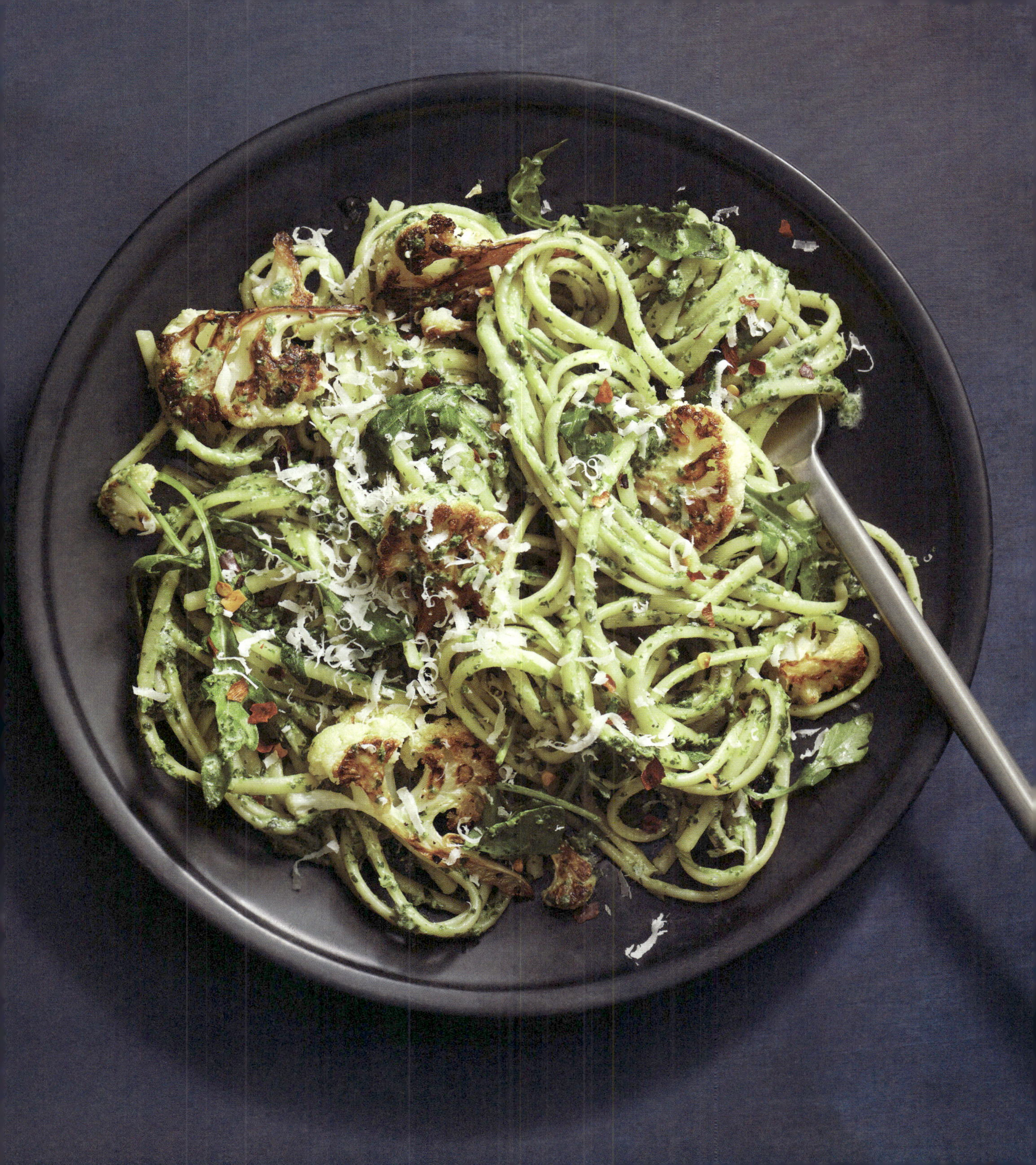

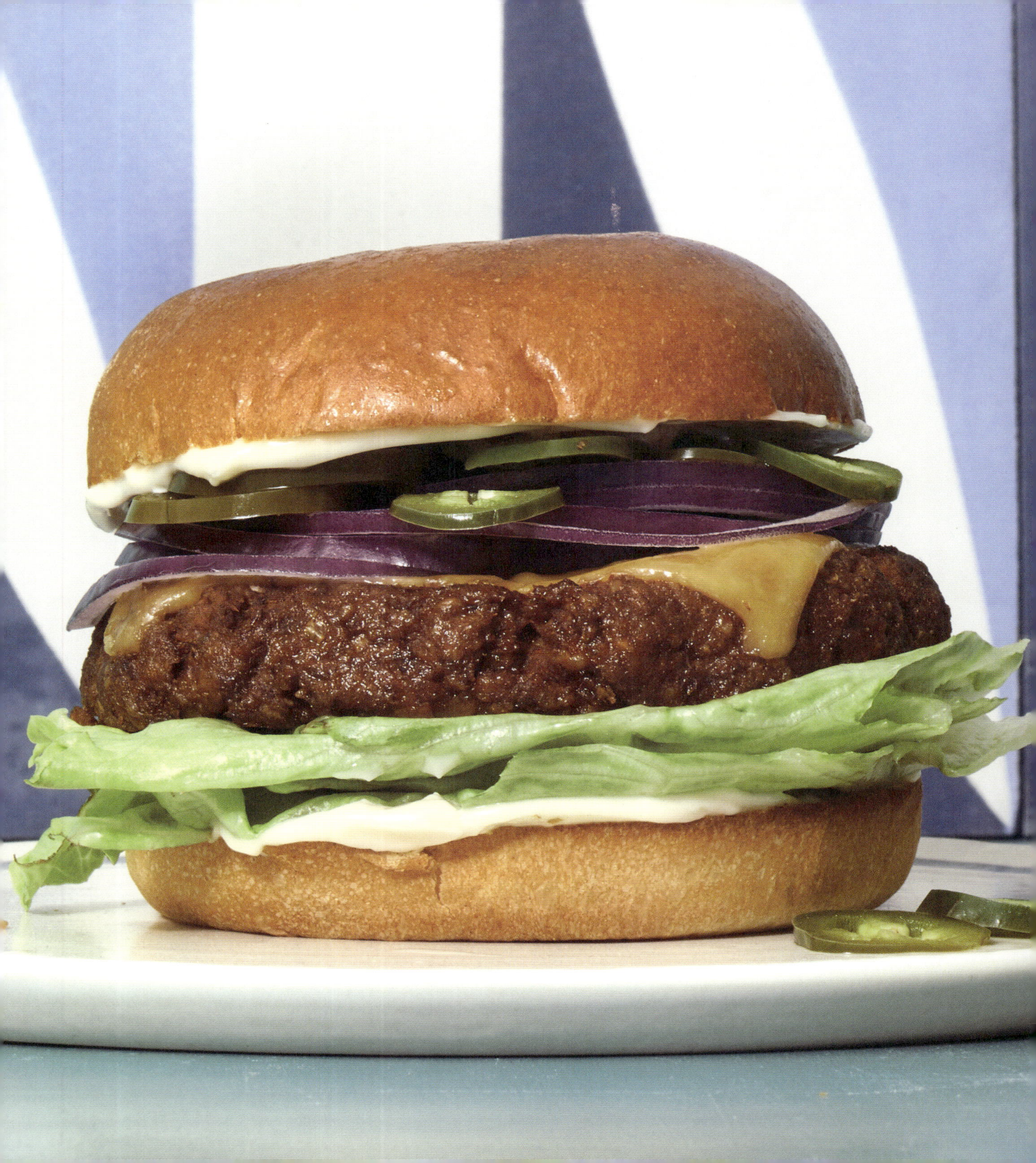

ROASTED EGGPLANT VEGGIE BURGER

ACTIVE 40 min. **TOTAL** 1 hr. **SERVES** 4

- 12-oz eggplant, halved lengthwise
- 3 Tbsp olive oil, divided
- Kosher salt and pepper
- 1 medium onion, chopped
- 2 cloves garlic, chopped
- 1 Tbsp paprika
- 1 tsp dried thyme
- 1 tsp dried oregano
- ½ cup quick-cooking oats
- ½ cup raw walnuts
- 15-oz can lentils, rinsed
- 1 large egg yolk
- 1 tsp Worcestershire sauce
- 4 slices American cheese (optional)
- 4 brioche buns
- Iceberg or romaine lettuce, mayonnaise, tomato, red onion, and pickled jalapeño, for topping

1. Heat oven to 375°F. Line a rimmed baking sheet with nonstick baking mat or parchment.
2. Score flesh side of each eggplant half in diamond pattern. Brush cut sides with 1 tablespoon oil and season with ¼ teaspoon salt. Roast until very tender, 25 to 30 minutes.
3. Meanwhile, heat remaining 2 tablespoons oil in a medium skillet over medium heat. Add onion, season with ½ teaspoon each salt and pepper, and cook, covered, stirring occasionally, 5 minutes. Stir in garlic, paprika, thyme, and oregano and cook, stirring, 2 minutes. Let cool.
4. In a food processor, pulse oats and walnuts until very finely chopped; transfer mixture to small bowl. Scoop eggplant into the food processor, discarding skin. Add lentils, egg yolk, Worcestershire sauce, and onion mixture and process until nearly smooth. Add walnut-oat mixture and pulse to combine.
5. Divide eggplant mixture in four and scoop onto the prepared pan, then gently shape mixture into round patties. Bake until browned, 10 to 13 minutes, adding cheese during last minute of cooking if using. Let cool 5 minutes before making sandwiches with buns and toppings.

PER SERVING *About 664 cal, 35 g fat (8.5 g sat), 90 mg chol, 1,012 mg sodium, 67 g carb, 13 g fiber, 15.5 g sugar (7 g added sugar), 21 g pro*

BUTTERNUT SQUASH WHITE BEAN SOUP

ACTIVE 20 min. **TOTAL** 45 min. **SERVES** 4

1 large butternut squash

2 Tbsp olive oil, divided

1 onion, chopped

2 cloves garlic, finely chopped

1-in. piece fresh ginger, finely chopped

6 cups low-sodium chicken broth

6 sprigs fresh thyme

15-oz can white beans, rinsed

15-oz can chickpeas, rinsed

½ cup couscous

¼ cup roasted pistachios, finely chopped

¼ cup dried apricots, finely chopped

¼ cup fresh cilantro, chopped

1 scallion, sliced

1. Cut neck off butternut squash (reserve base for another use). Peel and cut into ½-in. pieces. Heat 1 tablespoon oil in a nonstick skillet over medium heat. Add squash and cook, covered, stirring occasionally, 8 minutes.
2. Meanwhile, heat remaining tablespoon oil in a Dutch oven over medium heat. Add onion and cook, covered, stirring occasionally, 6 minutes. Stir in garlic and ginger and cook 1 minute.
3. Add broth, thyme, and butternut squash and bring to a boil. Using a fork, mash white beans and add to soup along with chickpeas.
4. Cook couscous per package directions; fluff with fork and fold in pistachios, apricots, cilantro, and scallion. Serve soup topped with couscous mixture.

PER SERVING *About 558 cal, 14.5 g fat (2.5 g sat), 0 mg chol, 386 mg sodium, 88 g carb, 19 g fiber, 10 g sugar (0 g added sugar), 26 g pro*

MAKE IT AHEAD

Refrigerate the soup and plain couscous in separate airtight containers for up to three days. Warm soup over medium heat. Reheat couscous in the microwave then fold in pistachios, apricots, cilantro, and scallion as directed.

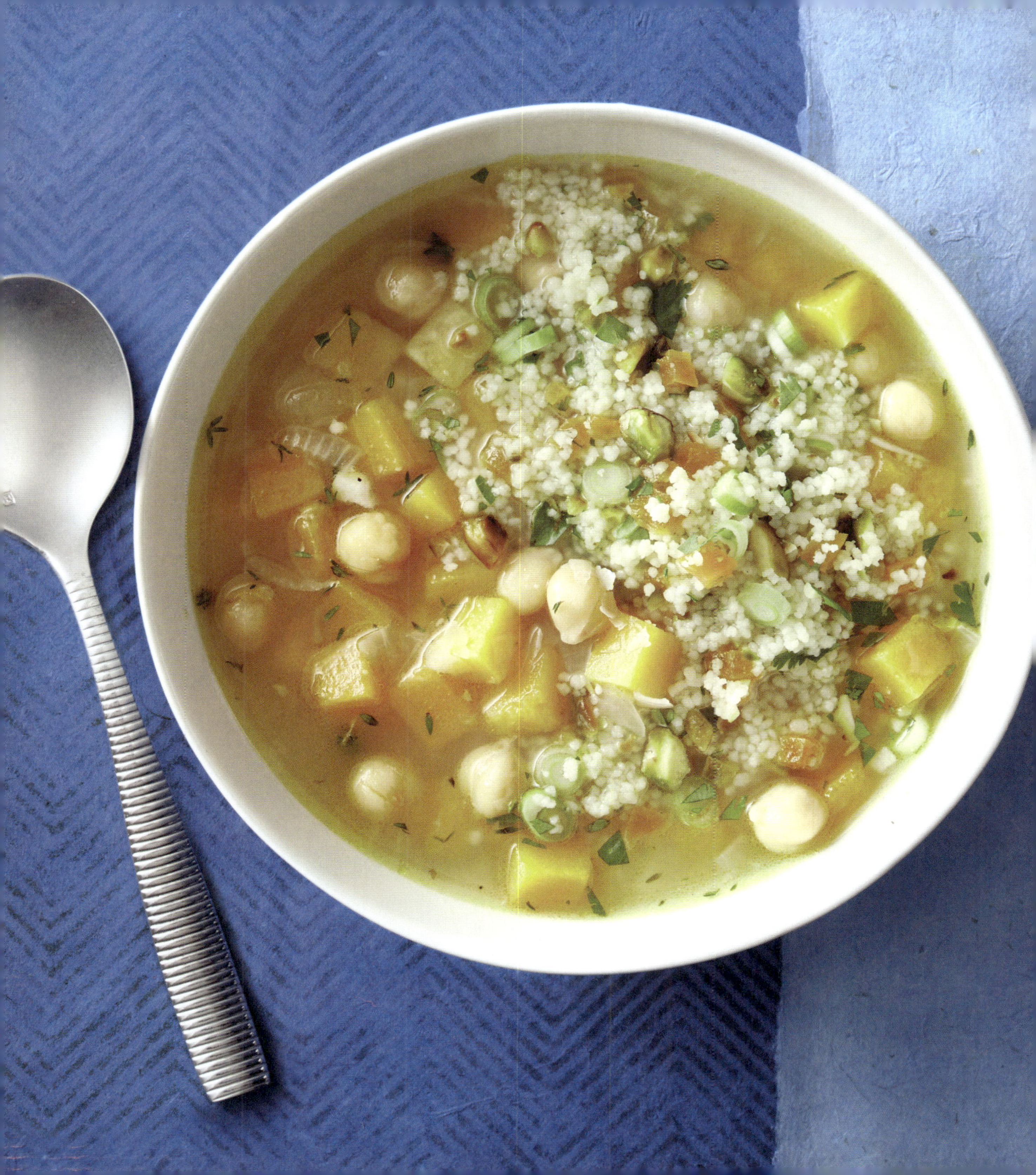

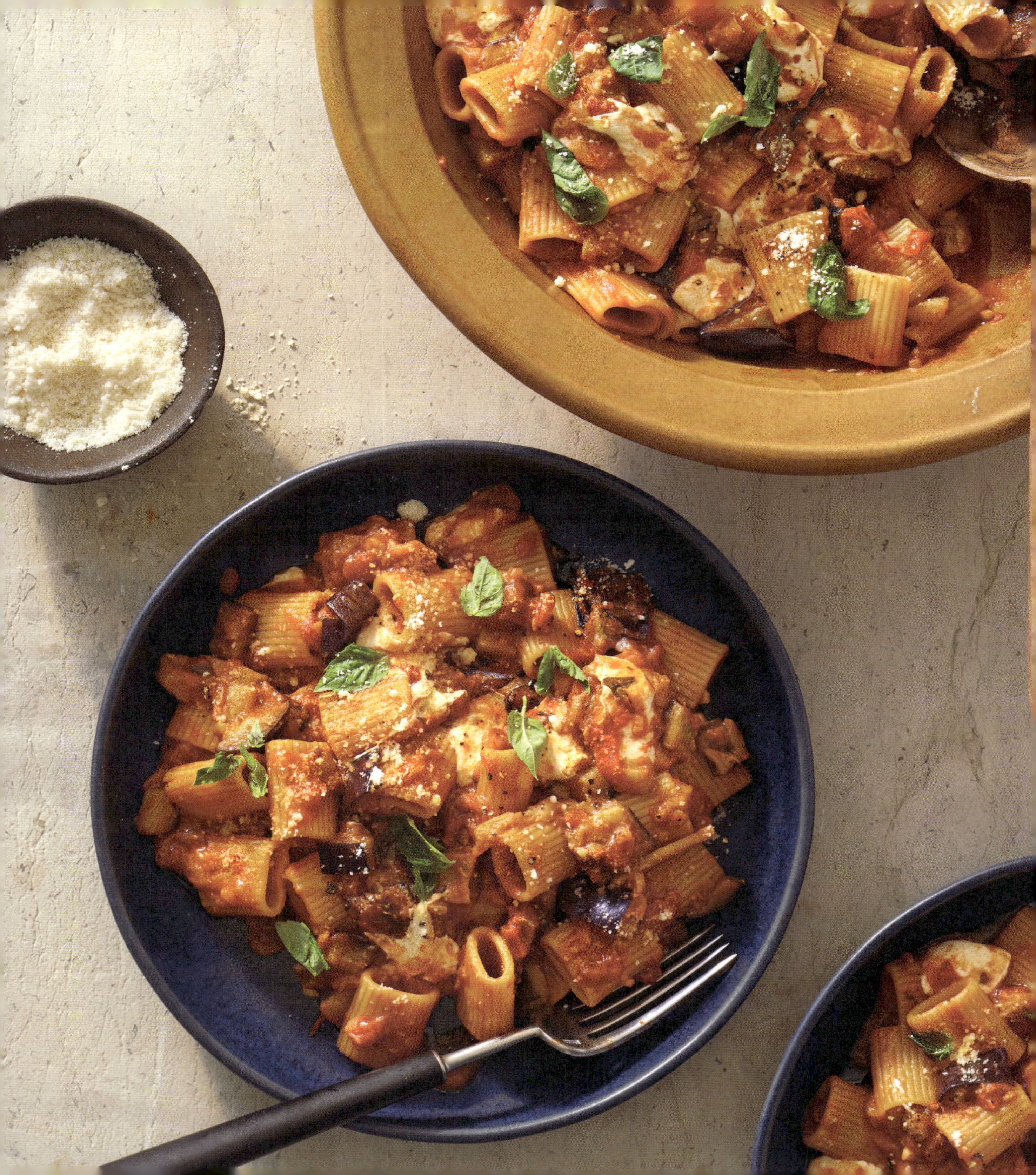

RIGATONI ALLA NORMA

ACTIVE 45 min. **TOTAL** 45 min. **SERVES** 4

8 oz fresh mozzarella, cut into ½-in. pieces

1¼ lb eggplant, cut into ½-in. pieces

¼ cup plus 2 Tbsp olive oil, divided

1 large shallot, finely chopped

4 cloves garlic, pressed

¼ tsp red pepper flakes

1 cup marinara sauce

14.5-oz can petite diced tomatoes

1 Tbsp vegetable bouillon base

12 oz rigatoni

1 Parmesan cheese rind (any you have is great), plus grated Parmesan for serving

½ cup basil leaves, torn

1. Freeze mozzarella until firm, at least 10 minutes. Meanwhile, heat oven to 425°F. On a large rimmed baking sheet, toss eggplant with ¼ cup oil. Roast 15 minutes. Toss and continue roasting until golden brown and tender, 15 to 18 minutes more.
2. Meanwhile, in a large Dutch oven, heat remaining 2 tablespoons oil and shallot over medium heat and cook, stirring occasionally, until sizzling, 2 minutes. Stir in garlic and red pepper flakes. Add marinara, tomatoes (and their juices), bouillon base, and 3 cups water, then stir in pasta and bring to a boil.
3. Stir in Parmesan rind and simmer vigorously, stirring frequently, until pasta is al dente, 12 to 15 minutes.
4. Remove Parmesan rind, fold eggplant and mozzarella into pasta and serve topped with basil and grated Parmesan if desired.

PER SERVING *About 764 cal, 36 g fat (11.5 g sat), 41 mg chol, 1,150 mg sodium, 85 g carb, 10 g fiber, 15.5 g sugar (2 g added sugar), 25 g pro*

KITCHEN TIP

When choosing a jarred marinara sauce, look for a short ingredient list with real foods like tomatoes, olive oil, and herbs. Skip sauces with added sugar and aim for under 400mg of sodium per serving.

TAHINI-LEMON QUINOA *with* ASPARAGUS RIBBONS

ACTIVE 45 min. **TOTAL** 45 min. **SERVES** 4

15-oz can chickpeas, rinsed

Zest and juice of 1 lemon

Kosher salt and pepper

1 cup quinoa

½ cup tahini

¼ cup fresh lime juice

1 Tbsp honey

1 cup packed fresh mint leaves

1 lb thick asparagus

¼ cup shelled pistachios, chopped

1. In a bowl, combine chickpeas, lemon zest, lemon juice, and a pinch of each salt and pepper. Let sit 20 minutes or refrigerate overnight, then drain.
2. Meanwhile, cook quinoa per package directions and season with a pinch of salt.
3. In a blender, purée tahini, lime juice, honey, mint, ½ cup water, and ¼ teaspoon salt until smooth, adding additional water if needed; set aside.
4. With vegetable peeler, shave asparagus into ribbons, peeling from woody end toward tip. In a bowl, combine cooked quinoa, asparagus ribbons, and marinated chickpeas. Sprinkle with pistachios and drizzle with tahini dressing.

PER SERVING *About 525 cal, 24 g fat (3.5 g sat), 0 mg chol, 313 mg sodium, 64 g carb, 14 g fiber, 11.5 g sugar (4.5 g added sugar), 21 g pro*

PROTEIN POWER
Pistachios are the only nut that are a complete protein, meaning that the little green gems contain all nine essential amino acids your body needs.

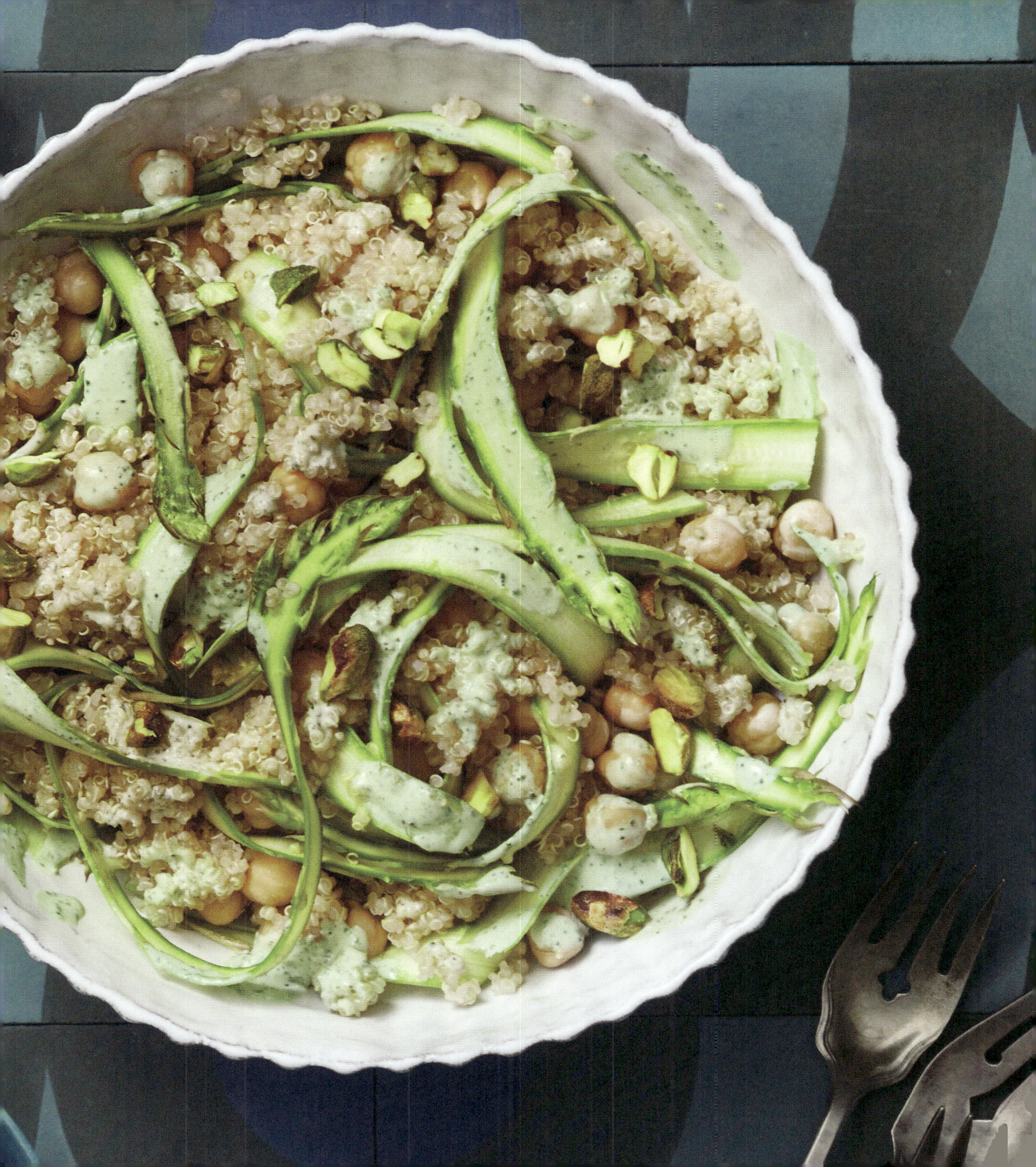

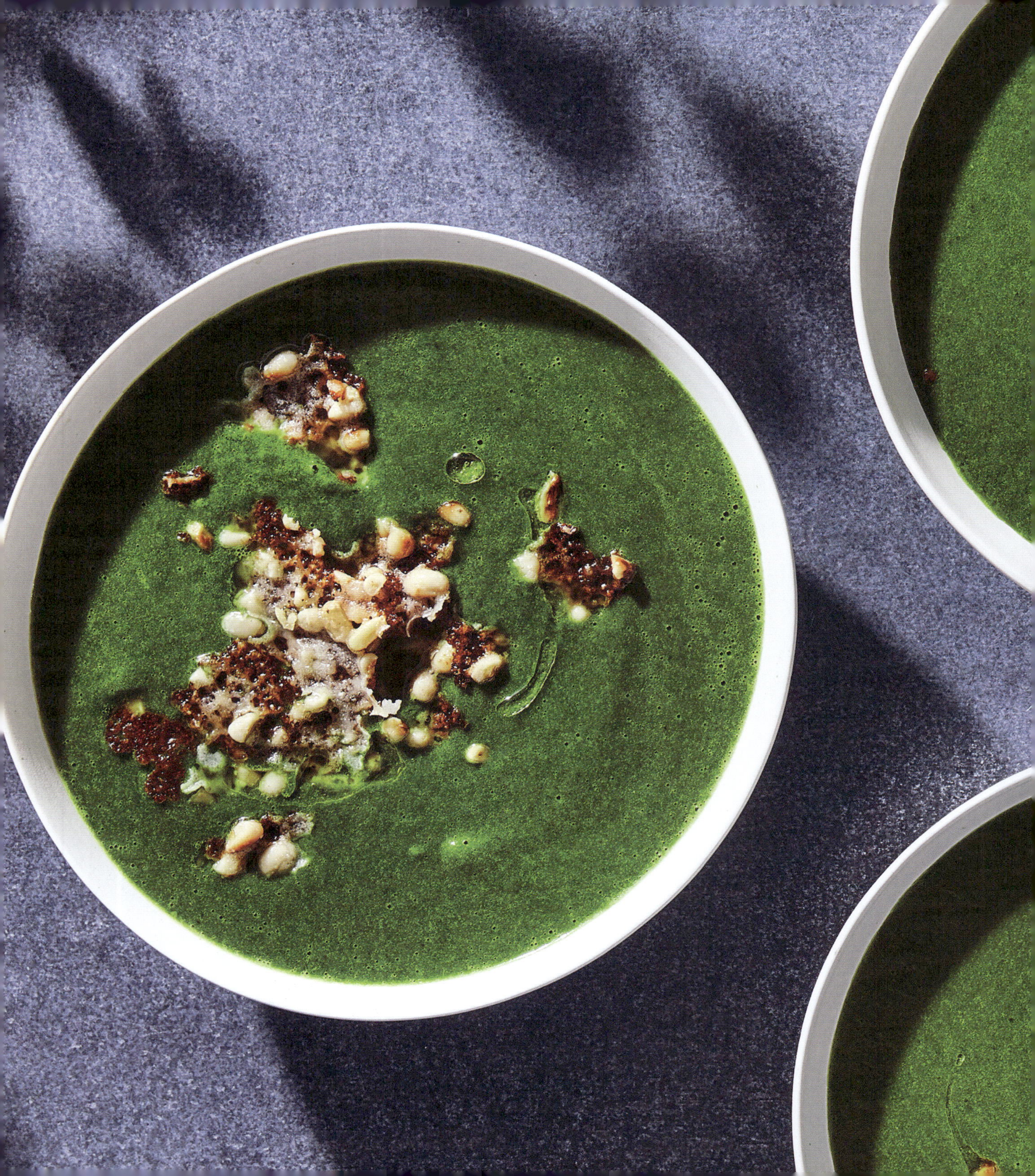

SUPER GREEN SOUP *with* PARM CRISPS

ACTIVE 40 min. **TOTAL** 1 hr. 10 min. **SERVES** 4

2 Tbsp pine nuts, roughly chopped

⅓ cup finely grated Parmesan

2 Tbsp olive oil

5 large shallots, chopped (2 to 3 cups)

6 large cloves garlic, smashed

Kosher salt and pepper

5 cups vegetable broth (homemade or low-sodium store-bought)

⅓ cup red lentils

1½ tsp freshly grated nutmeg

2 large bunches spinach (about 14 oz), thick stems removed (10 to 12 cups)

1½ cups fresh flat-leaf parsley leaves

1. Heat a medium nonstick skillet over medium heat. Add pine nuts and cook, tossing, until toasted, 2 to 3 minutes; transfer to small bowl. Sprinkle Parmesan in 7- to 8-inch rounds on skillet, sprinkle with pine nuts, and cook until golden brown, about 5 minutes. Remove from heat and let cook until slightly crisp, 45 seconds to 1 minute. Pry up edges and transfer to plate to cool completely, then break into shards.
2. Heat oil in a medium saucepan over medium-low heat. Add shallots, garlic, and 1 teaspoon salt and cook, stirring occasionally, until beginning to soften, 6 minutes. Stir in broth, lentils, and ½ teaspoon pepper and bring to a boil. Reduce heat and gently simmer, covered, stirring occasionally, until lentils are just tender 15 to 20 minutes.
3. Return to a boil, stir in nutmeg and half of spinach, and return to a boil. Stir in remaining spinach and parsley leaves, then immediately blend in batches until smooth.
4. Cool any soup for future use over ice bath. Serve soup with Parmesan crisps sprinkled on top.

PER SERVING *About 337 cal, 12.5 g fat (2.5 g sat), 8 mg chol, 1,026 mg sodium, 36 g carb, 8 g fiber, 8.5 g sugar (0 g added sugar), 25 g pro*

KITCHEN TIP

If using a regular blender, be sure to vent the lid and cover the opening with a kitchen towel to let steam escape safely. Or skip the transfer and use an immersion blender right in the pot—less mess, same silky results.

GRILLED LEEK, ZUCCHINI *and* RICOTTA PIZZA

ACTIVE 35 min. **TOTAL** 45 min. **SERVES** 4

- Flour, for surface
- 1 lb pizza dough
- 1 large leek, halved lengthwise
- 2 large zucchini, halved lengthwise
- 2 Tbsp olive oil, plus more for drizzling
- Kosher salt and pepper
- 2 tsp finely grated lemon zest plus 3 Tbsp lemon juice
- 2 cups ricotta cheese
- Mint, for serving

1. Heat oven to 425°F. Line a baking sheet with parchment paper. On a lightly floured surface, shape dough into a large rectangle. Place on prepared sheet and bake 10 minutes. Remove crust from oven and set aside. Reset oven temp to 475°F.
2. Meanwhile, heat grill over medium-high heat. Brush leek and zucchini with oil; season with salt and pepper. Grill until tender, turning once, 5 to 8 minutes. Thinly slice vegetables and toss with lemon juice.
3. In a small bowl, mix ricotta with lemon zest and ½ teaspoon salt. Spread ricotta on crust and top with vegetables. Bake until crust and toppings have browned, 5 to 8 minutes. Drizzle with olive oil and top with mint if desired.

PER SERVING *About 575 cal, 26.5 g fat (11.5 g sat), 63 mg chol, 1,235 mg sodium, 60 g carb, 4 g fiber, 4.5 g sugar (0 g added sugar), 22 g pro*

KITCHEN TIP
To clean leeks before cooking, slice them in half lengthwise, then rinse between the layers to remove any grit.

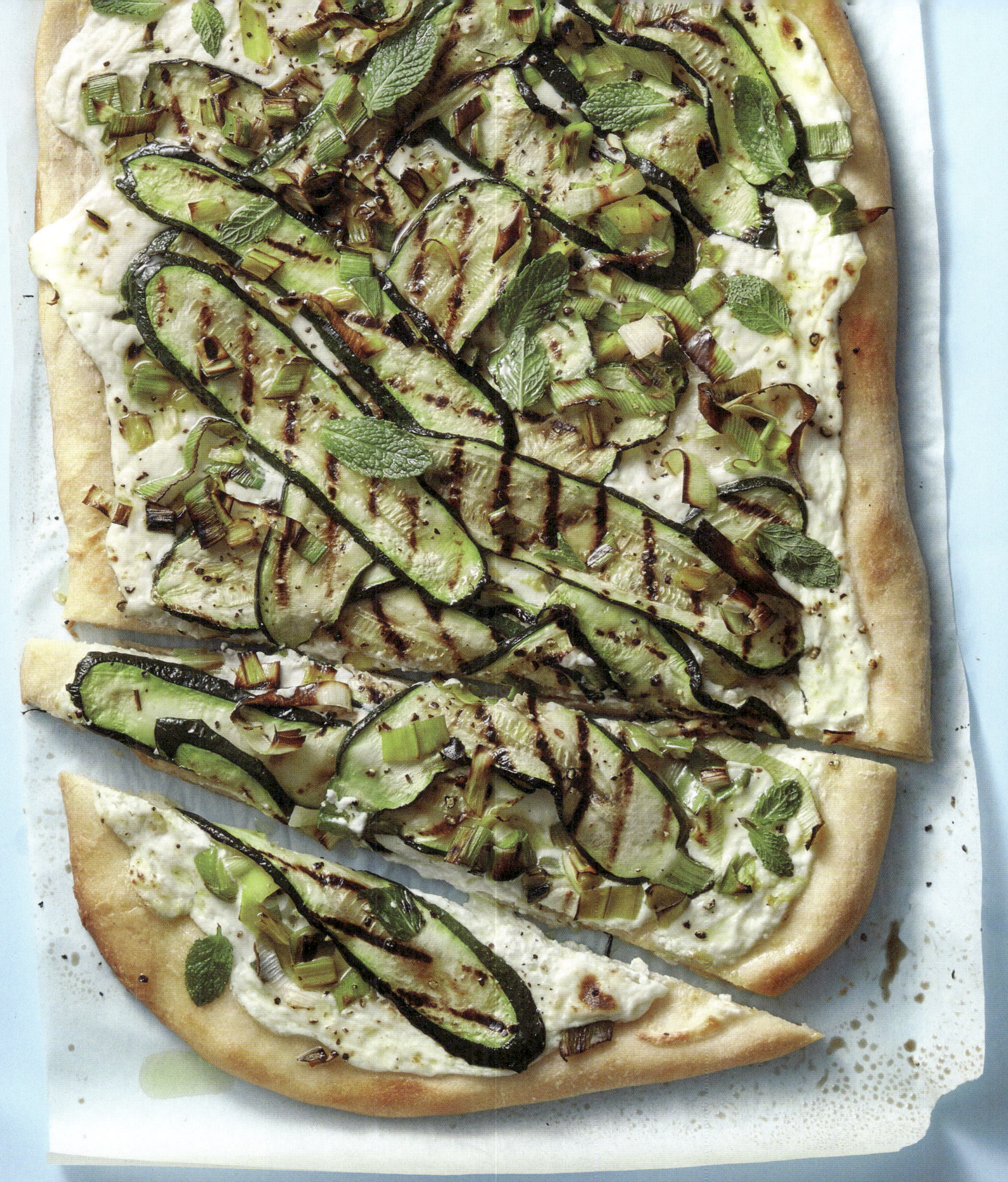

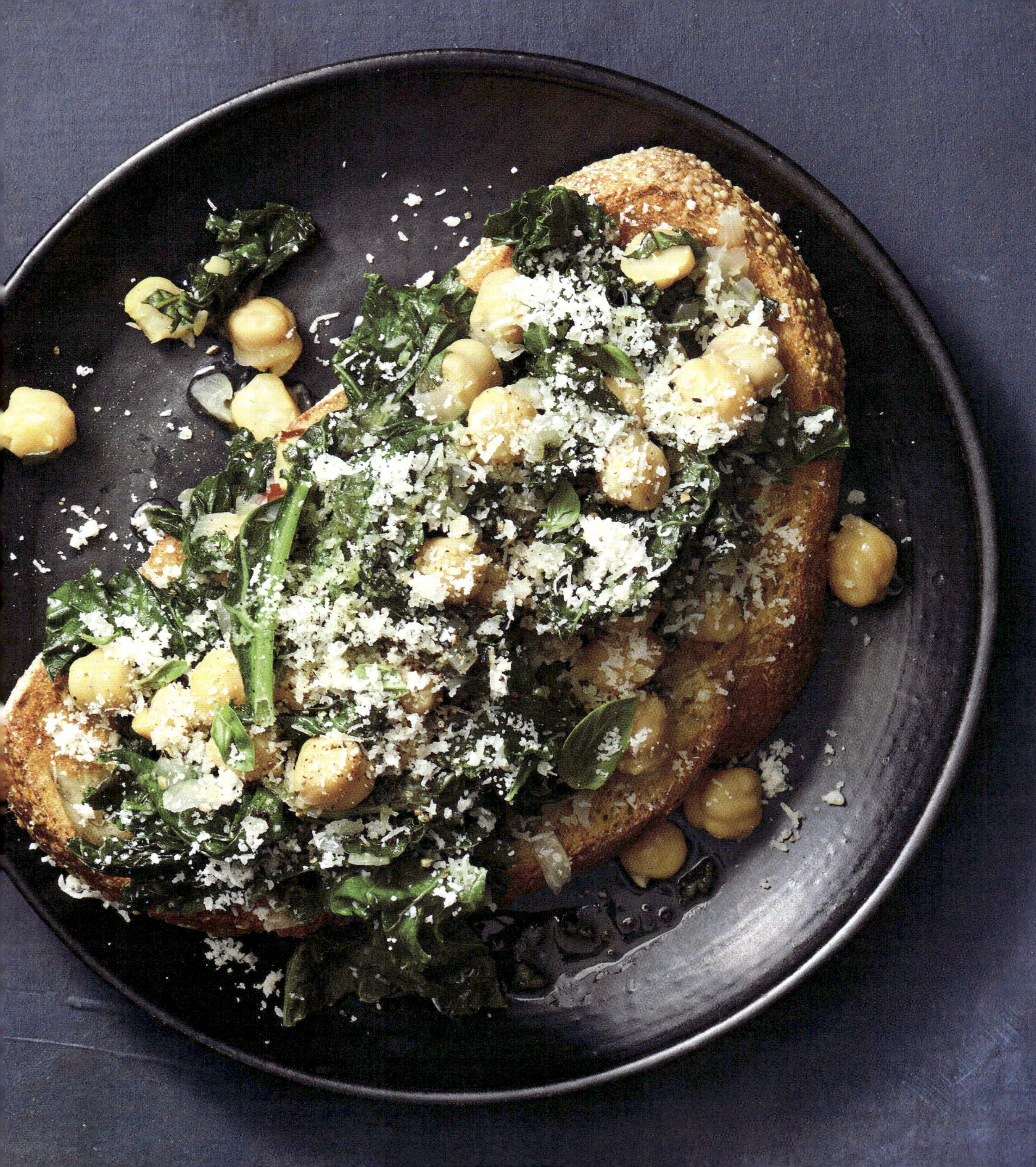

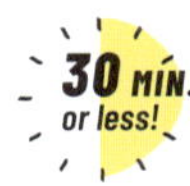

KALE and CHICKPEA TOASTS

ACTIVE 25 min. **TOTAL** 25 min. **SERVES** 4

2 Tbsp olive oil, plus more for drizzling

1 small onion, finely chopped

2 cloves garlic, thinly sliced

¼ tsp red pepper flakes

¼ cup dry white wine

19-oz can chickpeas

1 large bunch curly kale (about 14 oz), stems and ribs removed, leaves torn (about 12 cups)

Kosher salt and pepper

⅓ cup basil leaves, chopped

4 slices sourdough bread

1 lemon, halved

1 oz Parmesan cheese, finely grated

1. Heat broiler to high. Heat oil in a large skillet over medium heat. Add onion and cook, stirring occasionally, until just tender, 5 to 6 minutes. Stir in garlic and red pepper flakes and cook until fragrant, 1 minute. Add wine and simmer until mostly evaporated, 1 minute.

2. Add chickpeas and their liquid and simmer until slightly reduced, about 3 minutes. Add kale and ¼ teaspoon each salt and pepper and cook, tossing occasionally, until kale wilts, 3 to 4 minutes. Remove from heat and fold in basil.

3. Place bread on a baking sheet and broil until golden brown, about 1 minute per side. Immediately rub with cut side of lemon. Top with chickpea mixture and sprinkle with Parmesan.

PER SERVING *About 496 cal, 13.5 g fat (3 g sat), 5 mg chol, 884 mg sodium, 73 g carb, 15 g fiber, 10.5 g sugar (0 g added sugar), 24 g pro*

FIBER FIX

Kale is high in fiber—just one cup cooked delivers about 5 grams of fiber, helping to keep digestion smooth and you feeling full longer.

STUFFED QUINOA WRAPS

ACTIVE 30 min. **TOTAL** 30 min. (plus soaking) **SERVES** 1

FOR WRAPS
1 cup quinoa

¼ cup nutritional yeast

Kosher salt

Canola oil, for cooking

FOR FILLING
3 Tbsp beet hummus

½ Persian cucumber, sliced

Olive oil and lemon juice, for drizzling

1 hard-boiled egg, sliced

2 Tbsp crunchy chickpeas

½ oz feta, crumbled

⅓ cup microgreens

1 scallion, thinly sliced

1. Place quinoa in a medium bowl and add enough water to cover by 2 inches. Let soak at least 4 hours, up to overnight.

2. Drain and rinse quinoa in a fine-mesh sieve and shake off excess water. Transfer to a blender along with nutritional yeast and ½ teaspoon salt. Pour ¾ cup plus 2 tablespoons water down sides of the blender to loosen any quinoa that adhered. Starting on low speed, blend, slowly increasing to medium, 30 seconds. Increase to highest speed and blend until smooth and consistency of crepe batter, about 1 minute.

3. Brush a 10-inch nonstick skillet with oil and heat over medium heat. Measure heaping ⅓ cup batter and pour toward one side of pan, quickly tilting and swirling, until batter coats surface. Cook, reducing heat to medium-low as needed, until wrap is completely set and begins to brown, 2 minutes. Flip and cook 1 more minute. Transfer to wire rack to cool completely. Repeat cooking with oil and remaining batter.

4. Spread beet hummus on 1 quinoa wrap, top with cucumber, and drizzle with oil and lemon juice if desired. Top with egg, chickpeas, feta, microgreens, and scallion. Roll into cone for serving.

PER SERVING *About 474 cal, 26 g fat (5 g sat), 199 mg chol, 630 mg sodium, 41 g carb, 8 g fiber, 5 g sugar (0 g added sugar), 22 g pro*

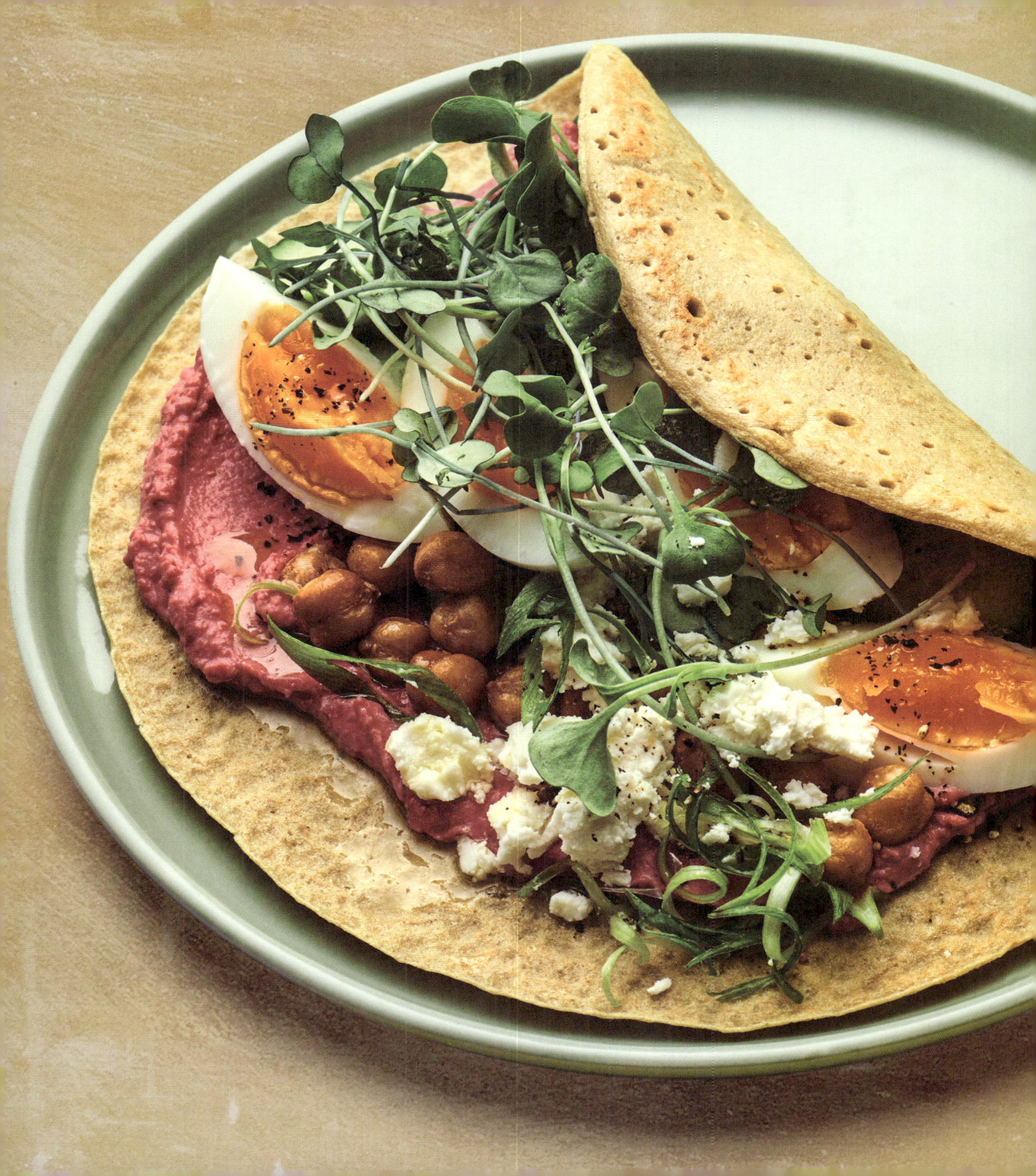

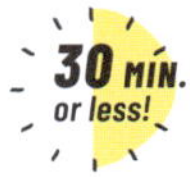

CHICKPEA SALAD SANDWICH

ACTIVE 10 min. **TOTAL** 10 min. **SERVES** 4

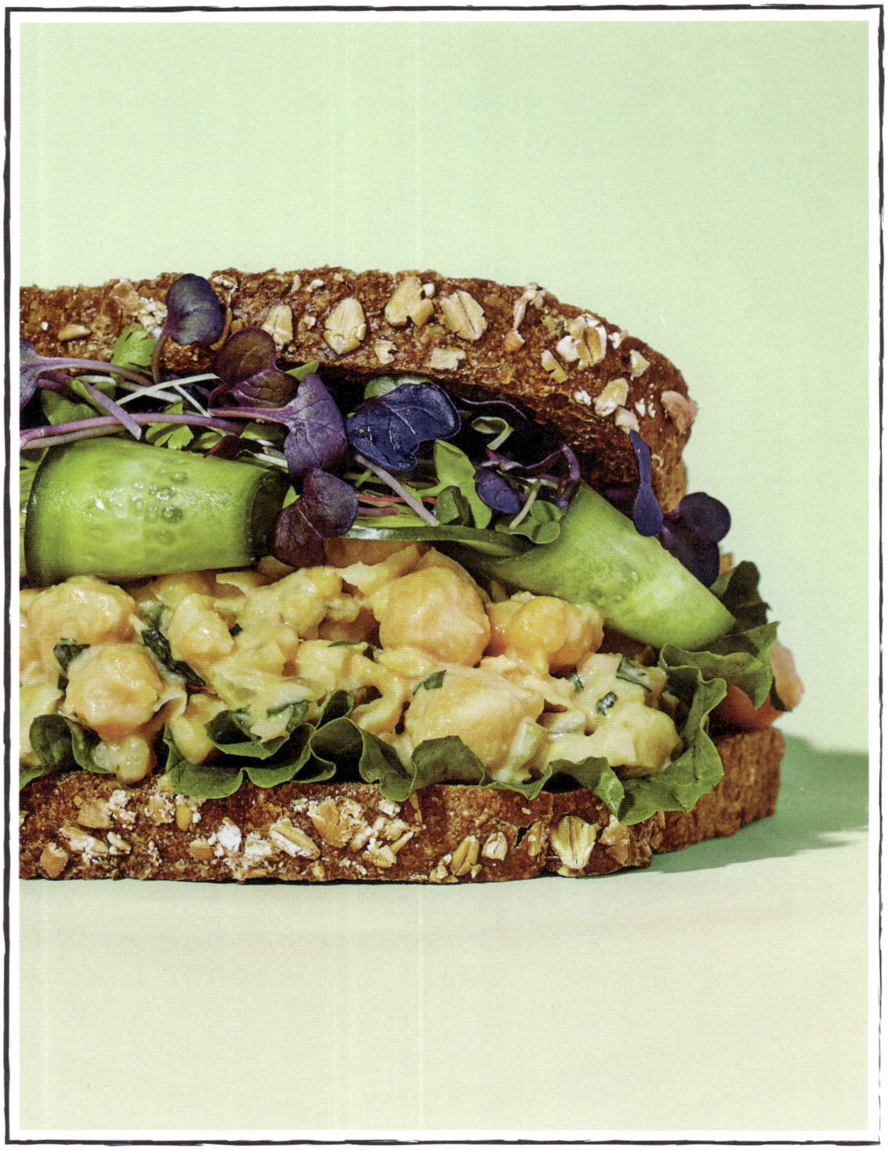

- 2 Tbsp fresh lemon juice
- 2 Tbsp vegan mayonnaise
- 1 Tbsp reduced-sodium soy sauce
- 1 Tbsp nutritional yeast
- 2 15-oz cans low-sodium chickpeas, drained and rinsed
- 2 stalks celery, thinly sliced
- 1 scallion, sliced
- ½ cup flat-leaf parsley, chopped
- 8 slices whole-grain bread
- 4 leaves green leaf lettuce
- 1 Persian cucumber or ½ seedless cucumber, peeled into ribbons
- 1 cup sprouts

1. In a large bowl, whisk together lemon juice, mayonnaise, soy sauce, and nutritional yeast.

2. Add chickpeas and mash, leaving some larger chunks. Fold in celery, scallion, and parsley.

3. Assemble sandwiches with bread, lettuce, chickpea mixture, cucumber, and sprouts.

PER SERVING *About 472 cal, 12 g fat (1.5 g sat), 3 mg chol, 905 mg sodium, 70 g carb, 16 g fiber, 11.5 g sugar (0 g added sugar), 23 g pro*

CHICKPEA PASTA SALAD

ACTIVE 10 min. **TOTAL** 10 min. **SERVES** 1

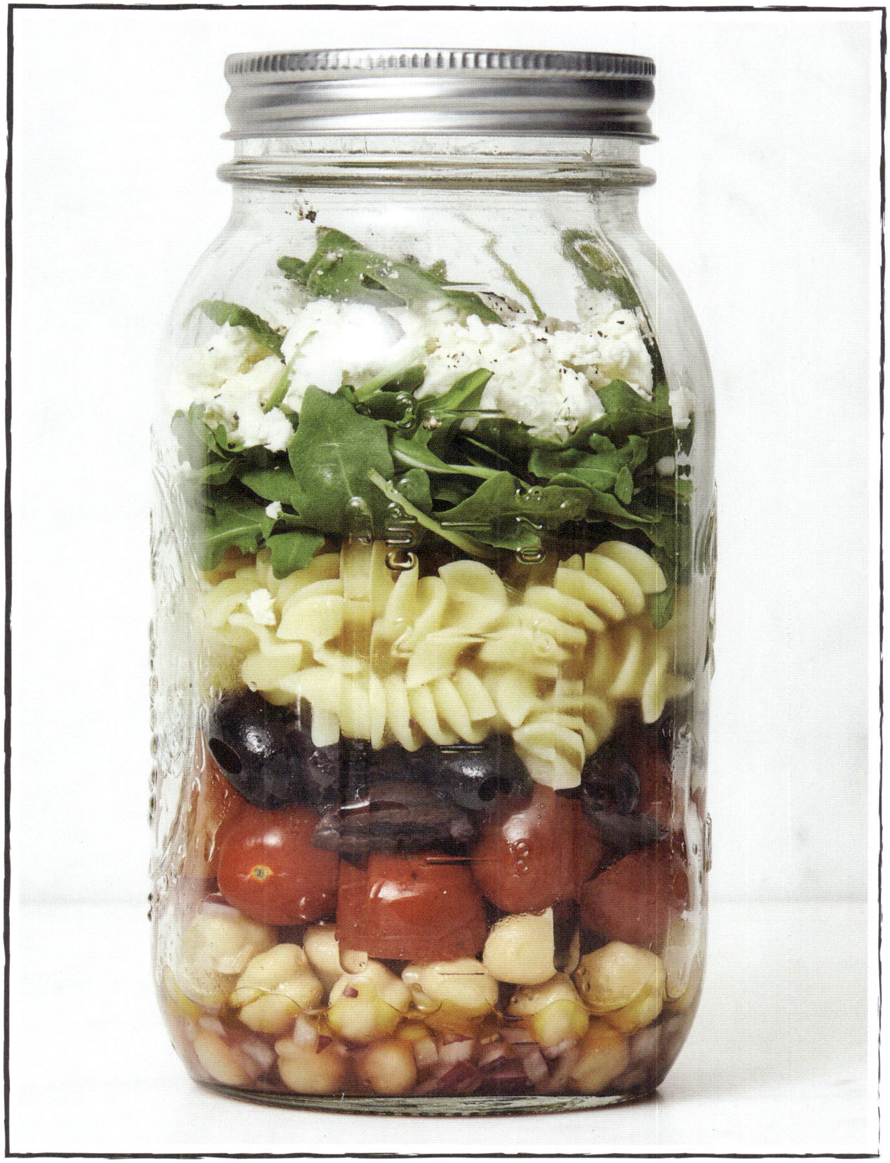

¼ very small red onion, finely chopped
2 Tbsp red wine vinegar
1½ Tbsp olive oil
Kosher salt and pepper
½ cup canned chickpeas, rinsed
1 cup grape tomatoes, halved
2 Tbsp Kalamata olives, halved
1 cup cooked protein plus rotini pasta
1½ cups baby arugula
2 Tbsp crumbled feta

In a 1-quart jar, shake onion, vinegar, oil, and a pinch each of salt and pepper. Add chickpeas and gently shake to coat. Top with tomatoes, olives, pasta, arugula, and feta. When ready to serve, turn upside down and let sit 2 minutes so dressing can run over rest of ingredients.

PER SERVING *About 610 cal, 32.5 g fat (6.5 g sat), 17 mg chol, 816 mg sodium, 71 g carb, 13 g fiber, 9.5 g sugar (0 g added sugar), 21 g pro*

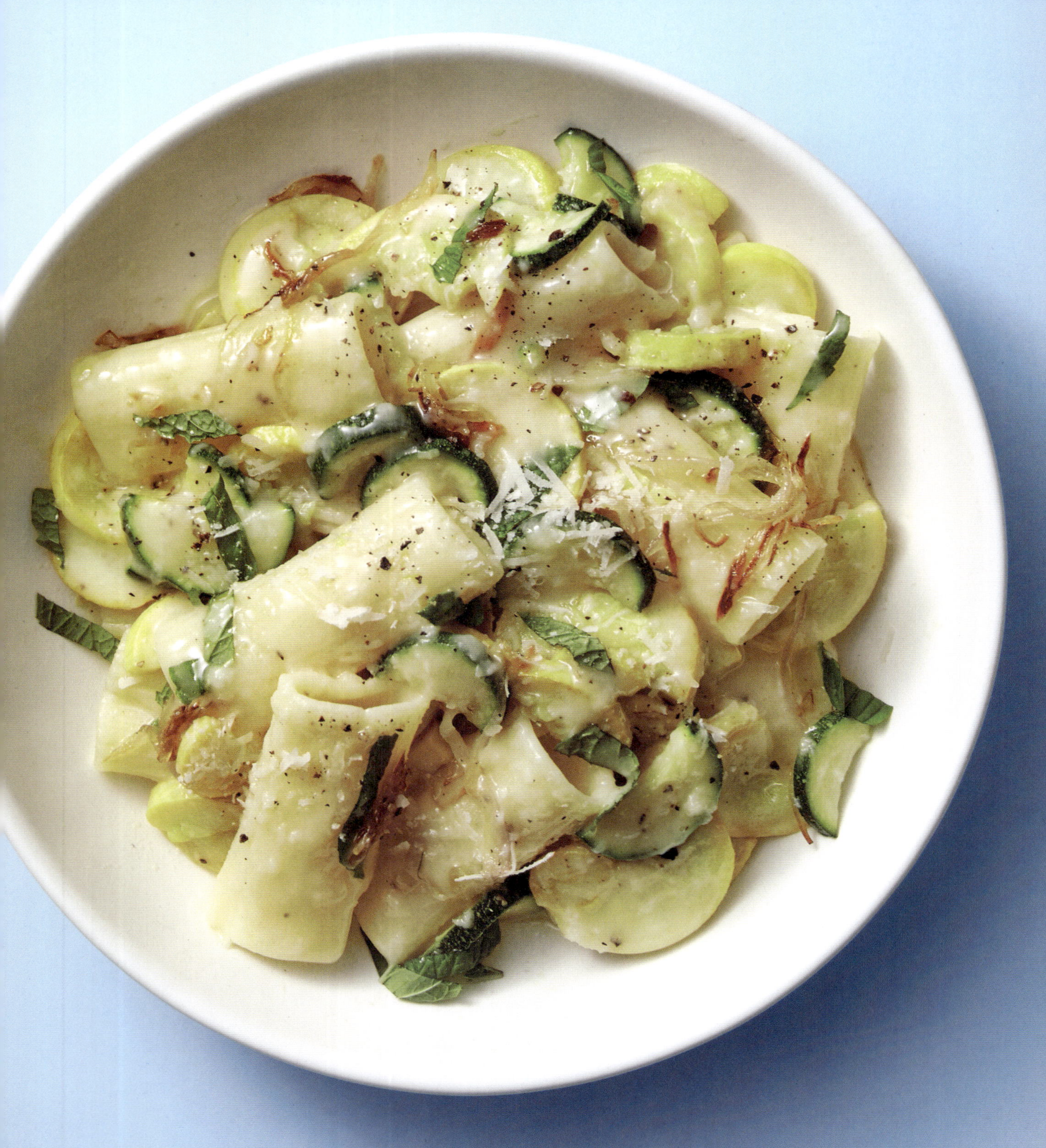

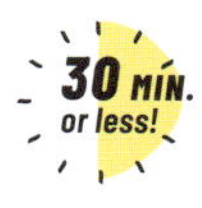

SUMMER SQUASH & PECORINO PASTA

ACTIVE 15 min. **TOTAL** 25 min. **SERVES** 4

12 oz rigatoni

2 Tbsp olive oil

1 shallot, halved and thinly sliced

1½ lb zucchini and summer squash (about 4 small), thinly sliced into half-moons

Kosher salt and pepper

3 oz pecorino cheese (about 1 cup), grated plus more for serving

⅓ cup mint, thinly sliced

1 Tbsp lemon juice

1. Cook pasta per package directions. Reserve ¾ cup cooking liquid then drain.
2. Meanwhile, heat oil in a large, deep skillet over medium heat. Cook shallot, stirring occasionally, until golden brown, 3 to 4 minutes. Add zucchini and squash and ½ teaspoon each salt and pepper and cook, tossing occasionally, until squash is very tender but still holds its shape, 10 to 12 minutes.
3. Add pasta to the skillet and toss with squash and cheese, adding reserved cooking liquid 2 tablespoons at a time, to form a sauce that coats pasta. Fold in mint and lemon juice. Top with additional cheese and black pepper if desired.

PER SERVING *About 487 cal, 13.5 g fat (5 g sat), 22 mg chol, 506 mg sodium, 71 g carb, 5 g fiber, 7.5 g sugar (0 g added sugar), 21 g pro*

KITCHEN TIP

Reserve some of the pasta cooking water before draining—its starch content helps emulsify and thicken sauces, creating a silky, smooth texture. If you forget, you can make a starchy substitute by stirring ¼ teaspoon cornstarch into 1 cup water, then use only what you need.

SPINACH SALAD *with* CRISPY LENTILS & AGED GOUDA

ACTIVE 35 min. **TOTAL** 55 min. **SERVES** 4

- 2 15-oz cans no-salt-added lentils, rinsed and drained well
- 4 Tbsp olive oil, divided
- Kosher salt and pepper
- ½ cup sliced almonds
- 1 tsp lightly crushed fennel seeds
- ¼ tsp red pepper flakes
- ¼ tsp granulated garlic (optional)
- 3 Tbsp sherry vinegar
- 1 medium shallot, finely chopped
- 1 Tbsp thyme leaves, chopped
- 5-oz pkg. baby spinach
- 2 large avocados, sliced
- 2 oz aged Gouda, shaved with vegetable peeler

1. Heat oven to 375°F. Spread lentils on a large rimmed baking sheet and blot dry with paper towels; transfer 1½ cups to bowl and refrigerate until ready to use.
2. Drizzle remaining lentils with 1 tablespoon oil, sprinkle with ½ teaspoon salt, and toss to coat; spread in even layer. Roast, stirring three times, until beginning to crisp but not completely crunchy, 22 to 25 minutes. Stir in almonds, fennel seeds, and red pepper flakes; roast until lentils are crisp and almonds are golden brown, 6 to 8 minutes. Toss with granulated garlic, if using, and let cool.
3. Meanwhile, in a large bowl, whisk together vinegar, shallot, thyme, ½ teaspoon each salt and pepper, and remaining 3 tablespoons oil; fold in reserved lentils, then spinach and avocado slices. Divide among plates. Top each plate with about ¼ cup crispy lentils, then Gouda. Leftover crispy lentils can be stored in airtight container at room temp up to 2 weeks.

PER SERVINGS *About 596 cal, 42 g fat (8 g sat), 18 mg chol, 701 mg sodium, 40 g carb, 24 g fiber, 4.5 g sugar (0 g added sugar), 20 g pro*

PROTEIN POWER

Lentils may be small, but they pack a serious protein punch—with about 18 grams per cup cooked, they're one of the easiest (and tastiest) ways to power up a plant-based plate.

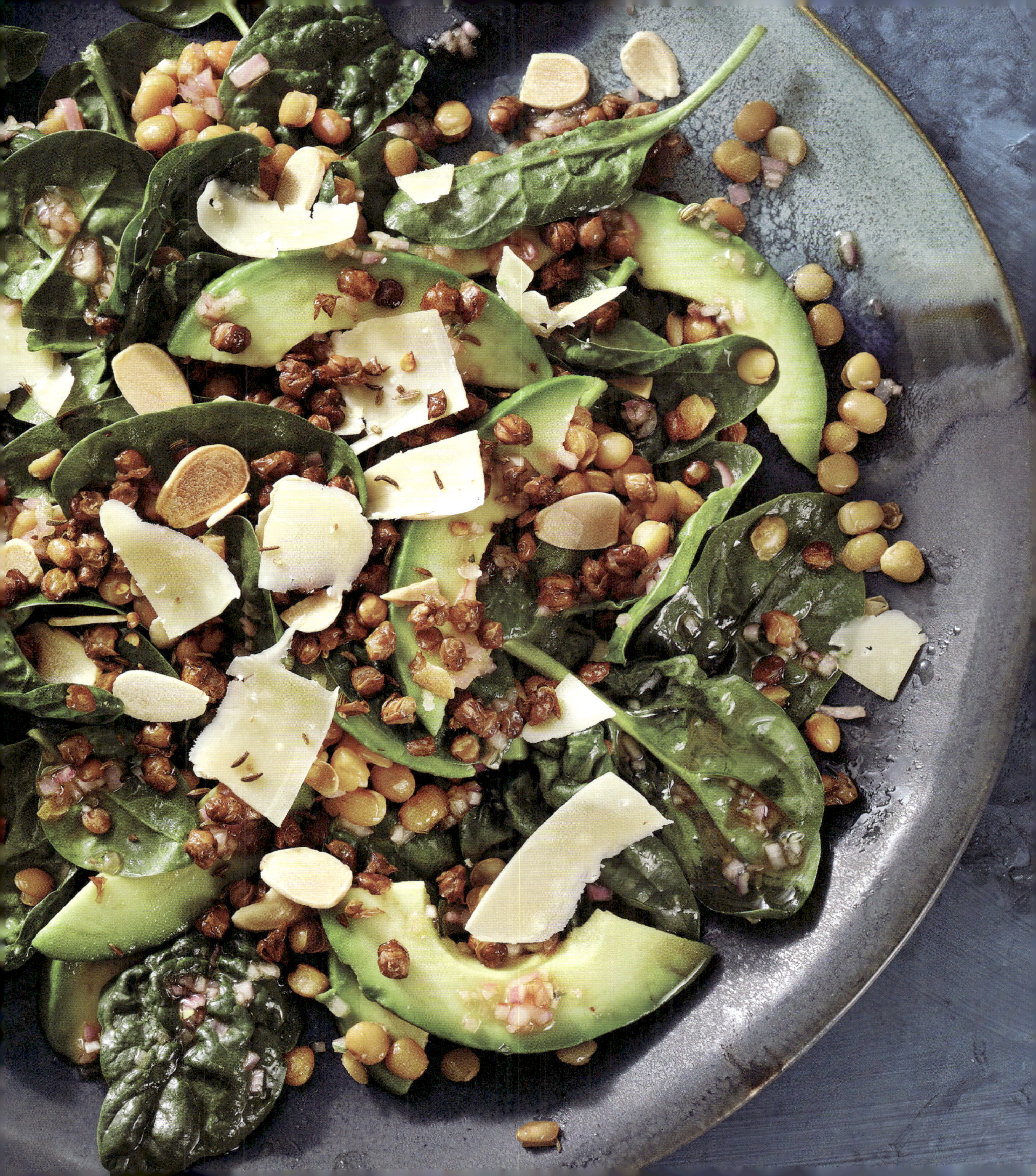

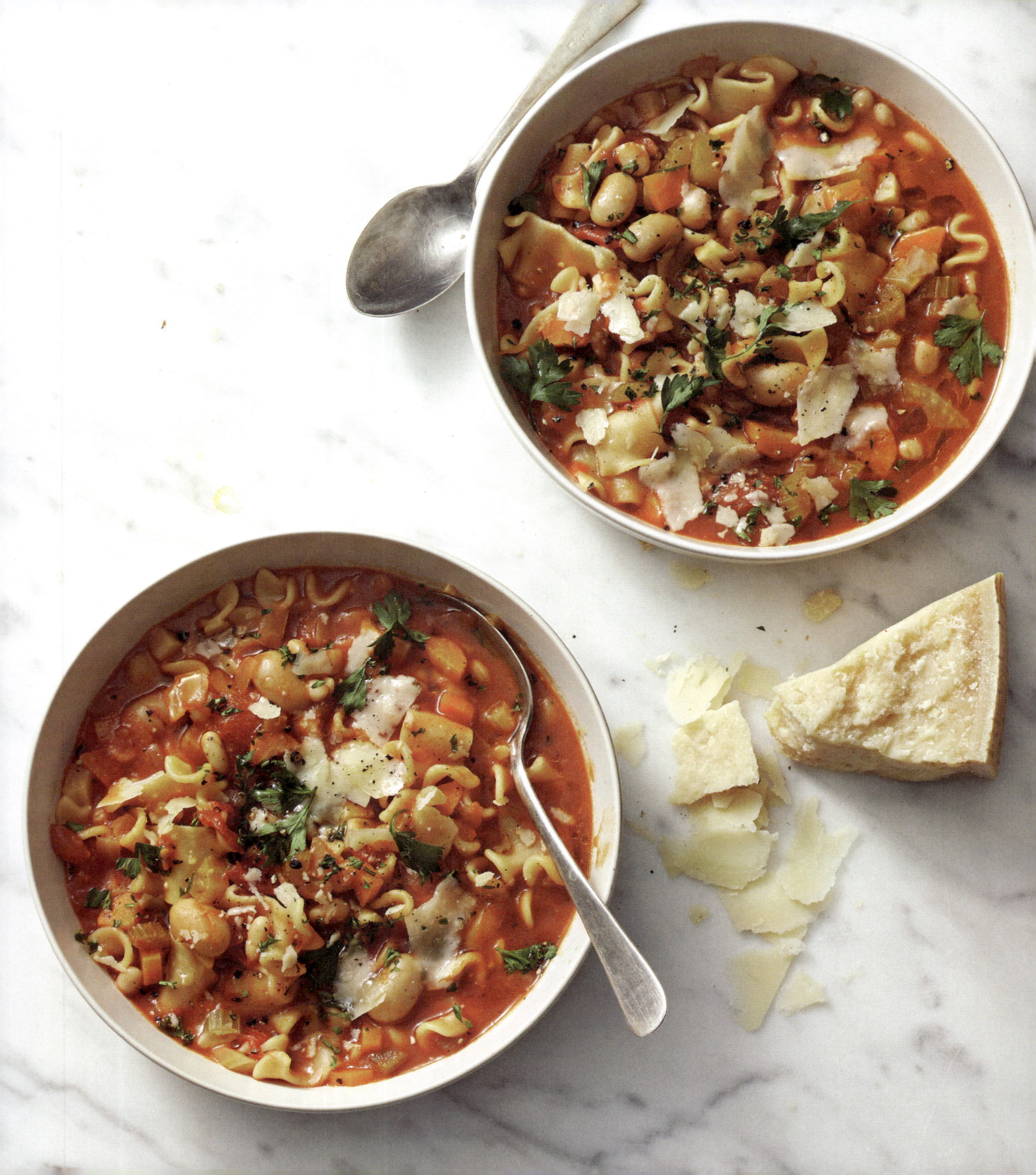

PASTA E FAGIOLI

ACTIVE 25 min. **TOTAL** 35 min. **SERVES** 5

2 Tbsp olive oil

1 large onion, chopped

2 medium carrots, cut into ¼-in. pieces

1 stalk celery, cut into ¼-in. pieces

1 small bulb fennel, cut into ¼-in. pieces

Kosher salt and pepper

2 large cloves garlic, finely chopped

6 sprigs fresh thyme

½ cup dry white wine

28-oz can whole peeled tomatoes

1 Tbsp vegetable base (optional)

8 oz orecchiette or other short pasta

2 15-oz cans white beans (cannellini, navy, butter, or a combination), rinsed

Chopped parsley and grated Parmesan, for serving

1. Heat oil in a large Dutch oven over medium heat. Add onion and cook, stirring occasionally, 5 minutes. Add carrots, celery, fennel, ¾ teaspoon salt, and ½ teaspoon pepper and cook, covered, stirring occasionally, until vegetables are beginning to soften, 6 to 8 minutes more. Stir in garlic and thyme and cook 2 minutes. Add wine and simmer until nearly evaporated, 1 to 2 minutes.

2. Add tomatoes and their juices, crushing into small pieces as you add to pot. Add 5 cups water and base (if using) and bring to a boil. Add pasta and simmer, stirring often, until barely tender, 8 to 12 minutes depending on type of pasta. Stir in beans and cook until heated through, about 2 minutes. Remove thyme and serve sprinkled with parsley and Parmesan.

PER SERVING *About 462 cal, 6.5 g fat (1.5 g sat), 3 mg chol, 819 mg sodium, 81 g carb, 18 g fiber, 11 g sugar (0 g added sugar), 20 g pro*

FIBER FIX

Beans are fiber all-stars. One hearty serving of this soup packs around 18 grams of fiber, getting you most of the way toward your daily 25 to 30 grams goal.

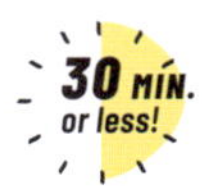

SKILLET PEPPER PASTA

ACTIVE 25 min. **TOTAL** 25 min. **SERVES** 4

4 Tbsp oil, divided

2 large peppers (red and yellow), halved and sliced crosswise

1 red onion, sliced

½ tsp red pepper flakes

Kosher salt

2 large cloves garlic, finely chopped

1½ tsp fennel seeds, crushed

2 Tbsp tomato paste

12 oz linguine

1 tsp lemon zest (plus more for serving), plus 1 Tbsp lemon juice

1 Tbsp capers, roughly chopped

3 oz Romano, grated, plus more for serving

Freshly cracked black pepper, for serving

Chopped parsley, for serving

1. Heat 1 tablespoon oil in a large skillet over medium heat. Add peppers, onion, red pepper flakes, and ¼ teaspoon salt and cook, tossing occasionally, until just tender, about 6 minutes; transfer to a bowl. Add remaining 3 tablespoons oil to skillet along with garlic and fennel seeds and cook, stirring, 1 minute. Stir in tomato paste and cook 1 minute.
2. Add linguine, 4½ cups water, lemon zest, and ¼ teaspoon salt and simmer, stirring often, 10 minutes. Fold in capers and continue cooking, stirring often, until pasta is just tender, 3 to 5 minutes more.
3. Toss with lemon juice and Romano until cheese is melted and a thick sauce is created, then fold in pepper-onion mixture and serve topped with cracked pepper, chopped parsley, and additional lemon zest and Romano if desired.

PER SERVING *About 564 cal, 22 g fat (6 g sat), 27 mg chol, 646 mg sodium, 73 g carb, 6 g fiber, 7 g sugar (0 g added sugar), 20 g pro*

KITCHEN TIP

Cooking pasta in a skillet with just enough water to cover it means faster cooking and starchier water—perfect for a creamy sauce without even draining.

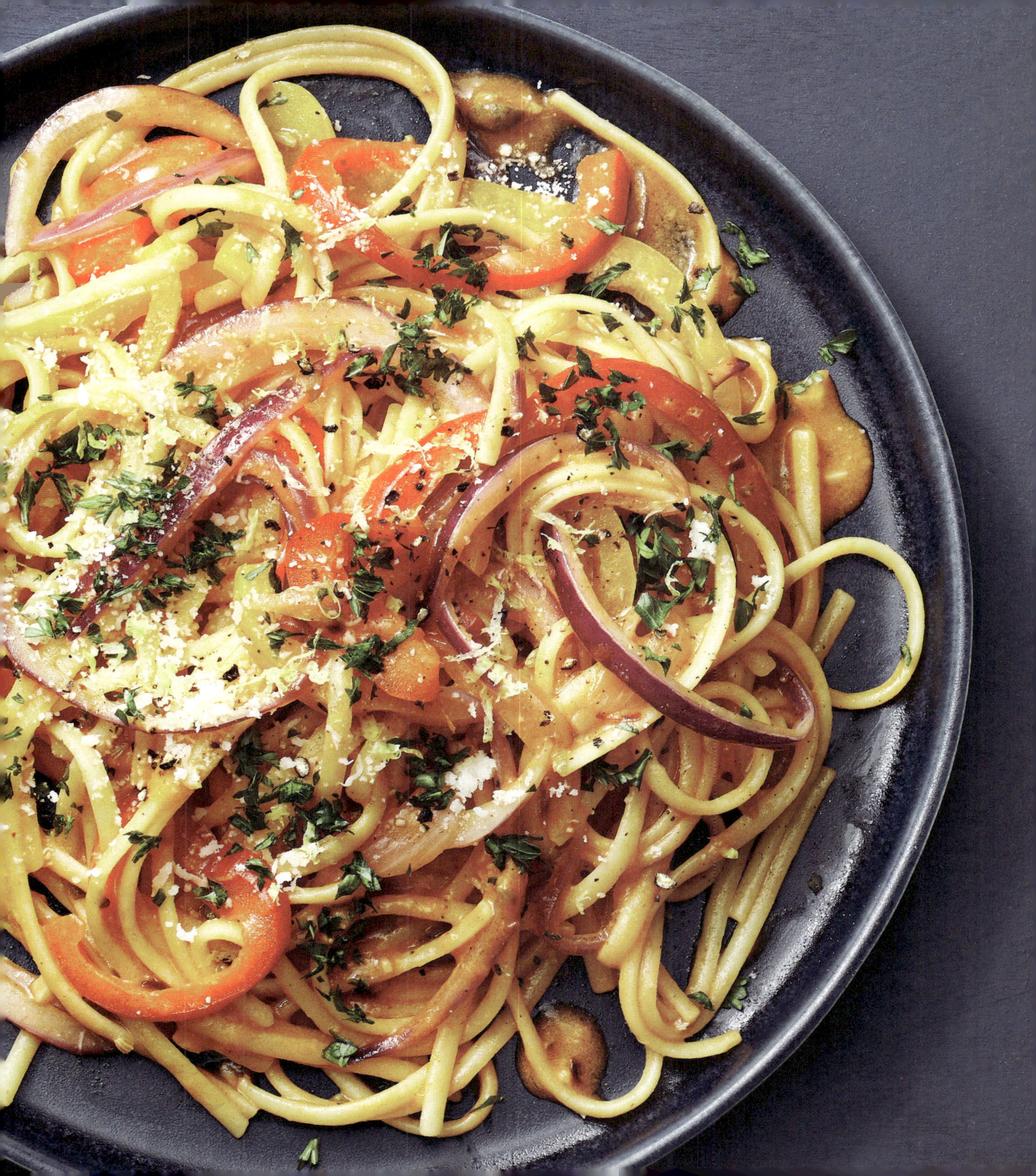

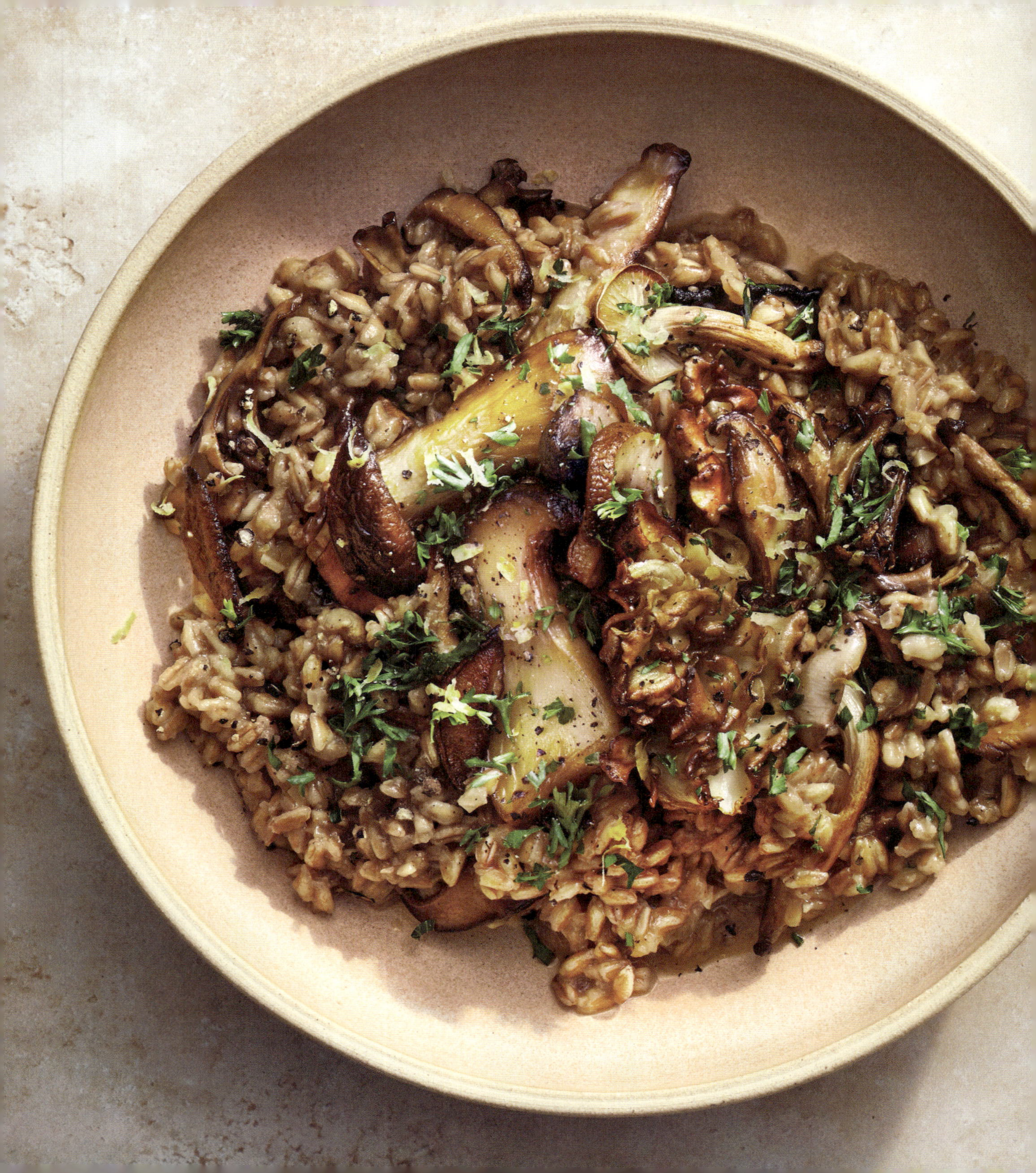

MUSHROOM FARROTTO

ACTIVE 50 min. **TOTAL** 50 min. **SERVES** 4

4 cups mushroom broth

3½ Tbsp olive oil, divided

1 large shallot, finely chopped

Kosher salt

2 cloves garlic, finely chopped

2 sprigs thyme

⅓ cup dry white wine

1½ cups quick-cooking farro

¾ cup grated Parmesan cheese

1½ lb mixed mushrooms (we used oyster, shiitake, beech, and cremini), torn, sliced, or quartered

Grated lemon zest, for sprinkling

½ cup sliced almonds, toasted and roughly chopped

2 Tbsp flat-leaf parsley leaves, chopped

1. Heat oven to 450°F. In a medium saucepan, combine mushroom broth with 1 cup water and bring to a gentle simmer.

2. Meanwhile, heat 1½ tablespoons oil in medium a Dutch oven over medium heat. Add shallot and ¼ teaspoon salt and cook, covered, stirring occasionally, until just tender, 3 to 4 minutes. Add garlic and thyme and cook, stirring constantly, 1 minute more. Add wine and cook, stirring constantly, until evaporated, 1 to 2 minutes.

3. Add farro and cook, stirring, 2 minutes. Add mushroom broth and bring to a boil. Reduce heat and simmer, stirring occasionally, until farro is tender and liquid is nearly all absorbed, 28 to 31 minutes. Remove from heat, discard thyme sprigs, then gradually add ½ cup Parmesan in batches, stirring constantly after each addition until incorporated before adding next batch (farro will continue to thicken as it stands).

4. While farro cooks, on a rimmed baking sheet, toss mushrooms with remaining 2 tablespoons oil. Roast, undisturbed, until starting to release some liquid, 12 to 15 minutes. Toss mushrooms, then continue roasting until golden brown, 8 to 10 minutes. Fold three-fourths of mushrooms into farrotto, then divide among bowls. Top with remaining mushrooms, then serve sprinkled with toasted almonds, parsley, remaining ¼ cup Parmesan and lemon zest, if desired.

PER SERVING *About 538 cal, 22 g fat (4.5 g sat), 13 mg chol, 876 mg sodium, 68 g carb, 8 g fiber, 4 g sugar (0 g added sugar), 21 g pro*

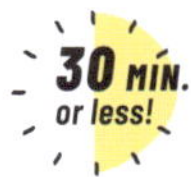

CREAMY KALE PASTA

ACTIVE 25 min. **TOTAL** 25 min. **SERVES** 4

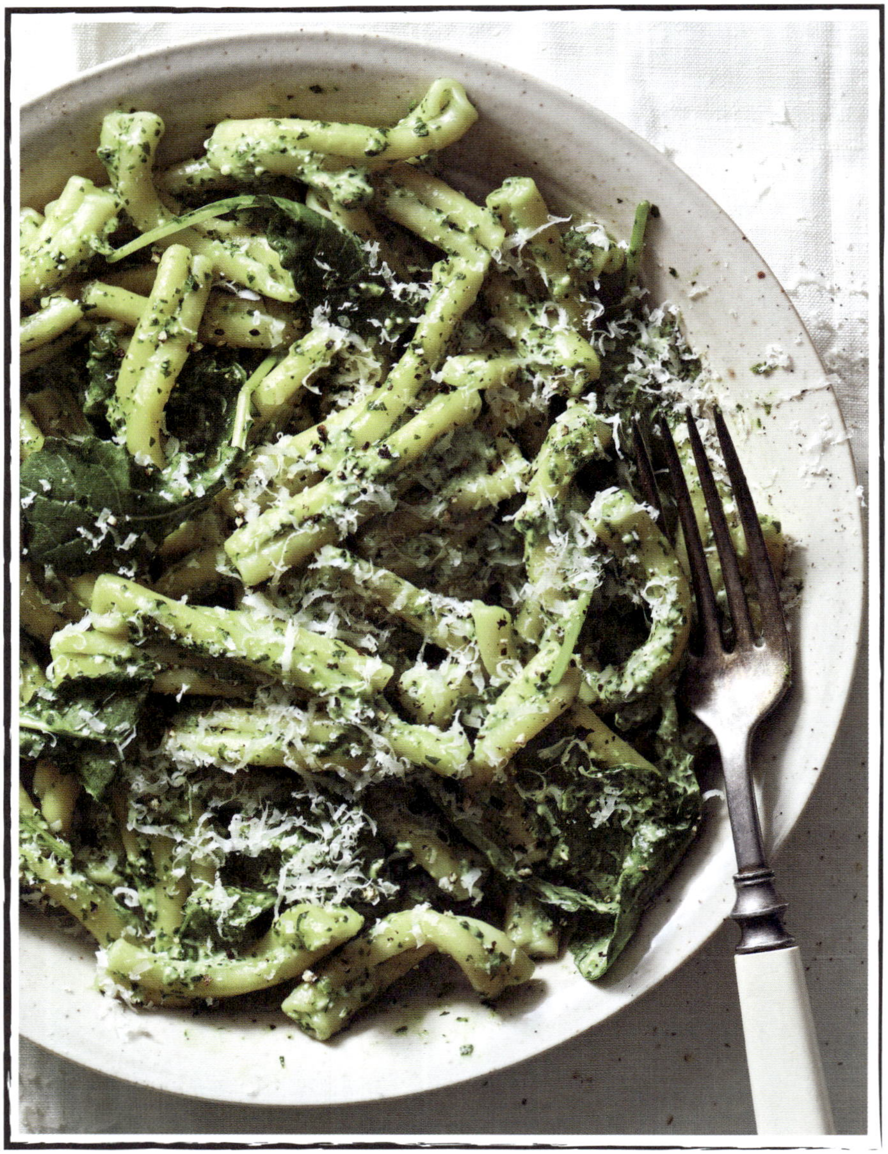

1. Cook 12 oz short **pasta** (like orecchiette or gemelli) per package directions. Reserve ½ cup **cooking water**, drain, and return pasta to pot.

2. While pasta cooks, in a food processor, pulse 2 **scallions** (roughly chopped) and 3 cups **baby kale** to finely chop.

3. Add ½ cup **cottage cheese**, ⅓ cup grated **Parmesan**, and ½ teaspoon each **kosher salt** and **pepper** and pulse to combine. Scrape down sides; then, with the machine running, gradually add 2 tablespoons **extra virgin olive oil** and puree until smooth.

4. Toss pasta with sauce to coat, then toss with another 3 cups **baby kale**, adding a couple of tablespoons of reserved pasta water as necessary to help kale wilt. Serve topped with additional Parmesan and freshly cracked **pepper**.

PER SERVING *About 462 cal, 14 g fat (3 g sat), 12 mg chol, 551 mg sodium, 62 g carb, 8 g fiber, 4 g sugar (0 g added sugar), 22 g pro*

BROTHY BEANS *with* HERB SAUCE

ACTIVE 5 min. **TOTAL** 1 hr. 25 min. **SERVES** 6

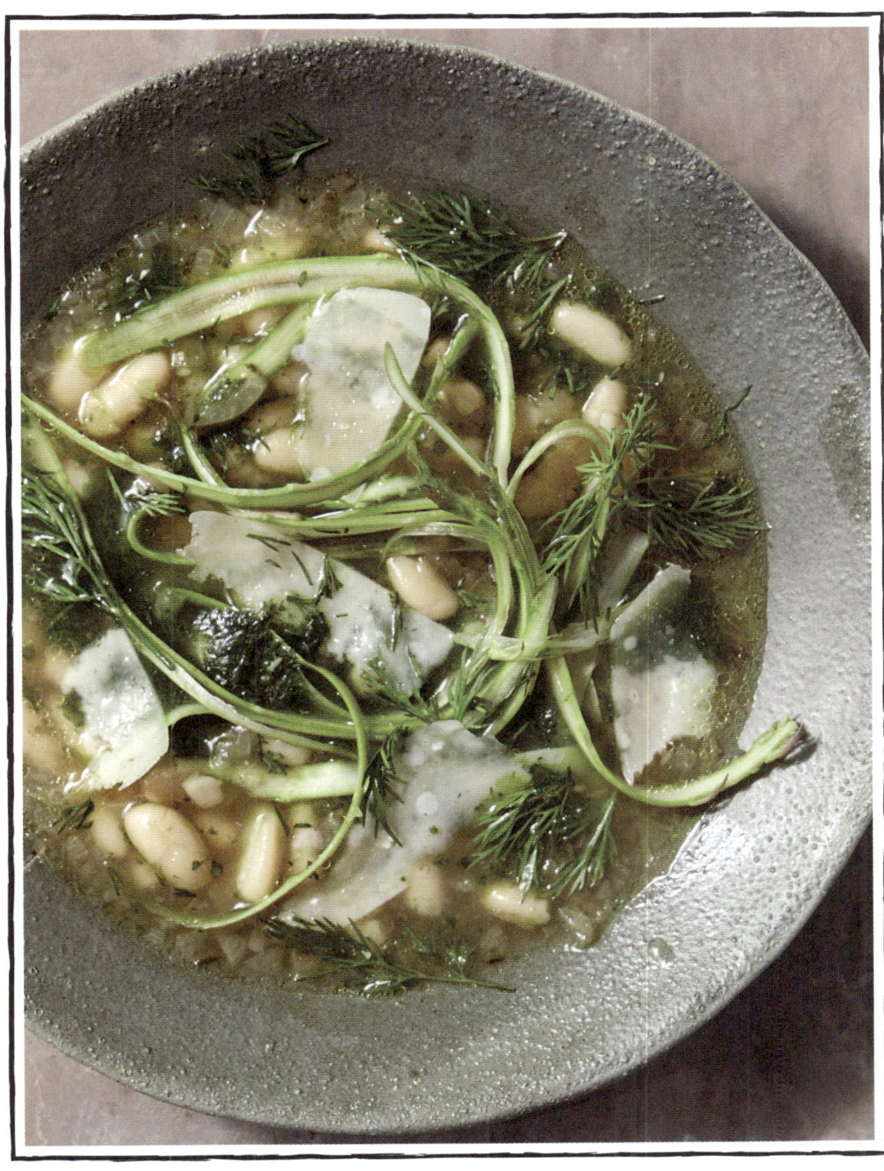

1. Set an Instant Pot to sauté on medium and heat 2 tablespoons **olive oil**. Add 2 cloves **garlic**, crushed, and sauté for 3 minutes. Stir in 1 pound dried **cannellini beans**, 2 **bay leaves**, and 10 cups **water**. Lock lid and cook on high pressure for 40 minutes.

2. Meanwhile, in a food processor, pulse 1 clove garlic, 1½ cups fresh **basil**, 1 bunch **chives**, and ¼ teaspoon **kosher salt**. With the machine running, slowly stream in ½ cup olive oil until smooth.

3. Let the Instant Pot pressure release naturally for 15 minutes, then manually release any remaining pressure. Open lid, discard bay leaves, stir in 1 tablespoon **vegetable bouillon base** and 1 teaspoon coarsely ground **pepper**.

4. Ladle beans into bowls. Swirl in herb sauce, top with **asparagus** ribbons (from 1 bunch trimmed and peeled asparagus), shaved **Parmesan** cheese (about 3 ounces), and small sprigs of fresh **dill**, if desired.

PER SERVING *About 534 cal, 27 g fat (5.5 g sat), 10 mg chol, 653 mg sodium, 50 g carb, 27 g fiber, 3.5 g sugar (0 g added sugar), 24 g pro*

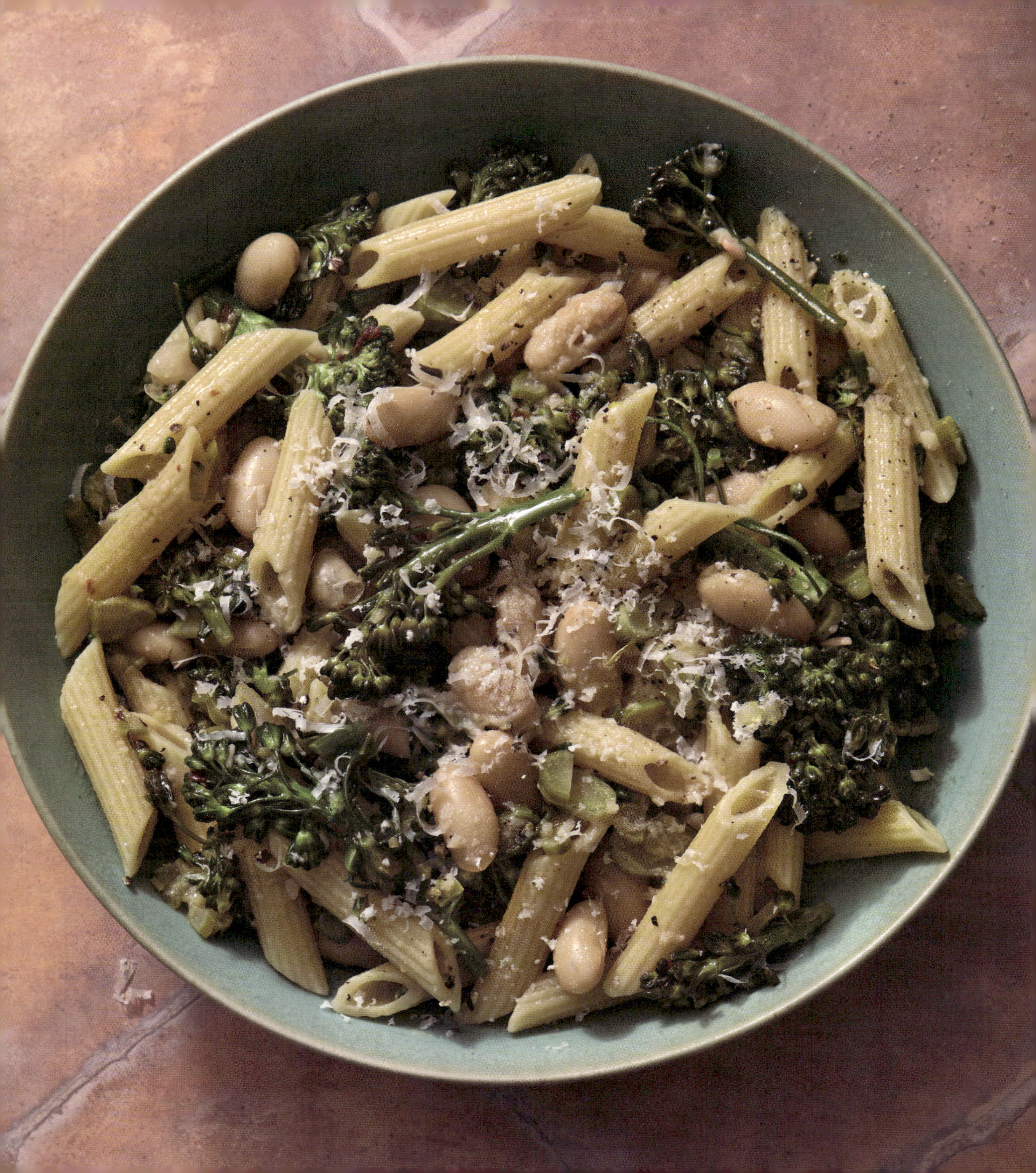

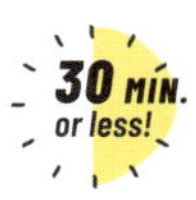

LEMONY BROCCOLINI PENNE

ACTIVE 20 min. **TOTAL** 20 min. **SERVES** 4

8 oz protein penne pasta

¼ cup olive oil, plus more for drizzling

5 anchovies, chopped

½ tsp red pepper flakes

3 large cloves garlic, finely chopped

1 lb broccolini, ends trimmed, finely chopped

Kosher salt

15.5-oz can cannellini beans, rinsed

2 tsp lemon zest plus 1 Tbsp lemon juice

4 Tbsp grated Parmesan cheese, divided

1. Cook pasta per package directions, reserving ½ cup pasta cooking water before draining.
2. In a large high-sided skillet or medium Dutch oven, heat oil, anchovies, and red pepper flakes over medium-low heat. Cook, stirring often, until anchovies start to break down, 3 to 4 minutes. Add garlic and cook, stirring often, until fragrant, 2 to 3 minutes.
3. Increase heat to medium and add broccolini and ¾ teaspoon salt; cook, stirring occasionally, until tender, 3 to 4 minutes.
4. Add beans, pasta, lemon zest and juice, and reserved pasta water; cook, stirring constantly, until warmed through, 3 minutes. Remove from heat and stir in 2 tablespoons Parmesan. Serve drizzled with oil and sprinkled with remaining 2 tablespoons Parmesan.

PER SERVING *About 541 cal, 20.5 g fat (3.5 g sat), 9 mg chol, 839 mg sodium, 71 g carb, 13 g fiber, 5.5 g sugar (0 g added sugar), 24 g pro*

PROTEIN POWER

Protein pasta is made with ingredients like lentils, chickpeas, or other added protein sources. While traditional pasta has about 7 grams of protein per serving, protein pasta can have up to 15 grams to 20 grams.

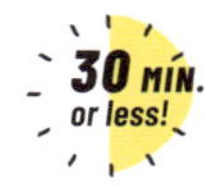

CAPONATA FLATBREAD

ACTIVE 20 min. **TOTAL** 25 min. **SERVES** 4

- Flour, for surface
- 1 lb pizza dough, thawed if frozen
- 2 Tbsp red wine vinegar
- 1 tsp honey
- 2½ Tbsp olive oil, divided
- 2 plum tomatoes, halved lengthwise
- 1 small eggplant (about 12 oz), halved lengthwise
- 1 red pepper, quartered
- Kosher salt and pepper
- 1 Tbsp capers, chopped
- ¼ cup flat-leaf parsley, roughly chopped
- 1 cup part-skim ricotta

1. Heat oven to 425°F and heat grill to medium-high. On a lightly floured surface, shape pizza dough into large rectangle, transfer to a parchment-lined baking sheet, and bake 10 minutes. Remove from oven, then increase heat to 475°F.
2. Meanwhile, in a large bowl, whisk together vinegar, honey, and 1 tablespoon oil.
3. Brush tomatoes, eggplant, and red pepper with 1 tablespoon oil and season with ¼ teaspoon each salt and pepper. Grill, turning occasionally, until just tender, 2 to 4 minutes per side; transfer to a cutting board and cut into large pieces.
4. Add vegetables and capers to vinegar mixture and toss to combine; fold in parsley. Spread ricotta on crust, leaving a ½-in. border all the way around, then top with vegetables. Brush crust with remaining ½ tablespoon oil and bake until crust is deep golden brown, 4 to 6 minutes.

PER SERVING *About 600 cal, 44 g fat (7.5 g sat), 15 mg chol, 1,139 mg sodium, 42 g carb, 9 g fiber, 24.5 g sugar (0 g added sugar), 21 g pro*

KITCHEN TIP
If you can't find pizza dough in your supermarket's freezer aisle or refrigerated section, see if your local pizza shop will sell you some of their fresh dough.

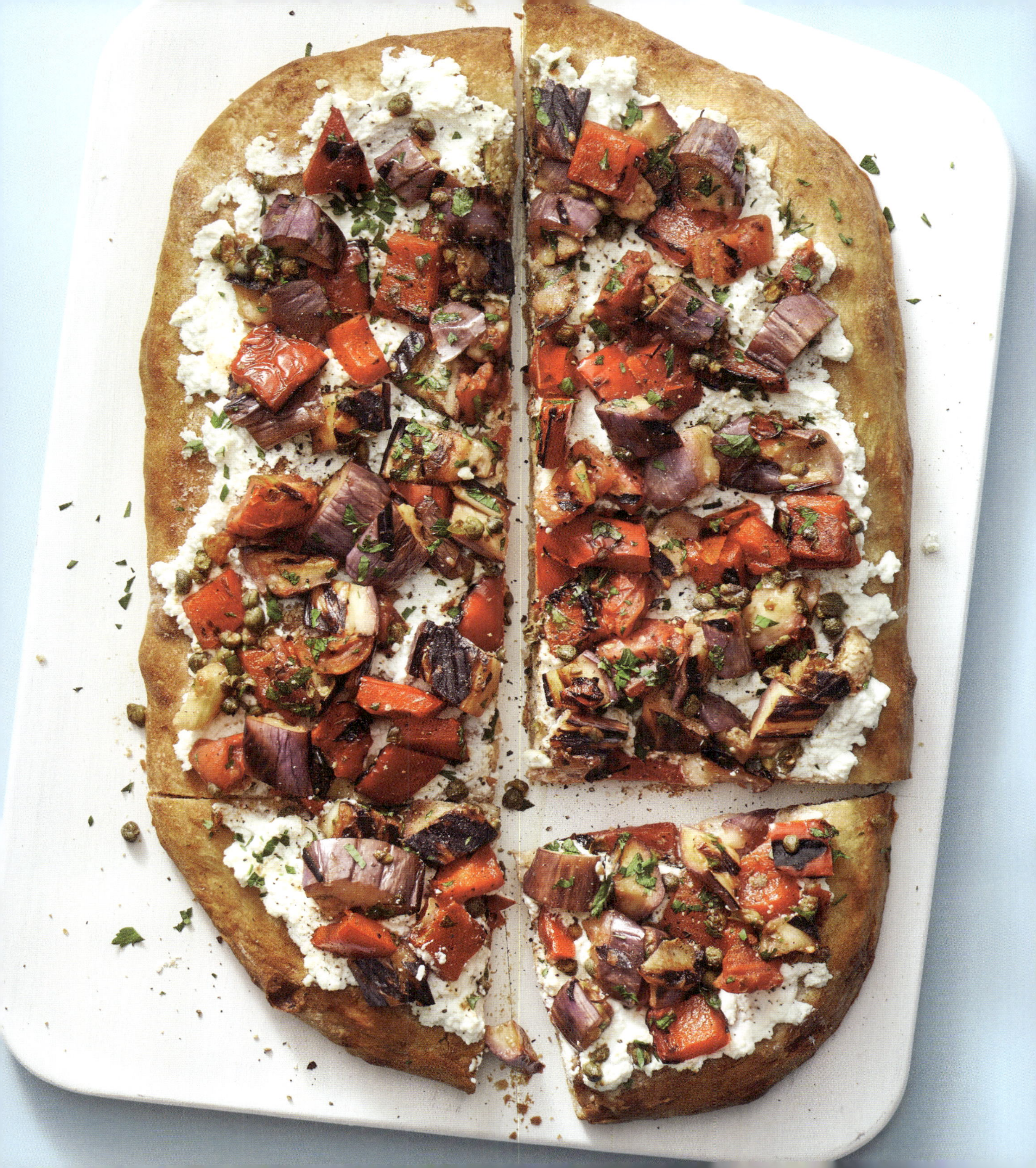

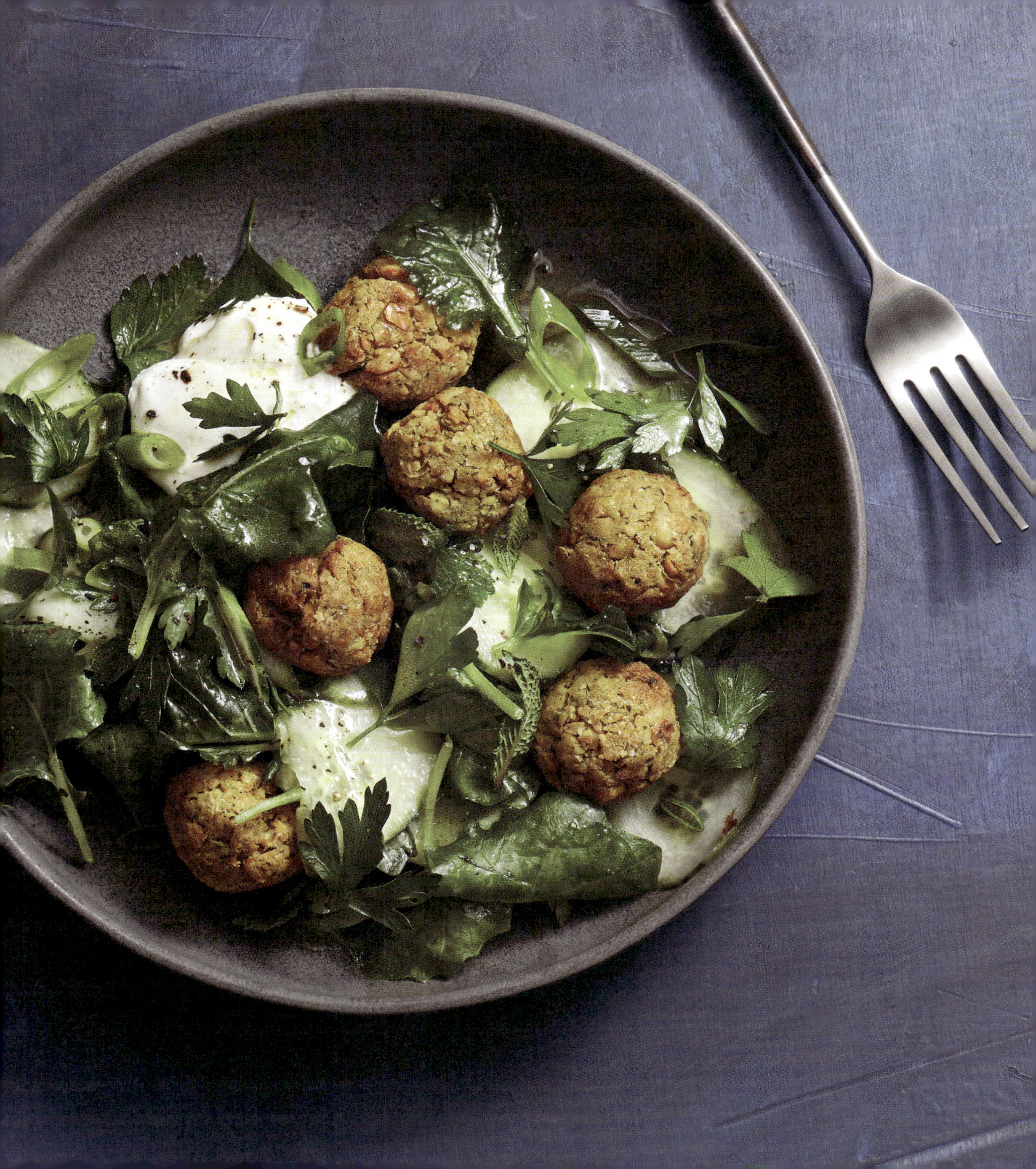

AIR FYER FALAFEL SALAD

ACTIVE 25 min. **TOTAL** 35 min. **SERVES** 4

- 2 cloves garlic
- 4 scallions, whites and greens, thinly sliced, separated
- 6½ cups baby kale, divided
- 2 15-oz cans chickpeas, drained and rinsed
- 1 tsp grated lemon zest
- 2 Tbsp all-purpose flour
- 1 tsp ground cumin
- 1 tsp ground coriander
- Kosher salt
- 3 Tbsp olive oil, divided, plus more for basket
- 2 Tbsp lemon juice
- ½ English cucumber, thinly sliced on bias
- ½ cup flat-leaf parsley leaves
- ¼ cup fresh mint leaves
- ¾ cup Greek Yogurt

1. In a food processor, pulse garlic, scallion whites, and ½ cup baby kale until very finely chopped. Add chickpeas, lemon zest, flour, cumin, coriander, and ½ teaspoon salt and pulse to combine (chickpeas should be chopped but coarse). Form mixture into twenty-four 2-tablespoon balls.
2. Heat the air fryer to 325°F. Brush insert of basket with oil and add 12 falafel. Air-fry 15 minutes. Brush falafel with 1 tablespoon oil and increase air fryer temperature to 400°F. Air-fry until deeply golden, 4 more minutes. Repeat with remaining falafel.
3. In a large bowl, whisk together lemon juice and remaining 2 tablespoons olive oil. Add cucumbers and marinate, 5 minutes. Add remaining 6 cups baby kale, parsley, and mint leaves, scallion greens, and ½ teaspoon salt and toss. Top with falafel and dollop with yogurt.

PER SERVING *About 394 cal, 18.5 g fat (4 g sat), 12 mg chol, 818 mg sodium, 41 g carb, 12 g fiber, 8.5 g sugar (0 g added sugar), 21 g pro*

LOVE YOUR LEFTOVERS

Refrigerate any unsauced falafel in an airtight container for up to four days. (You can also freeze in a single layer on a baking sheet first, then transfer to a freezer bag.) To keep them crispy, reheat falafel in a 375°F oven or air fryer for 5-10 minutes.

ROASTED SQUASH & COUSCOUS SALAD

ACTIVE 15 min. **TOTAL** 35 min. **SERVES** 4

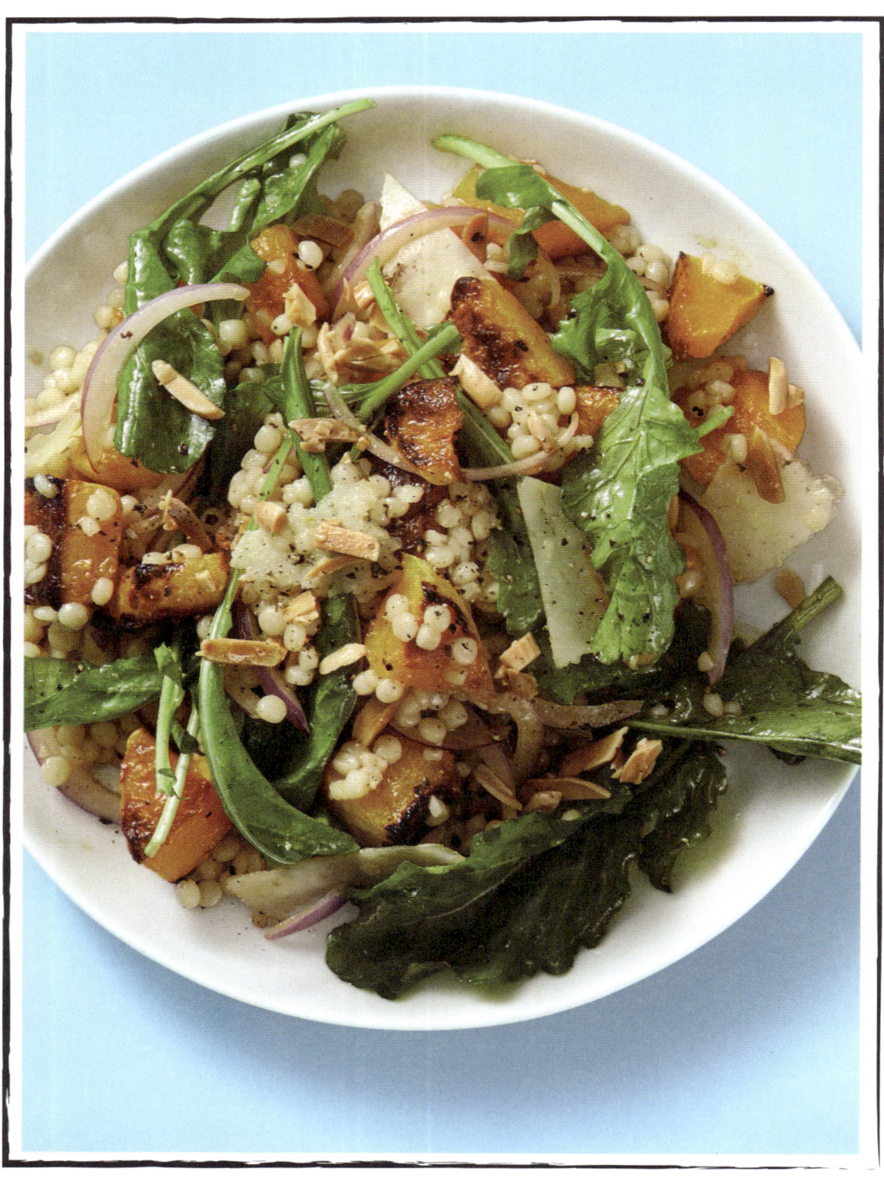

1. Heat oven to 450°F. On a rimmed baking sheet, toss 1 medium **butternut squash** (about 2¼ lb), peeled and cut into ½-in. pieces with 1 tablespoon **olive oil** and ½ teaspoon each **kosher salt** and **pepper**. Roast until golden brown and tender, 20 to 25 minutes.

2. Meanwhile, cook 1½ cups **Israeli (pearl) couscous** per package directions. Drain and refrigerate until ready to use.

3. In a large bowl, whisk together 2 tablespoons **balsamic vinegar,** 1½ tablespoon olive oil, 2 teaspoon **honey**. Toss in ½ small **red onion**, thinly sliced, and let sit 5 minutes.

4. Toss couscous with onion mixture, then fold in squash, 4 cups **baby arugula**, ½ cup blanched **almonds**, toasted and roughly chopped, and 2 oz **pecorino cheese**, shaved with a peeler.

PER SERVING *About 619 cal, 21.5 g fat (4.5 g sat), 15 mg chol, 437 mg sodium, 89 g carb, 10 g fiber, 12.5 g sugar (2.5 g added sugar), 21 g pro*

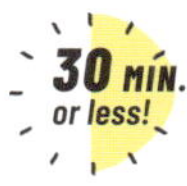

GREEN GODDESS SANDWICHES

ACTIVE 15 min. **TOTAL** 15 min. **SERVES** 4

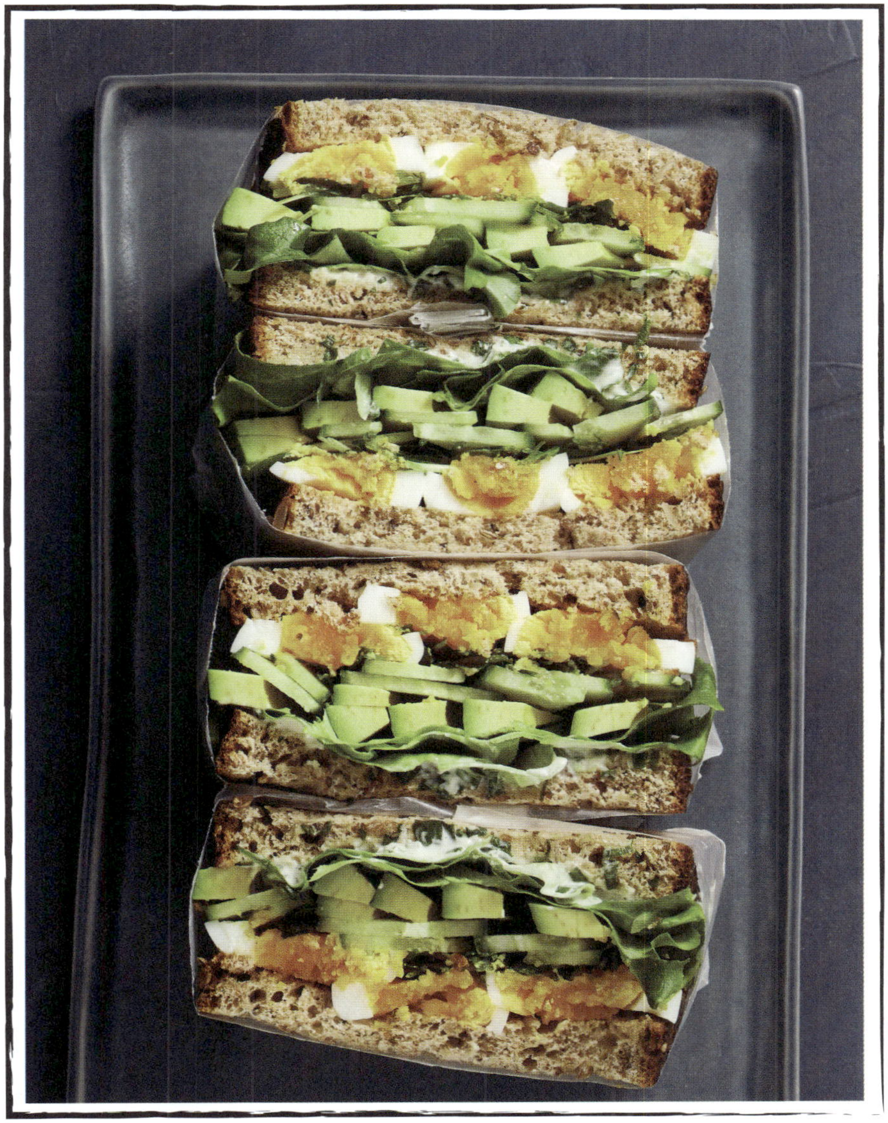

1. In a small bowl, combine ⅓ cup **mayonnaise**, ½ tablespoon **lemon juice**, ½ small clove **garlic** (finely grated), and ¼ teaspoon each **kosher salt** and **pepper**; fold in ¼ cup **basil** (chopped) and 2 tablespoons chopped **chives**.

2. Spread basil mayo on 8 slices **whole-grain bread**, then create sandwiches with 2 cups **salad greens** or favorite lettuce, 1 **avocado** (sliced), ½ seedless **cucumber** (halved crosswise and thinly sliced lengthwise), 1 cup **sprouts**, and 4 **hard-boiled eggs** (sliced).

PER SERVING *About 549 cal, 28.5 g fat (5.5 g sat), 194 mg chol, 624 mg sodium, 55 g carb, 10 g fiber, 9.5 g sugar (6 g added sugar), 21 g pro.*

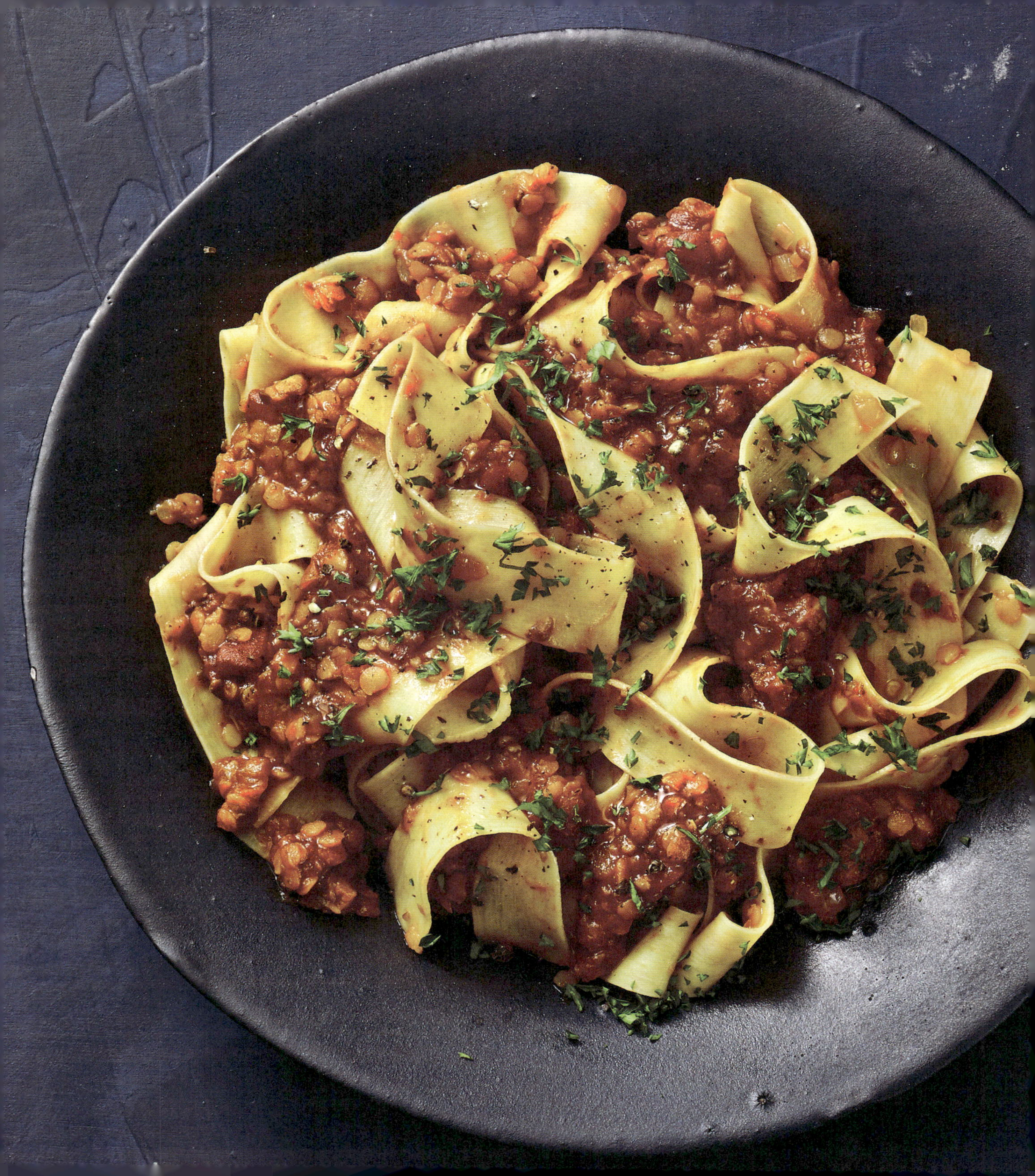

VEGAN BOLOGNESE

ACTIVE 20 min. **TOTAL** 55 min. **SERVES** 6

3 Tbsp olive oil

1 onion, finely chopped

Kosher salt and pepper

8 oz cremini mushrooms, trimmed and chopped in food processor

2 large cloves garlic, finely chopped

¼ to ½ tsp red pepper flakes

3 Tbsp tomato paste

½ cup dry white wine

1 cup red lentils

14.5-oz can crushed tomatoes

1 Tbsp mushroom bouillon base

1 lb pappardelle, linguine, or fettuccine

Chopped chervil or parsley, for serving

1. Heat oil in a Dutch oven over medium heat. Add onion, season with ½ teaspoon each salt and pepper, and cook, covered, stirring occasionally, 4 minutes. Increase heat to medium-high, add mushrooms, and cook, stirring occasionally, until deep brown and beginning to stick, 8 to 10 minutes.
2. Reduce heat to medium, stir in garlic and red pepper flakes, and cook 1 minute. Stir in tomato paste and cook, stirring, until dark brown, 2 minutes.
3. Stir in wine, scraping up any browned bits, then stir in lentils, tomatoes, 2 cups water, and bouillon base. Bring to a boil, then simmer until lentils are tender, 30 to 35 minutes.
4. Meanwhile, cook pasta per package directions. Serve bolognese over pasta, topped with chervil if desired.

PER SERVING *About 531 cal, 10 g fat (1.5 g sat), 41 mg chol, 792 mg sodium, 88 g carb, 8 g fiber, 7.5 g sugar (0 g added sugar), 22 g pro*

MAKE IT AHEAD

Refrigerate the bolognese and pasta in separate airtight containers for up to four days. When ready to serve, bring a pot of water to a boil and reheat the pasta. Warm the bolognese in a skillet over medium heat. You can also freeze the bolognese in an airtight container for up to three months. Thaw in the refrigerator overnight.

SAUCY BEANS & FARRO

ACTIVE 30 min. **TOTAL** 40 min. **SERVES** 4

⅔ cup quick-cooking farro

1½ Tbsp olive oil, plus more for drizzling

1 tsp fennel seeds, crushed

¼ to ½ tsp red pepper flakes

1 medium yellow onion, chopped

1 medium bulb fennel, cored and chopped

Kosher salt and pepper

3 cloves garlic, finely chopped

3 Tbsp double concentrated tomato paste

14-oz can whole peeled tomatoes (pulsed with immersion blender until crushed)

1 Tbsp low-sodium vegetable bouillon base

15.5-oz can no-salt cannellini beans, rinsed

15.5-oz can low-sodium chickpeas, rinsed

2-in. piece Parmesan rind, plus ½ cup grated Parmesan

1. Cook farro per package directions. Drain; set aside.
2. Meanwhile, in a large high-sided skillet over medium heat, heat oil, fennel seeds, and red pepper flakes, stirring occasionally, until fragrant and golden brown, 4 to 5 minutes.
3. Add onion, fennel, and ¼ teaspoon each salt and pepper and cook, covered, stirring occasionally, until vegetables are tender, 7 to 9 minutes. Add garlic and cook, stirring occasionally, until fragrant, 1 minute more.
4. Add tomato paste and cook, stirring constantly, until caramelized and vegetables are coated, 2 minutes. Add tomatoes, bouillon base, cannellini beans, chickpeas, and 3 cups water, then stir in Parmesan rind and bring to a simmer. Simmer, stirring occasionally, until saucy and thickened, 10 to 13 minutes. Stir in cooked farro and cook 1 minute more. Remove Parmesan rind.
5. Serve in bowls, sprinkled with grated Parmesan and black pepper. Drizzle with oil if desired.

PER SERVING *About 515 cal, 13 g fat (8 g sat), 9 mg chol, 887 mg sodium, 80 g carb, 14 g fiber, 11.5 g sugar (0 g added sugar), 21 g pro*

LOVE YOUR LEFTOVERS

Refrigerate any leftovers in an airtight container for up to four days. Reheat gently on the stove or in the microwave, adding a splash of water or broth. You can also freeze in an airtight container for up to three months. Thaw in the refrigerator overnight.

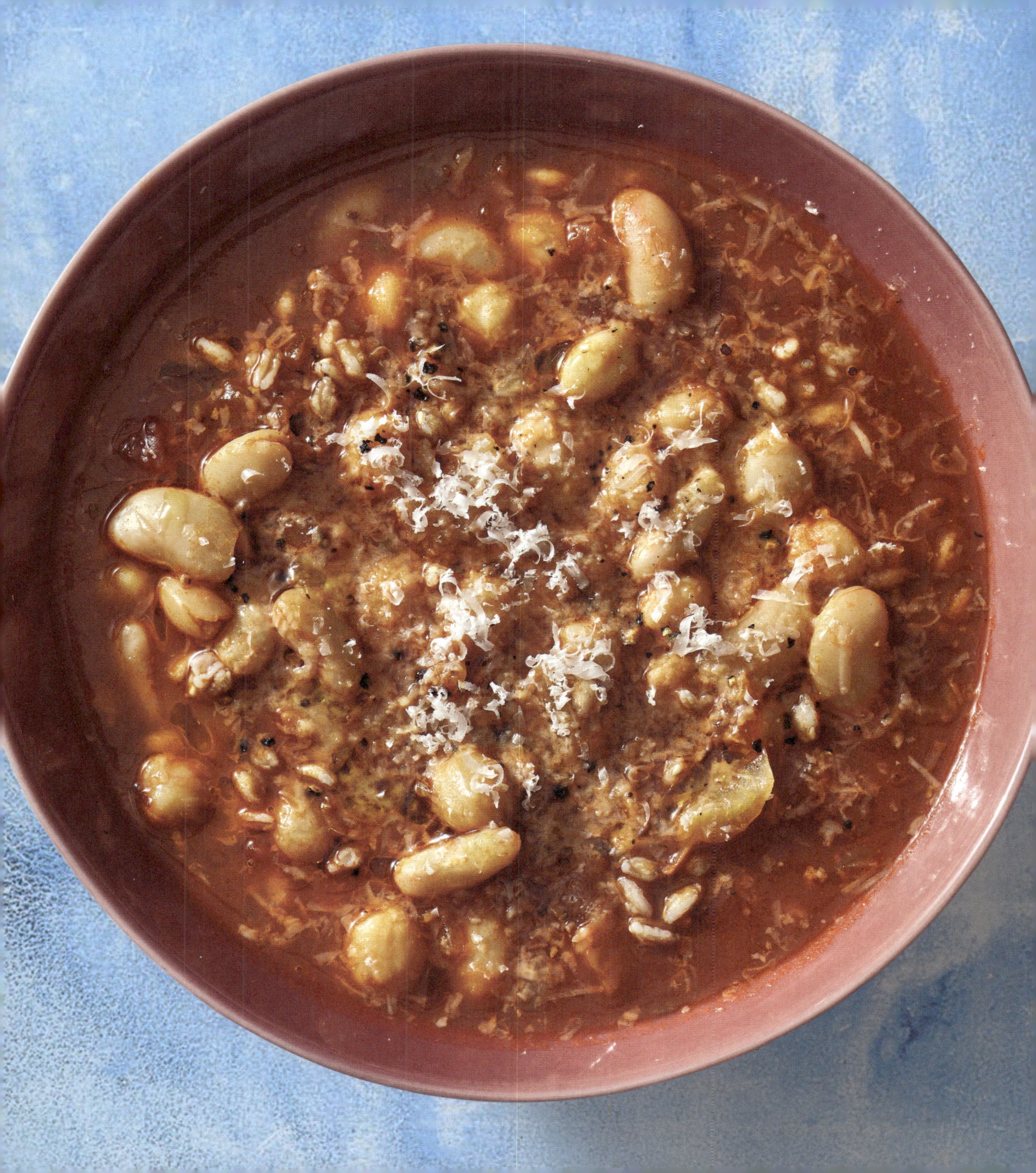

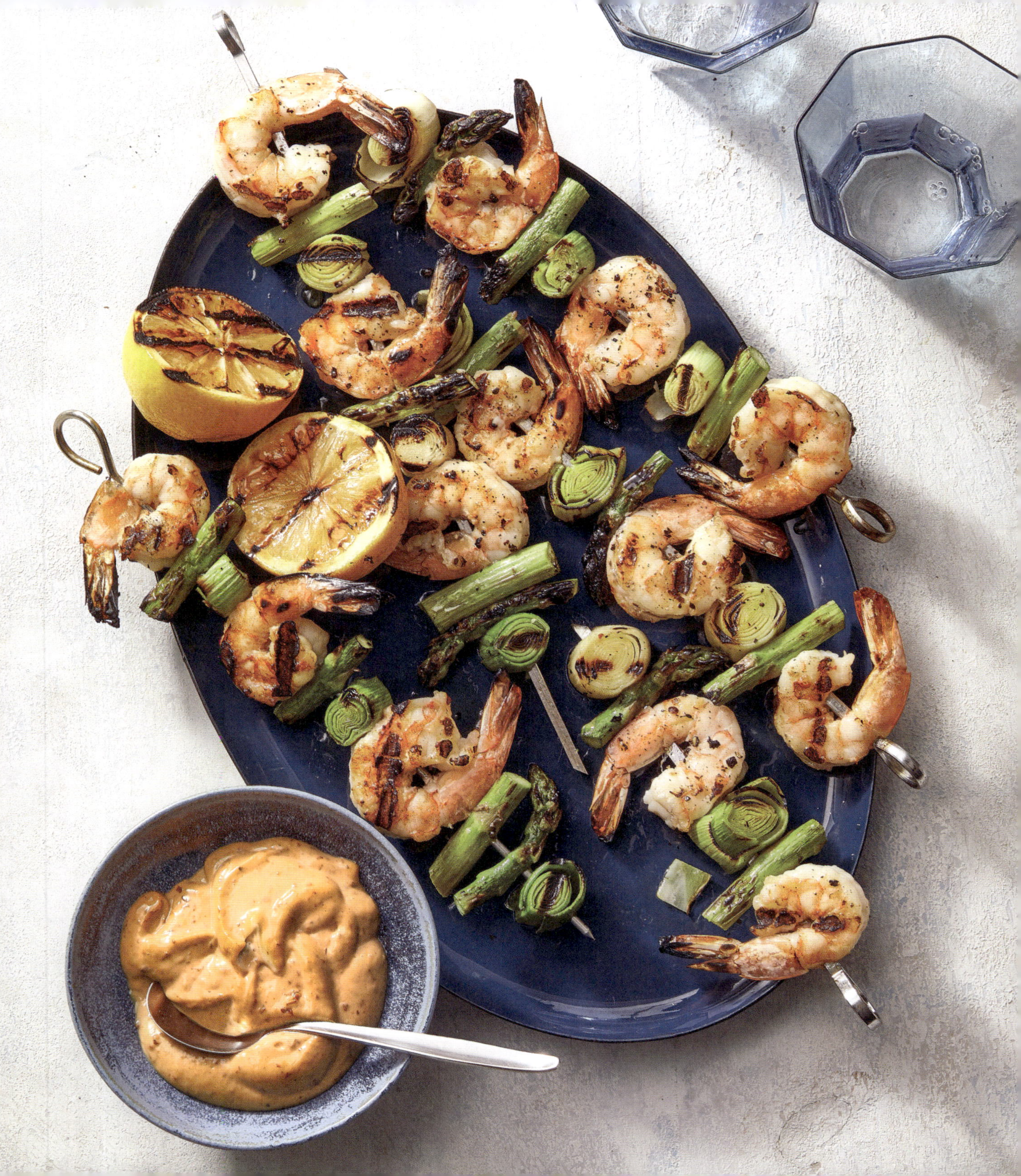

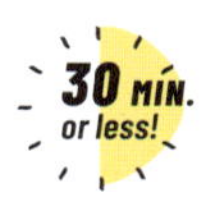

CHARRED SHRIMP, LEEK *and* ASPARAGUS SKEWERS

ACTIVE 30 min. **TOTAL** 30 min. **SERVES** 4

¾ cup bulgur

2½ cups baby spinach

1¼ cups flat-leaf parsley leaves

1 small bunch chives, roughly chopped (about ¼ cup)

½ tsp ground cumin

⅓ cup roasted almonds

3 Tbsp olive oil, plus more for brushing

Kosher salt and pepper

1 lb (21- to 25-count) peeled and deveined shrimp

1 lb asparagus, trimmed and cut into 2-in. pieces

2 medium leeks, white and light green parts only, cut into ¾-in.-thick rounds

2 lemons, halved

½ cup mayonnaise

1½ Tbsp harissa paste

1. In a medium saucepan, bring 1¼ cups water to a boil. Stir in bulgur and simmer, covered, until nearly tender, 9 minutes. Remove from heat and let sit, covered, 3 minutes, then fluff with fork and transfer to a large bowl.
2. Meanwhile, in a food processor, pulse spinach, parsley, chives, and cumin until finely chopped. Add almonds, oil, and ½ teaspoon salt and pulse to finely chop nuts. Fold into bulgur.
3. Heat grill to medium-high heat. Thread shrimp, asparagus, and leek rounds onto skewers. Brush lightly with oil and season with ½ teaspoon each salt and pepper.
4. Grill skewers until vegetables are tender and shrimp are opaque throughout, 3 to 4 minutes per side.
5. Place lemons on the grill alongside skewers, cut sides down, and grill until charred, about 4 minutes.
6. Into a small bowl, squeeze 2 teaspoons juice from 1 charred lemon half. Stir in mayonnaise and harissa to combine. Serve skewers with harissa mayo, remaining charred lemon halves, and herbed bulgur salad.

PER SERVING *About 581 cal, 39 g fat (5.5 g sat), 154 mg chol, 1,374 mg sodium, 37 g carb, 8.5 g fiber, 4.5 g sugar (0 g added sugar), 25 g pro*

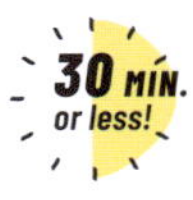

ROASTED FISH *with* CUMIN-ROASTED TOMATOES & CHICKPEAS

ACTIVE 15 min. **TOTAL** 30 min. **SERVES** 4

- 1 Tbsp coriander seeds
- 2 tsp cumin seeds
- ¼ to ½ tsp red pepper flakes
- 1¼ tsp ground sumac, divided
- Kosher salt and pepper
- 2 pints grape tomatoes
- 6 cloves garlic, smashed
- 3 Tbsp olive oil, divided
- 15-oz can chickpeas, rinsed
- 1¼ lb firm white fish (see Tip)
- 4 sprigs fresh thyme, leaves stripped

1. Heat oven to 425°F. With a mortar and pestle, coarsely crush coriander and cumin seeds. Stir in red pepper, 1 teaspoon sumac, and ½ teaspoon salt.
2. On a rimmed baking sheet, toss tomatoes and garlic with 2 tablespoons oil and spices. Roast 10 minutes.
3. Toss tomato mixture with chickpeas. Nestle fish in center, then drizzle with remaining tablespoon oil, season with remaining ¼ teaspoon sumac and ¼ teaspoon each salt and pepper, and sprinkle with thyme.
4. Roast until fish is just opaque throughout, about 15 minutes depending on thickness.

PER SERVING *About 328 cal, 13 g fat (2 g sat), 54 mg chol, 627 mg sodium, 32 g carb, 7 g fiber, 4.5 g sugar (0 g added sugar), 30 g pro*

KITCHEN TIP
Thin, lean fillets like tilapia or flounder cook faster than thicker, meatier fillets like cod, haddock, or halibut.

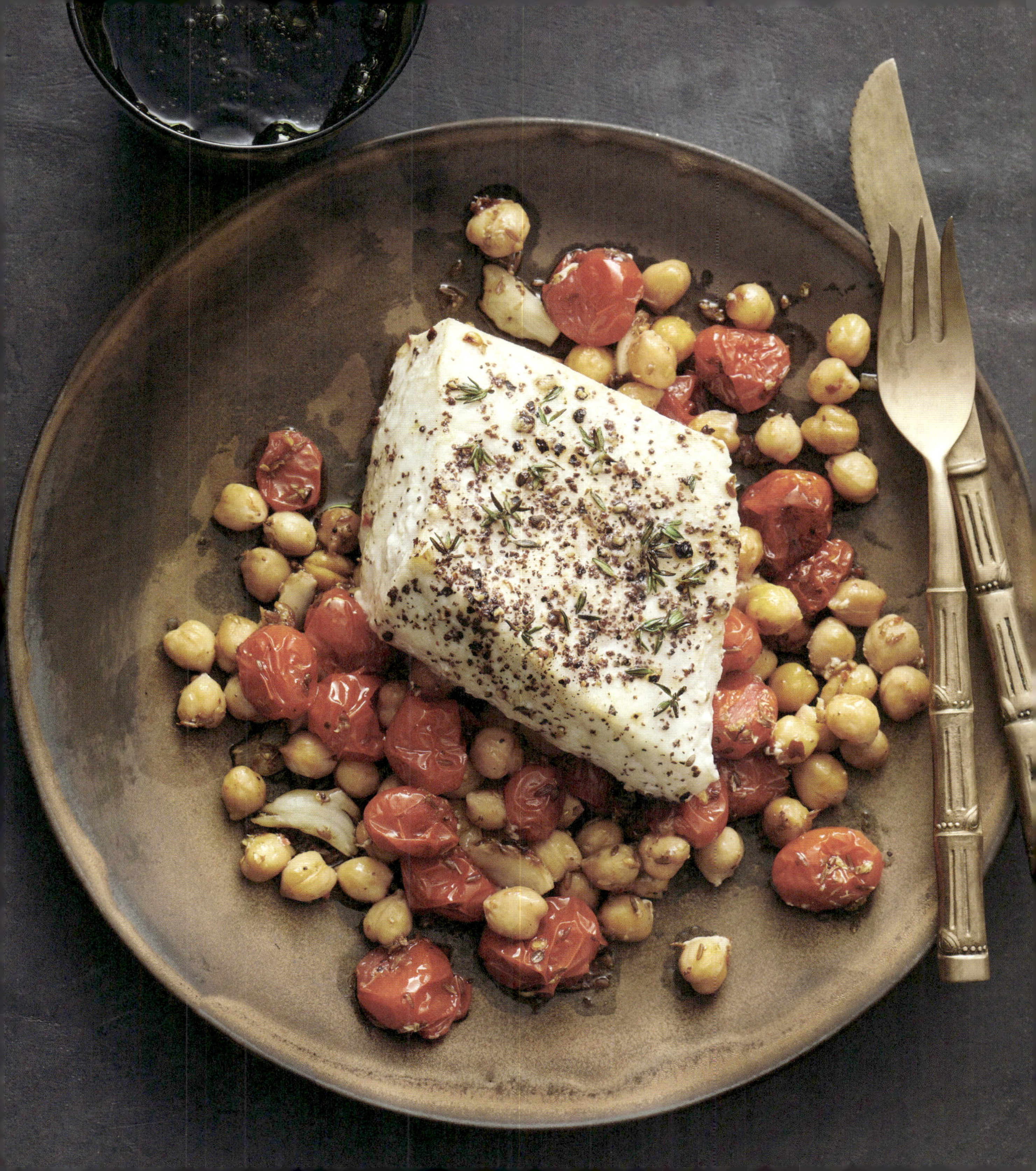

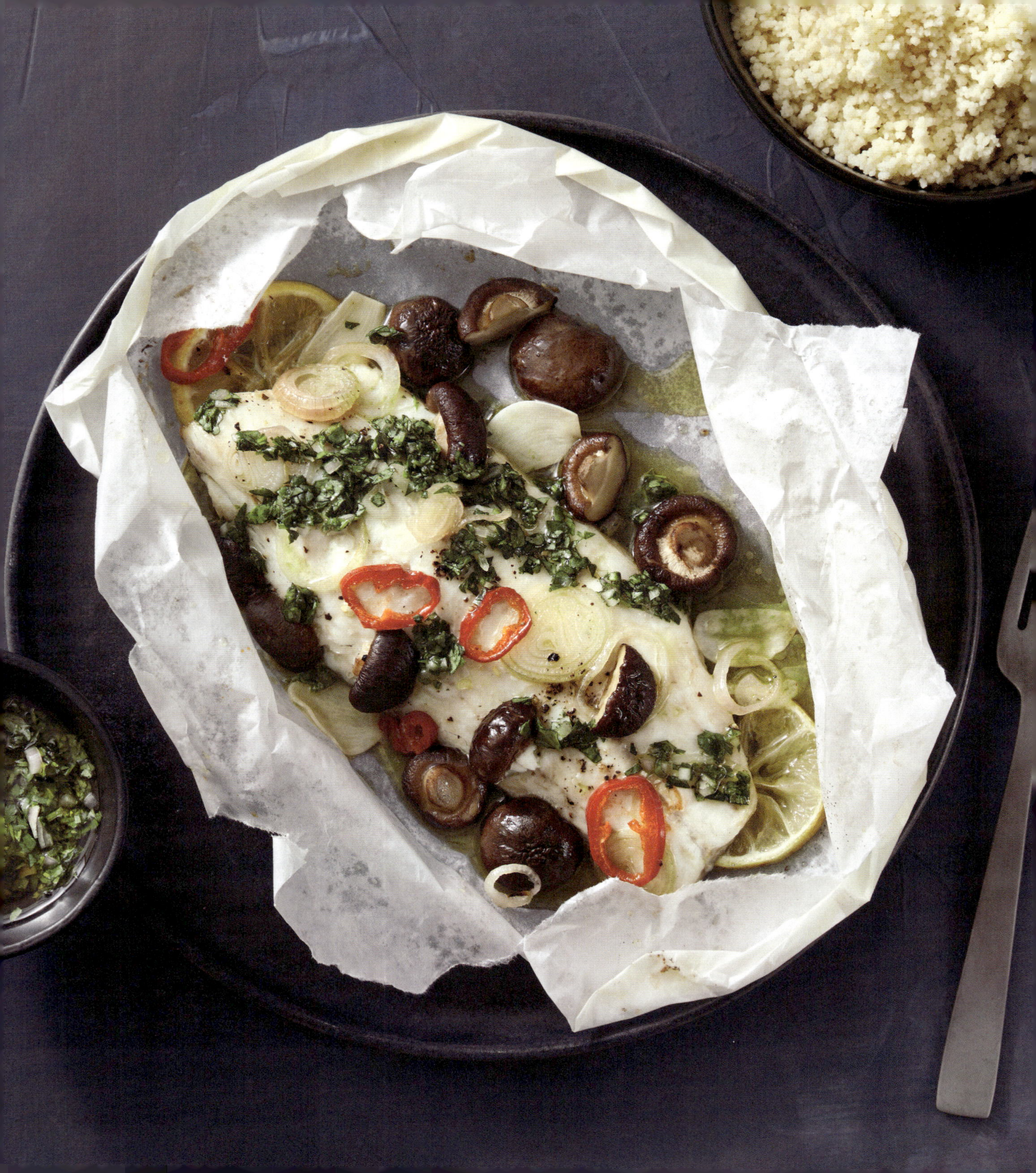

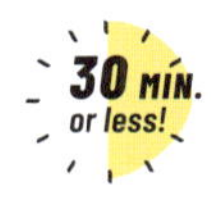

SEA BASS *in* PARCHMENT *with* WATERCRESS CHIMICHURRI

ACTIVE 30 min. **TOTAL** 30 min. **SERVES** 4

1 cup couscous

1 lemon, sliced into 8 rounds, plus 2 tablespoons lemon juice

2 cloves garlic, sliced

4 6-oz skinless sea bass fillets

12 oz baby shiitake mushrooms, whole and trimmed if small (stemmed and halved if large)

1 medium shallot, ½ thinly sliced and ½ finely chopped

1 Fresno chile, sliced

5 Tbsp olive oil, divided

Kosher salt and pepper

2 cups hydroponic watercress, finely chopped

½ cup cilantro, finely chopped

1. Arrange racks in upper and lower thirds of oven and heat oven to 400°F. In a medium bowl, stir together couscous and 1¼ cups water. Let sit until water is absorbed, about 15 minutes. Fluff with fork.

2. Meanwhile, fold four 12- by 16-inch sheets parchment paper in half crosswise and unfold. Place 2 lemon rounds near crease of 1 side of each sheet and top with sliced garlic; top with sea bass fillets along crease. Arrange mushrooms around fish. Top fish with sliced shallot and chile. Drizzle everything with 2 tablespoons oil and season with ¼ teaspoon each salt and pepper.

3. Fold parchment over fish and vegetables and, starting at bottom edge of parchment at the crease, make small overlapping, concentric folds to create half-moon-shaped package and completely seal sides, folding final corner slightly underneath. Divide between 2 rimmed baking sheets and roast, rotating position of pans halfway through, until fish is cooked through and mushrooms are tender, 10 to 12 minutes.

4. Meanwhile, in a medium bowl, stir together chopped shallot and lemon juice; let sit 5 minutes. Stir in watercress and cilantro, ⅛ teaspoon each salt and pepper, and remaining 3 tablespoons oil.

PER SERVING *About 521 cal, 21 g fat (3.5 g sat), 70 mg chol, 317 mg sodium, 43 g carb, 5 g fiber, 3.5 g sugar (0 g added sugar), 40 g pro*

KITCHEN TIP

Fold parchment over fish and vegetables and, starting at bottom edge of parchment at the crease, make small overlapping, concentric folds to create half-moon-shaped package and completely seal sides, folding final corner slightly underneath.

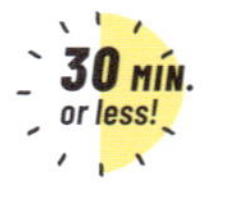

TOMATO-POACHED COD *with* OLIVES AND CAPERS

ACTIVE 10 min. **TOTAL** 20 min. **SERVES** 4

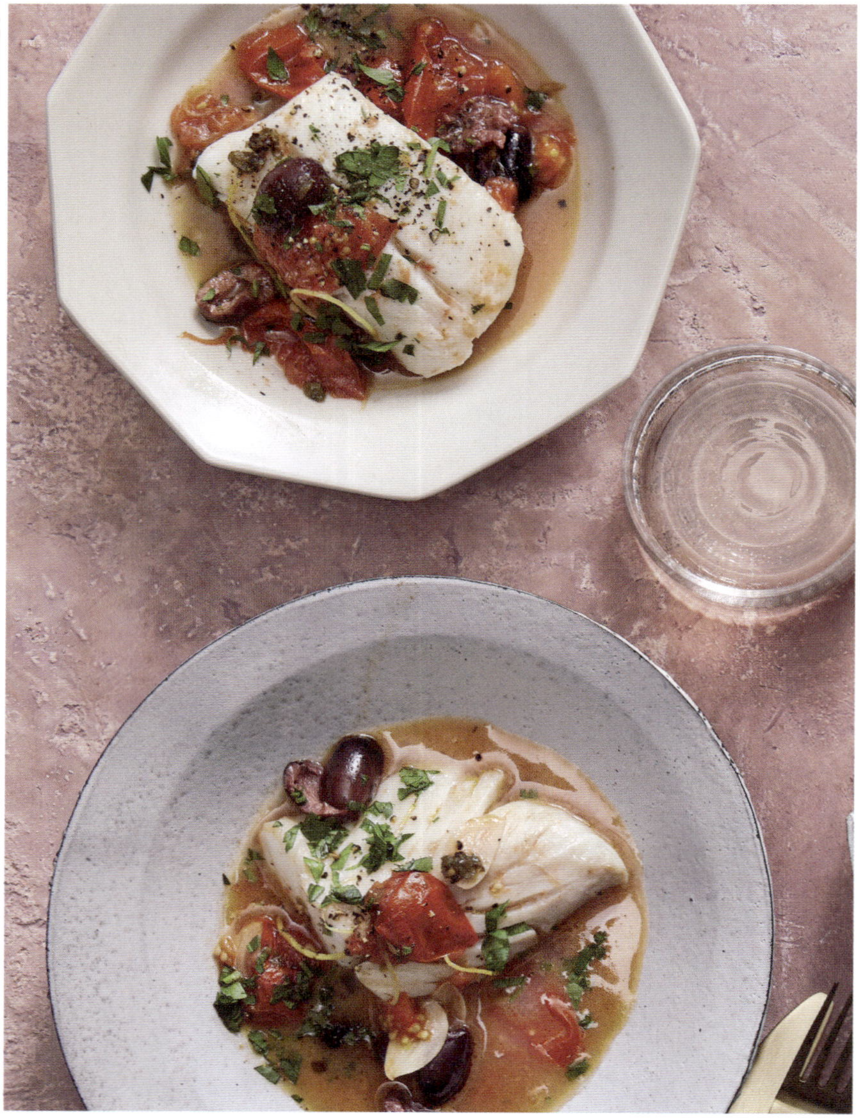

- 2 Tbsp olive oil
- 2 cloves garlic, thinly sliced
- 1 Tbsp capers, rinsed
- 1 strip lemon zest, thinly sliced
- ¾ cup dry rosé
- ½ lb Campari tomatoes, quartered
- ¼ cup pitted kalamata olives, halved
- Kosher salt and pepper
- 4 6-oz skinless cod fillets
- Chopped flat-leaf parsley, for serving

1. Heat oil, garlic, capers, and lemon zest in a large skillet on medium, stirring occasionally, until garlic is lightly golden brown, about 2 minutes.

2. Add wine and simmer 2 minutes. Stir in tomatoes, olives, and ¼ teaspoon each salt and pepper. Nestle fish in tomatoes and simmer, covering skillet during last 3 minutes of cooking, until cooked and opaque throughout, 6 to 8 minutes. Sprinkle with parsley.

PER SERVING *About 229 cal, 10 g fat (1.5 g sat), 67 mg chol, 381 mg sodium, 5 g carb, 1 g fiber, 2 g sugar (0 g added sugar), 28 g pro*

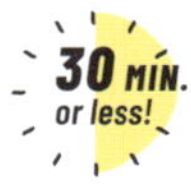

SCALLION-LEMON ARUGULA SALAD *with* ROASTED SALMON

ACTIVE 25 min. **TOTAL** 25 min. **SERVES** 4

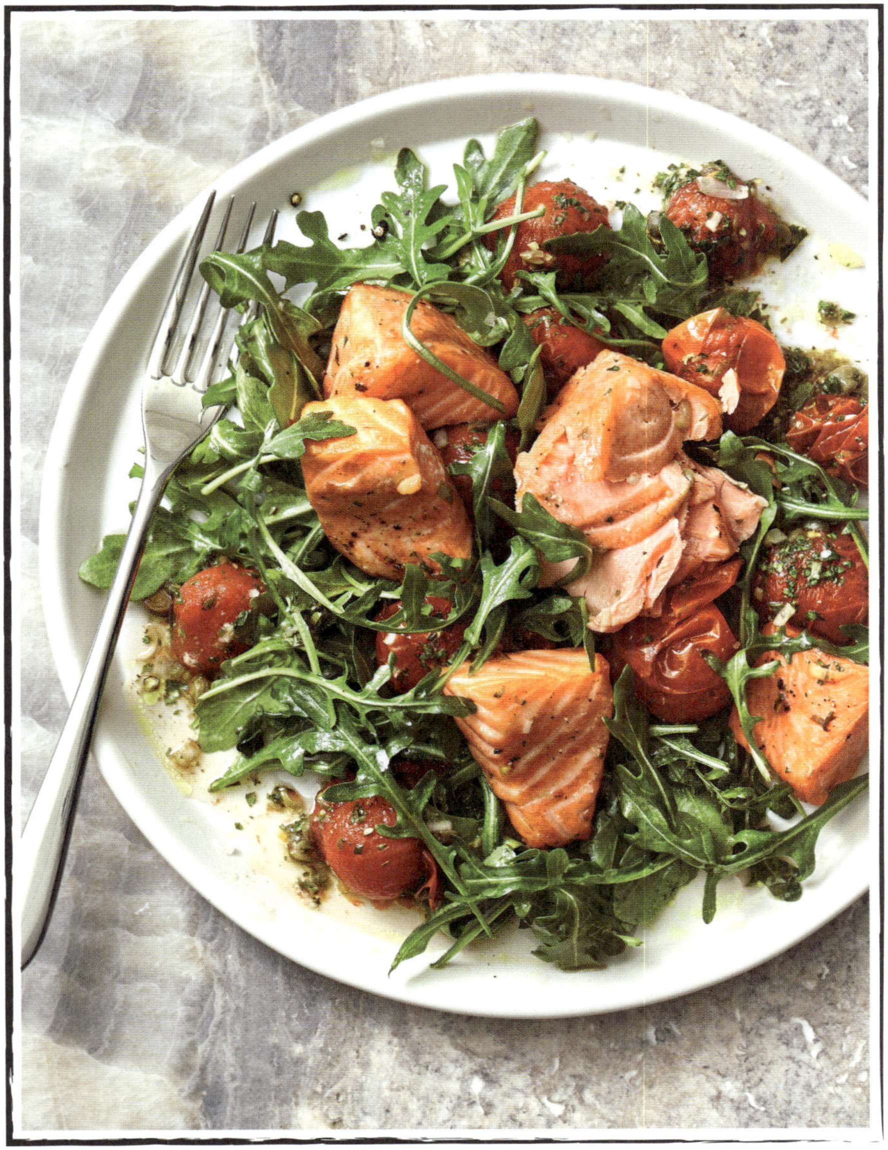

1. Heat oven to 425°F. On a large rimmed baking sheet, toss 1 pint **grape tomatoes** with 1 tablespoon **olive oil** and a pinch each of **kosher salt** and **black pepper**. Roast for 12 minutes.

2. Season 1 pound skinless **salmon filet**, cut into 1½-inch pieces, with ¼ teaspoon each salt and pepper. Push tomatoes to one side of the sheet pan, place salmon on the other side. Roast until salmon is opaque throughout, 6 to 8 minutes more.

3. Meanwhile, in bowl, combine 1 tablespoon chopped **capers**, 1 thinly sliced **scallion**, 1 tablespoon oil, 1 tablespoon **red wine vinegar**, and ¼ teaspoon black pepper. Add tomatoes; toss to combine.

4. In a large bowl, whisk 1 tablespoon oil, 1 tablespoon red wine vinegar, ½ teaspoon **honey**, and a pinch each of salt and pepper. Toss with a 5-ounce package of **arugula**. Serve topped with tomatoes and salmon.

PER SERVING *About 254 cal, 14.5 g fat (2.5 g sat), 53 mg chol, 313 mg sodium, 10 g carb, 1.5 g fiber, 2.5 g sugar (0.5 g added sugar), 25 g pro*

ROASTED PEPPER BULGUR *with* FENNEL-SPICED SALMON

ACTIVE 25 min. **TOTAL** 35 min. **SERVES** 4

- 1 cup medium-grind red bulgur
- 1½ cups boiling water
- 3½ Tbsp red wine vinegar
- 4 Tbsp olive oil, divided
- Kosher salt and pepper
- 4 scallions, whites, roughly chopped; greens, sliced and kept separate
- 2 peppers (1 red, 1 yellow), seeded and quartered
- 1½ lb skinless salmon fillet
- ½ tsp fennel seeds, crushed
- ½ tsp cumin seeds, crushed
- 1 cup baby arugula

1. Heat broiler with oven rack 4 inches from heat source. Place bulgur in a medium heatproof bowl, add boiling water, cover, and let sit until water is absorbed, about 30 minutes. Drain.
2. Meanwhile, in a large bowl, whisk together vinegar, 3½ tablespoons oil, ½ teaspoon salt, and ¼ teaspoon pepper. Stir in scallion whites and let sit.
3. On a rimmed baking sheet, toss peppers with remaining ½ tablespoon oil and ¼ teaspoon salt, arrange cut sides down, and broil until charred in spots and slightly tender, 4 to 9 minutes. Transfer to a cutting board and roughly chop on bias into ½-inch pieces, then fold into dressing. Adjust oven temperature to 450°F.
4. Place salmon on the foil-lined rimmed baking sheet. Season with fennel and cumin seeds and ¼ teaspoon salt. Roast until opaque throughout, 14 to 16 minutes.
5. Add bulgur to marinated peppers and toss together, then fold in arugula and scallion greens. Serve with salmon.

PER SERVING *About 510 cal, 20.5 g fat (3.5 g sat), 80 mg chol, 573 mg sodium, 41 g carb, 1 g fiber, 2 g sugar (0 g added sugar), 39 g pro*

FIBER FIX

Red bulgur is a whole grain that has a slightly nuttier flavor and a deeper color than regular (usually golden) bulgur. It's quick-cooking, high in fiber, and great in salads, grain bowls, or as a hearty side.

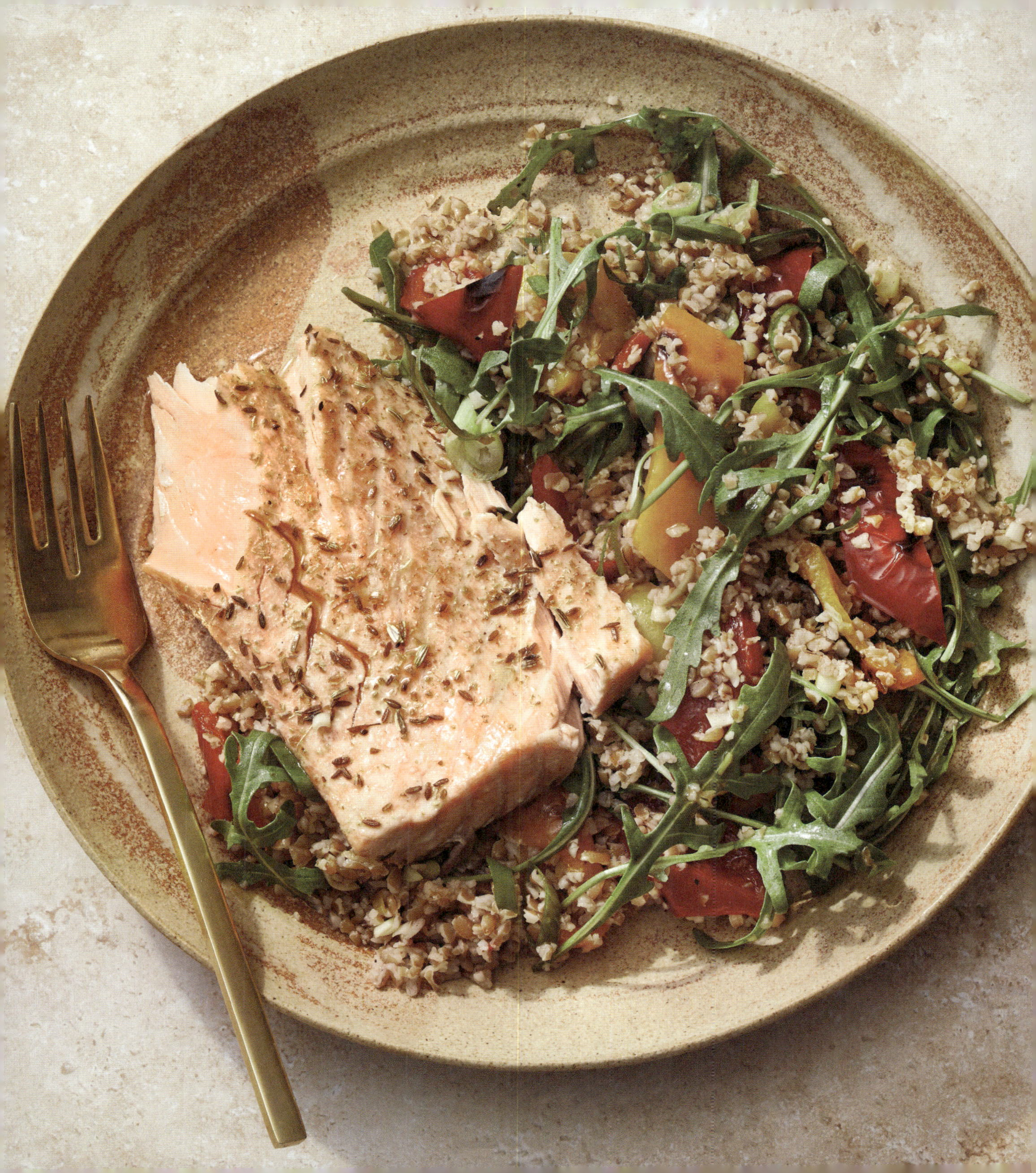

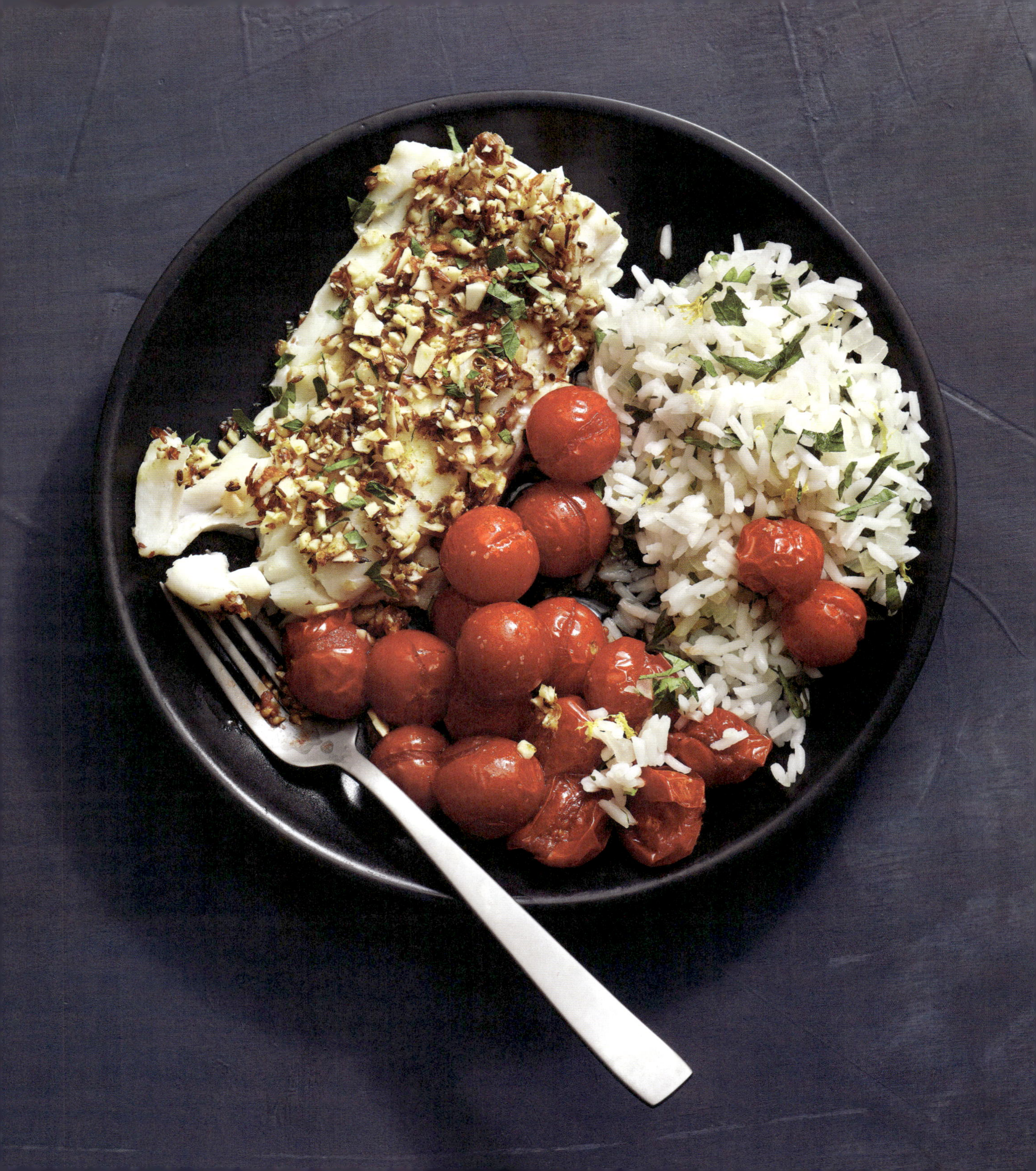

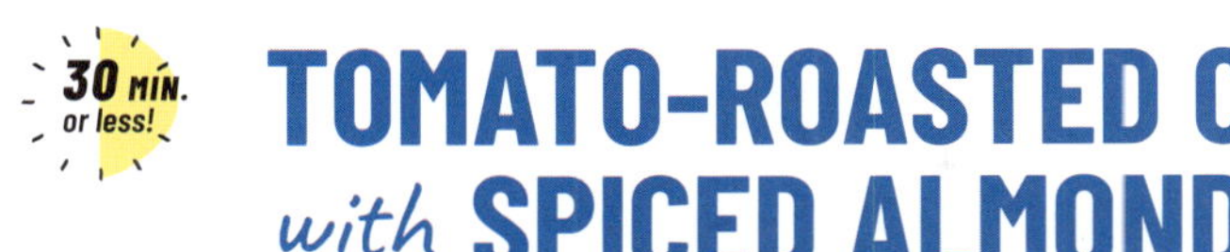

TOMATO-ROASTED COD *with* SPICED ALMONDS

ACTIVE 25 min. **TOTAL** 30 min. **SERVES** 4

- 1 tsp plus 2½ Tbsp olive oil, divided
- 1 small onion, chopped
- Kosher salt
- 1¼ cups jasmine rice
- 2-in. piece ginger, sliced
- 1 clove garlic, smashed
- 1 lb cherry tomatoes
- ¼ cup sliced almonds, chopped
- 1 tsp cumin seeds, crushed
- ¾ tsp coriander seeds, crushed
- 2 tsp lemon zest, divided
- 4 6-oz skinless cod fillets
- ¼ cup flat-leaf parsley leaves, roughly chopped, plus more for sprinkling

1. Heat oven to 400°F. Heat 1 teaspoon oil in a medium saucepan on medium. Add onion and ¼ teaspoon salt and cook, covered, stirring occasionally, until just tender, 3 to 4 minutes. Add rice, ginger, garlic, and 1¾ cups water and bring to a boil. Reduce heat and simmer, covered, until rice is just tender, 12 to 14 minutes. Remove from heat and let sit, covered, until ready to serve.
2. Meanwhile, on a large rimmed baking sheet, toss tomatoes with ½ tablespoon oil and ¼ teaspoon salt. Roast undisturbed until tomatoes begin to soften, 9 to 10 minutes.
3. While tomatoes roast, in a medium bowl, stir together almonds, cumin seeds, coriander seeds, half of lemon zest, ¼ teaspoon salt, and remaining 2 tablespoons oil. Dividing evenly, spoon mixture on top of cod fillets. Nestle cod fillets among roasted tomatoes and roast until cod is opaque and just cooked through, 6 to 9 minutes.
4. Discard garlic and ginger from rice and fluff with fork. Fold in parsley and remaining lemon zest.
5. Serve rice topped with fish and tomatoes and sprinkled with additional chopped parsley.

PER SERVING *About 488 cal, 14 g fat (2 g sat), 73 mg chol, 461 mg sodium, 51 g carb, 4 g fiber, 4 g sugar (0 g added sugar), 37 g pro*

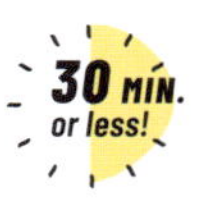

HALIBUT *with* LEMON-ANCHOVY SAUCE

ACTIVE 20 min. **TOTAL** 20 min. **SERVES** 4

- 1¼ cups couscous
- 3 Tbsp plus 2 tsp olive oil, divided
- 2 tsp lemon zest plus 3 Tbsp lemon juice
- 8 anchovy fillets, thinly sliced (about 2 Tbsp)
- ½ shallot, finely chopped
- ½ Fresno chile, finely chopped, plus more for serving
- ½ small clove garlic, grated
- Kosher salt
- ¼ cup flat-leaf parsley, chopped, plus more for serving
- 4 6-oz halibut fillets

1. Cook couscous per package directions. Fluff with a fork.
2. In a small bowl, combine 3 tablespoons olive oil, lemon zest and juice, anchovy fillets, shallot, Fresno chile, garlic, and a pinch of salt. Stir in parsley.
3. Heat remaining 2 teaspoons olive oil in a large cast-iron or nonstick skillet on medium-high. Season halibut with ½ teaspoon salt and cook, flesh side down, until golden brown, 4 minutes. Flip and cook until just opaque throughout, 2 to 3 minutes more. Transfer to a platter and spoon sauce over top. Sprinkle with additional chiles and parsley if desired and serve with couscous.

PER SERVING *About 487 cal, 15.5 g fat (2.5 g sat), 88 mg chol, 701 mg sodium, 44 g carb, 3 g fiber, 1 g sugar (0 g added sugar), 40 g pro*

MAKE IT A MEAL

Serve this savory sauced fish with a side like steamed asparagus, cucumber salad, or an herbed quinoa.

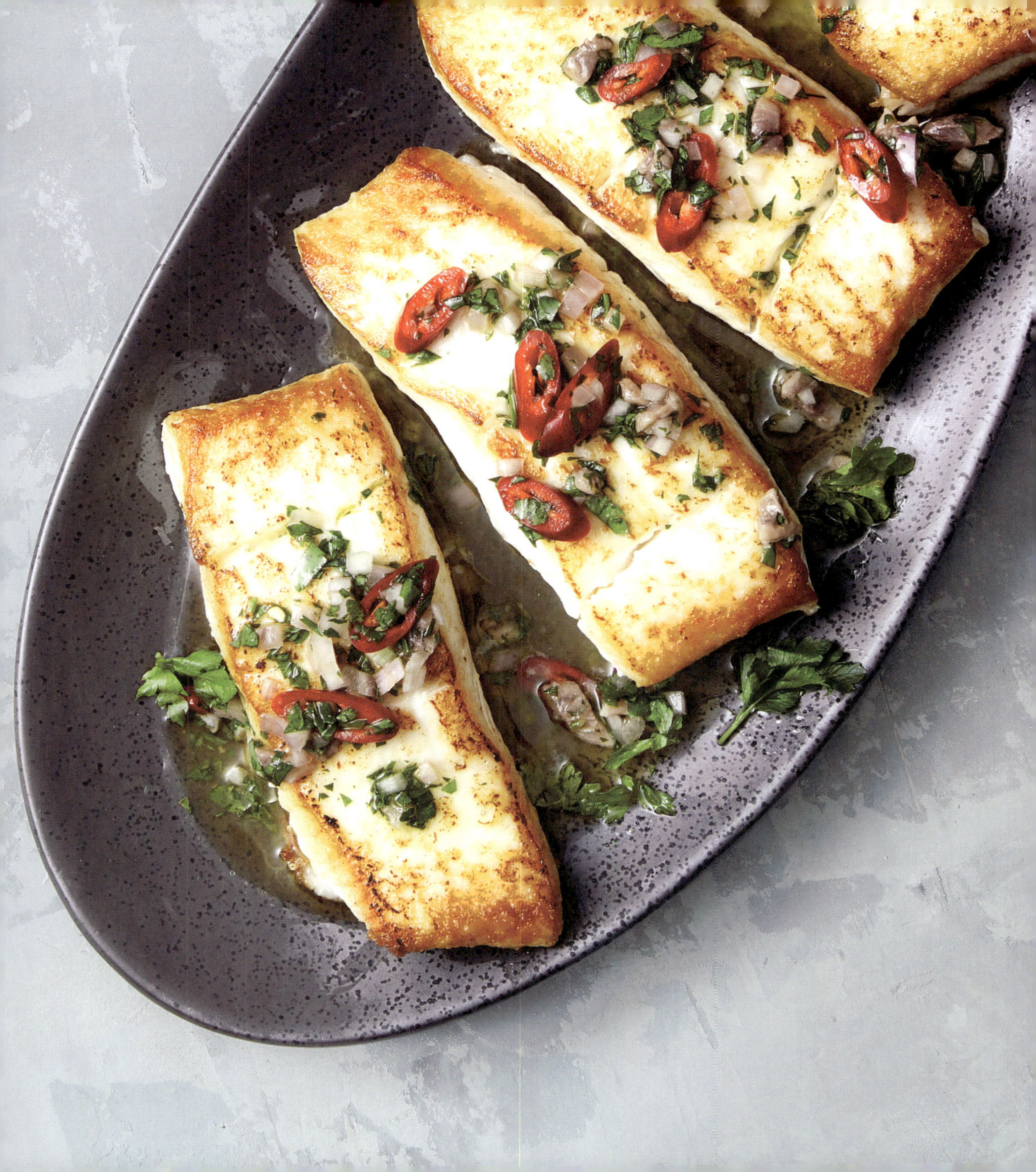

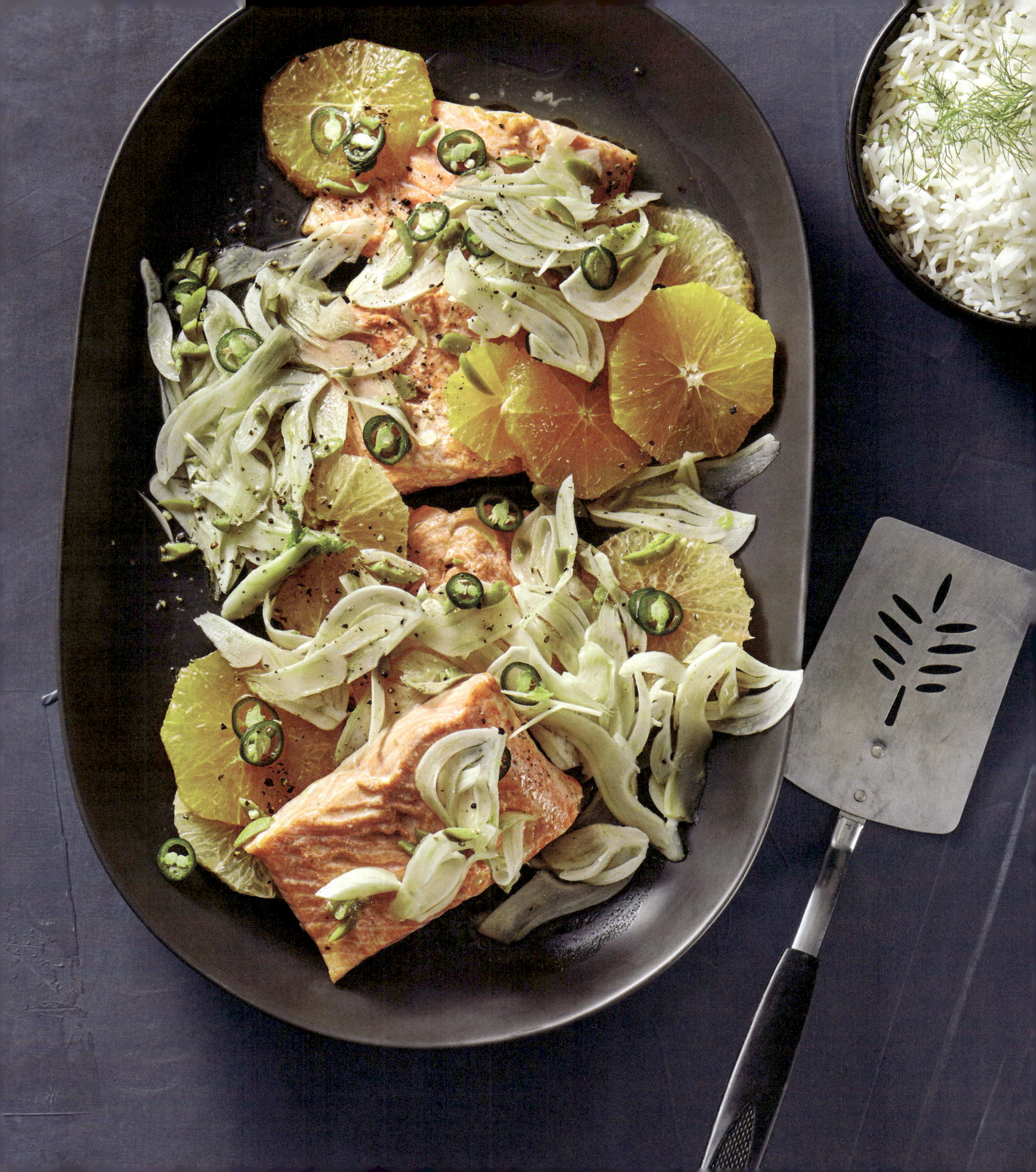

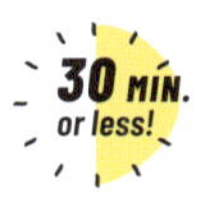

ARCTIC CHAR *with* CITRUS-FENNEL SALAD

ACTIVE 30 min. **TOTAL** 30 min. **SERVES** 4

- 1¼ cups basmati rice, rinsed
- 1 bay leaf
- Kosher salt and pepper
- 1 tsp orange zest plus 2 Tbsp orange juice
- 2 Tbsp olive oil, plus more for brushing
- 4 5-oz skin-on arctic char fillets
- 1 Tbsp fresh lemon juice
- 2 Tbsp olive oil, plus more for brushing
- 5 Castelvetrano olives, pitted, quartered, and thinly sliced
- 1 serrano chile, thinly sliced
- 1 fennel bulb (12 oz), cored and thinly sliced, fronds reserved for serving
- 1 grapefruit, peel removed, flesh thinly sliced into rounds
- 1 navel orange, peel removed, flesh thinly sliced into rounds

1. In a medium saucepan, bring to a boil rice, bay leaf, ¼ teaspoon salt, and 1¾ cups water. Reduce heat and simmer, covered, until rice is just tender, 12 to 14 minutes. Remove from heat and let sit, covered, until ready to serve. Discard bay leaf, then fluff rice and fold in orange zest.

2. Heat broiler with oven rack 6 inches from heat source. Brush a rimmed baking sheet with olive oil. Place arctic char skin side down on pan and season with ½ teaspoon salt. Broil until just opaque throughout, 4 to 6 minutes (depending on thickness).

3. Meanwhile, in a small bowl, whisk orange juice and lemon juice with 2 tablespoons oil. Stir in olives and serrano chile; transfer 1 tablespoon to a large bowl, add sliced fennel and ¼ teaspoon each salt and pepper; toss to coat.

4. Arrange fish on a platter, top with fennel salad, grapefruit, and orange and drizzle with remaining dressing. Serve with rice sprinkled with reserved fennel fronds.

PER SERVING *About 565 cal, 22.5 g fat (6.5 g sat), 50 mg chol, 747 mg sodium, 58 g carb, 5 g fiber, 6 g sugar (0 g added sugar), 36 g pro*

KITCHEN TIP

When buying fish, look for the thickest fillets you can find and make sure they're all comparable sizes for similar cooking times.

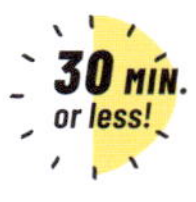

BROILED MACKEREL *with* AGRODOLCE TOMATOES

ACTIVE 25 min. **TOTAL** 25 min. **SERVES** 4

⅓ cup dry white wine

3 Tbsp golden raisins

1 Tbsp olive oil, plus more for brushing

1 medium onion, chopped

Kosher salt and pepper

12 oz cherry tomatoes, cut in half

2 cloves garlic, finely chopped

2 Tbsp balsamic or red wine vinegar

¼ cup flat-leaf parsley leaves, roughly chopped

4 6-oz skin-on mackerel fillets

Flaky sea salt, for serving

1. Measure wine in a liquid measuring cup, add raisins, and let soak 10 minutes.
2. Meanwhile, heat oil in a large skillet on medium. Add onion and ¼ teaspoon each salt and pepper, and cook, covered, stirring occasionally, until tender, 5 to 7 minutes. Add tomatoes and garlic and cook, stirring occasionally, until tomatoes start to soften, 3 to 4 minutes. Add raisins and soaking liquid. Bring to a simmer and cook until liquid is reduced by three-fourths, 2 to 3 minutes. Stir in vinegar and cook 30 seconds. Remove from heat and sprinkle with parsley.
3. Meanwhile, heat broiler with oven rack 6 inches from heat source. Brush small rimmed baking sheet with oil. Season mackerel with ½ teaspoon salt. Place skin side up on a prepared baking sheet. Broil until fish is just cooked through and skin is slightly charred, 6 to 8 minutes.
4. Divide tomatoes among plates and top with fish. Sprinkle with flaky sea salt if desired.

PER SERVING *About 486 cal, 31 g fat (7 g sat), 110 mg chol, 493 mg sodium, 14 g carb, 2 g fiber, 9 g sugar (0 g added sugar), 36 g pro*

MAKE IT AHEAD

These tomatoes are cooked agrodolce-style—a classic Italian sweet-and-sour sauce made with vinegar and a touch of sweetness (like golden raisins). Refrigerate the tomatoes and mackerel in separate airtight containers for up to four days. Give the tomatoes a stir before serving.

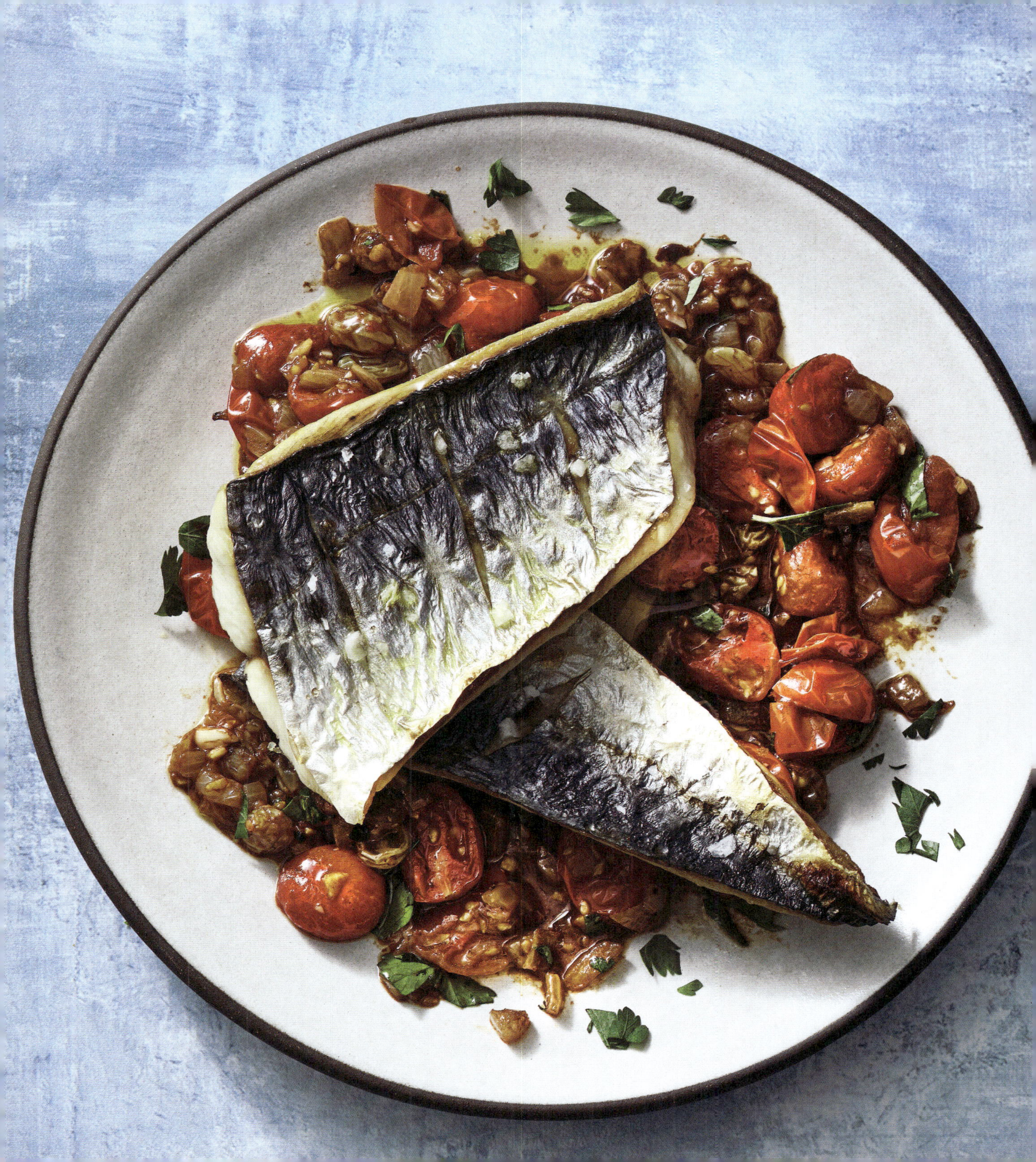

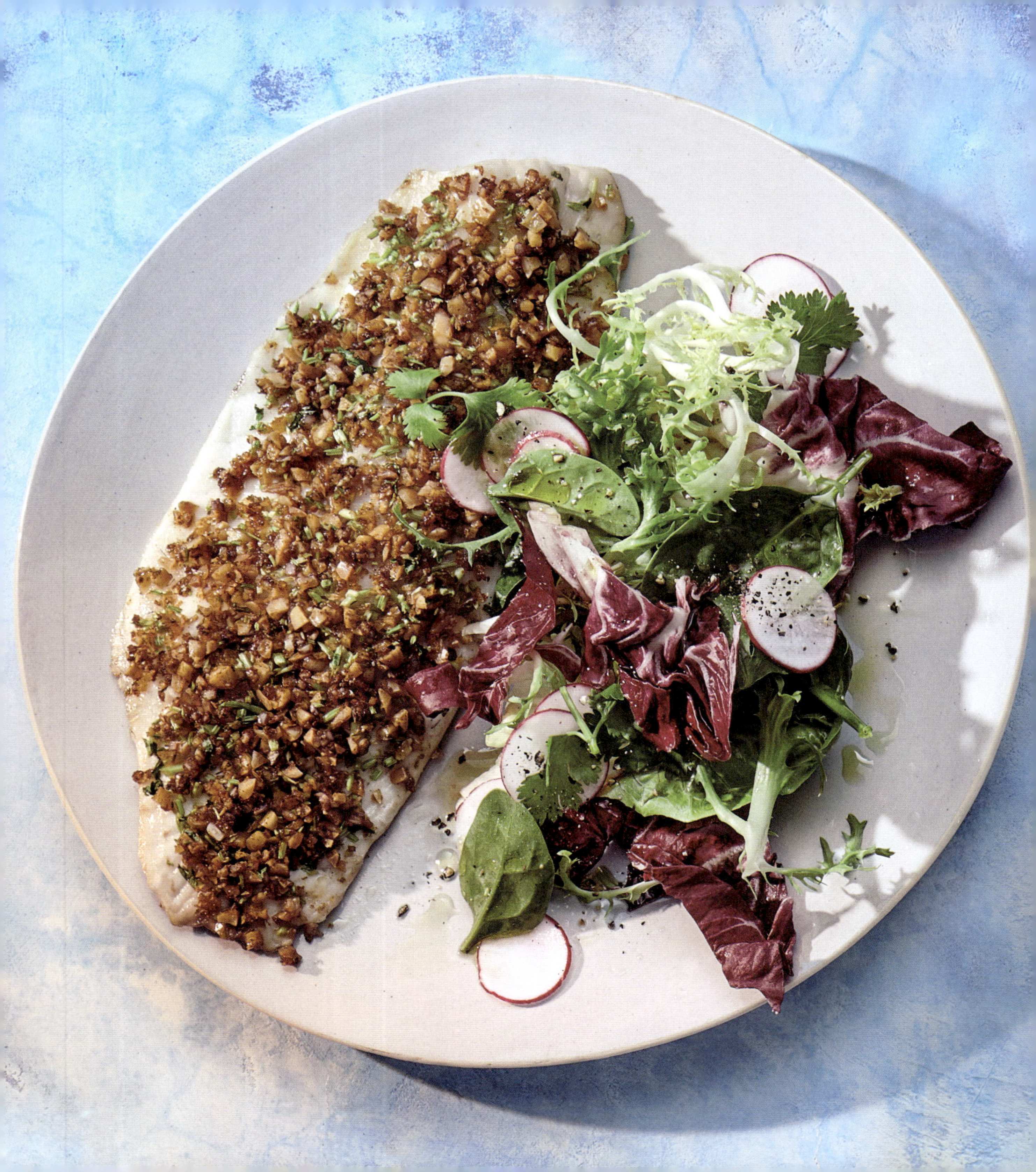

ALMOND-CRUSTED STRIPED BASS

ACTIVE 25 min. **TOTAL** 35 min. **SERVES** 4

2 Tbsp olive oil, divided

4 5-oz boneless, skinless striped bass fillets

¼ bunch fresh cilantro

⅔ cup blanched slivered almonds, toasted and roughly chopped

1 medium shallot, finely chopped

2 tsp grated lime zest plus 1 Tbsp lime juice, plus lime wedges for serving

1¼ tsp smoked paprika

1 tsp ground cumin

½ tsp ground cinnamon

¼ tsp ground allspice

Kosher salt and pepper

6 cups mixed greens

4 small radishes, thinly sliced

1. Heat oven to 375°F. Line a rimmed baking sheet with parchment paper and brush with 1 teaspoon oil. Pat fillets dry with paper towels and lay on parchment.

2. From cilantro, finely chop stems to equal ⅓ cup and set aside ½ cup leaves for salad. In a medium bowl, toss together cilantro stems, almonds, shallot, lime zest, smoked paprika, cumin, cinnamon, allspice, ½ teaspoon salt, and 2 teaspoons oil. Season fish with ¼ teaspoon each salt and pepper and divide almond mixture among fillets, spreading to coat surface of fish and pressing to adhere. Roast until fish is just opaque throughout, 10 to 14 minutes.

3. Meanwhile, in a large bowl, combine lime juice with remaining tablespoon oil. Add greens, radishes, reserved cilantro leaves, and a pinch each of salt and pepper and toss to coat. Serve with lime wedges if desired.

PER SERVING *About 339 cal, 19.8 g fat (2.5 g sat), 117 mg chol, 502 mg sodium, 11 g carb, 4.5 g fiber, 3 g sugar (0 g added sugar), 31 g pro*

KITCHEN TIP

White fish like striped bass, cod, and halibut have a mild flavor and firm texture, making them super versatile for all kinds of dishes. For a crusted recipe like this, choose skinless fillets—it's the best way to help nuts or breadcrumbs stick.

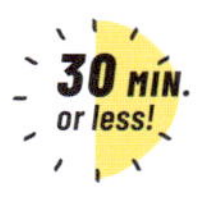

ROASTED SHRIMP *and* ASPARAGUS PASTA

ACTIVE 20 min. **TOTAL** 20 min. **SERVES** 4

12 oz whole-wheat spaghetti

1½ lb asparagus, trimmed, cut into thirds

2 cloves garlic, chopped

2 Tbsp olive oil, divided

Kosher salt and pepper

1 lemon

1 lb large peeled and deveined shrimp

½ tsp red pepper flakes, plus more for serving

½ cup flat-leaf parsley, chopped

Grated Parmesan, for serving

1. Heat oven to 425°F. Cook pasta per package directions. Reserve 1 cup pasta cooking water; drain pasta and return to pot.
2. On a rimmed baking sheet, toss asparagus and garlic with 1 tablespoon oil and ¼ teaspoon each salt and pepper. Zest lemon and set zest aside. Halve lemon and place on a baking sheet, cut sides down; roast 4 minutes.
3. Meanwhile, toss shrimp with remaining tablespoon oil, then red pepper, ½ teaspoon salt, and ¼ teaspoon pepper. Nestle shrimp on a tray with asparagus and continue roasting until shrimp are opaque throughout and asparagus is just tender, 5 to 7 minutes more.
4. Transfer lemons to a plate, then transfer vegetables, shrimp, and any pan juices to pot with pasta. Squeeze roasted lemon halves over top and toss to combine, adding some reserved pasta water if pasta seems dry. Toss with parsley and serve sprinkled with reserved lemon zest, grated Parmesan, and additional red pepper if desired.

PER SERVING *About 524 cal, 13 g fat (2 g sat), 145 mg chol, 1,073 mg sodium, 77 g carb, 11 g fiber, 3.5 g sugar (0 g added sugar), 33 g pro*

FIBER FIX

Asparagus is a good source of fiber—one cup cooked has 3 to 4 grams, making it great for digestion and supporting steady blood sugar. Plus, it's low in calories and rich in folate and vitamin K.

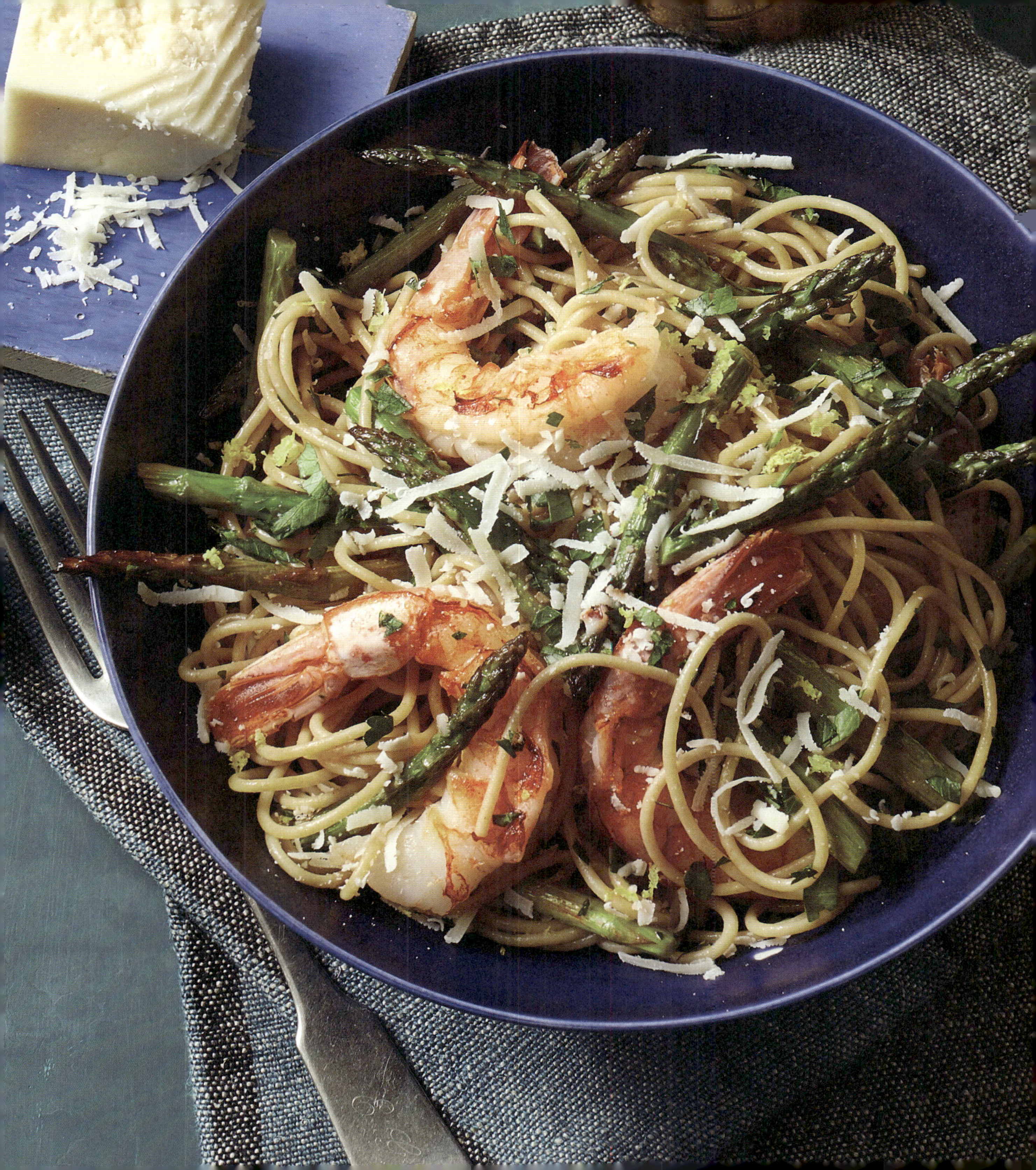

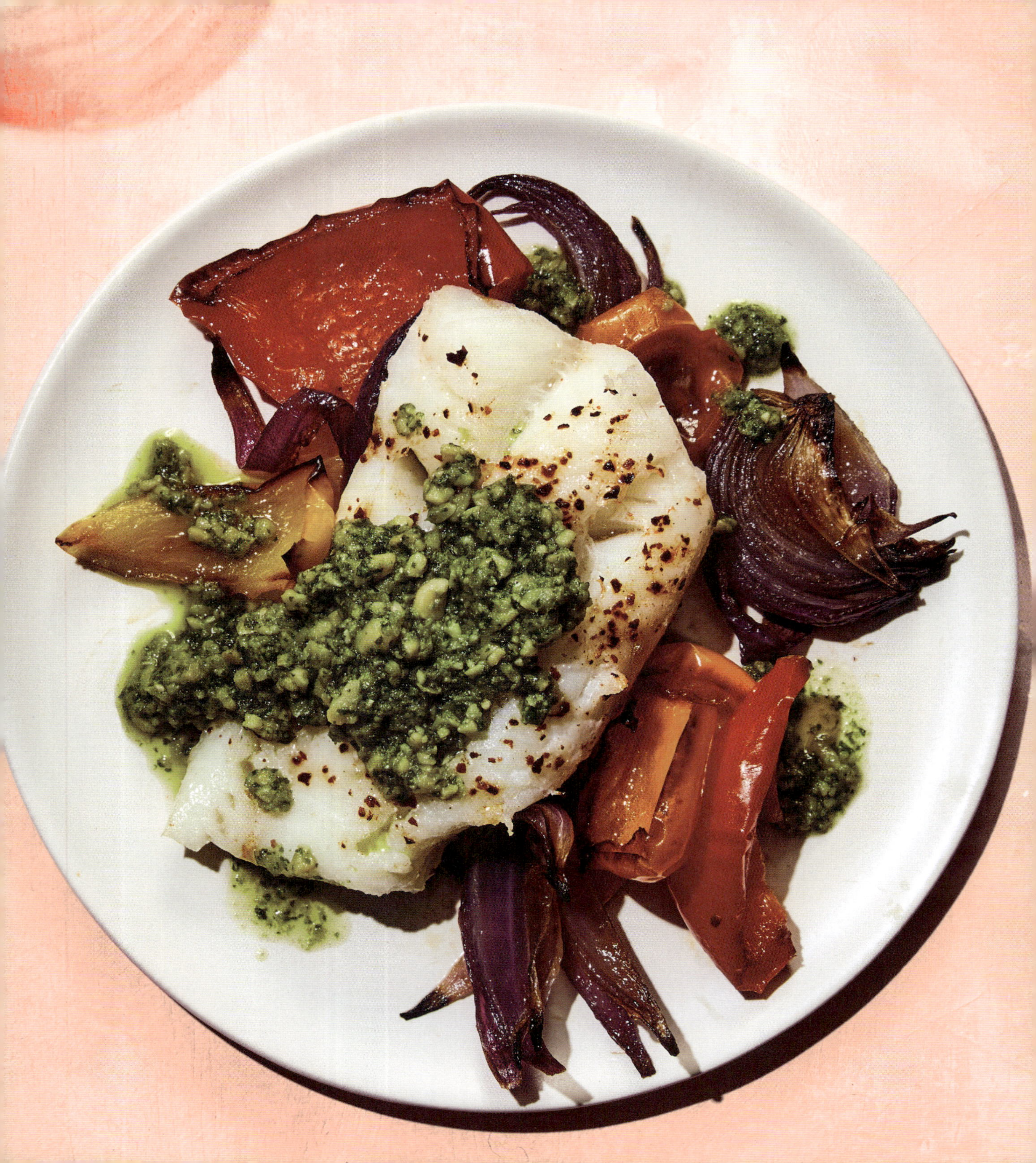

ROASTED FISH *and* PEPPERS *with* CHICKPEA PESTO

ACTIVE 25 min. **TOTAL** 45 min. **SERVES** 1

3 small peppers, cut into 2-in. pieces

1 medium red onion, cut into ½-inch-thick wedges

½ cup plus 1 Tbsp olive oil, divided

Kosher salt and pepper

4 6-oz firm white fish fillets (we used cod)

½ tsp Aleppo pepper

3 cups basil leaves

1½ Tbsp grated lemon zest plus 3 Tbsp juice (from 1 large lemon)

2 small cloves garlic

15-oz can low-sodium chickpeas, rinsed

1. Heat oven to 425°F. On a rimmed baking sheet, toss peppers and onion with 1 tablespoon oil and ¼ teaspoon each salt and pepper. Roast until tender and beginning to brown, 20 to 22 minutes.

2. Season fish with Aleppo pepper and ½ teaspoon salt; nestle amid vegetables and roast until vegetables are golden brown and tender and fish is opaque throughout, 10 to 12 minutes more.

3. Meanwhile, in a food processor, pulse basil, lemon zest and juice, garlic, and ¼ teaspoon salt until finely chopped. Add remaining ½ cup oil and process until smooth. Add chickpeas and pulse until chopped but still slightly chunky. Serve pesto with fish and vegetables.

PER SERVING *About 521 cal, 33.5 g fat (4.5 g sat), 65 mg chol, 646 mg sodium, 23 g carb, 6.5 g fiber, 5.5 g sugar (0 g added sugar), 34 g pro*

KITCHEN TIP

Aleppo pepper is a mildly spicy, fruity chili from Syria and Turkey with rich red color and sweet, smoky kick. Can't find it? Sub in paprika plus a pinch of cayenne for a similar flavor.

SALMON BURGERS

ACTIVE 25 min. **TOTAL** 45 min. **SERVES** 4

1 large egg

1 lb skinless salmon fillet, finely chopped

2 scallions, chopped

1 jalapeño, finely chopped

3 Tbsp cilantro, chopped and divided

Kosher salt and pepper

1 Tbsp olive oil

½ cup Greek yogurt

1 tsp lime zest plus 2 Tbsp juice

4 brioche buns, toasted

8 Bibb lettuce leaves

2 Persian cucumbers or ½ English cucumber, shaved lengthwise

2 cup broccoli or radish sprouts

1. In a medium bowl, beat egg until frothy. Fold in salmon, scallions, jalapeño, 2 tablespoons cilantro, ½ teaspoon salt, and ¼ teaspoon pepper.
2. Heat oil in a large nonstick skillet on medium. Spoon 4 mounds of salmon mixture (about ½ cup each) into skillet and flatten into ½-inch thick patties. Cook until golden brown, 2 minutes per side.
3. Meanwhile, in a bowl, combine yogurt, lime zest and juice, remaining tablespoon cilantro, and ¼ teaspoon each salt and pepper and spread on buns. Top bottom buns with lettuce, salmon patties, cucumber, and sprouts; sandwich with top buns.

PER SERVING *About 379 cal, 13.2 g fat (3.5 g sat), 134 mg chol, 580 mg sodium, 32 g carb, 3 g fiber, 8.5 g sugar (0 g added sugar), 34 g pro*

KITCHEN TIP
If your patties are having a hard time holding together, pop them in the fridge for 15 to 30 minutes before cooking to help them firm up and hold their shape in the skillet.

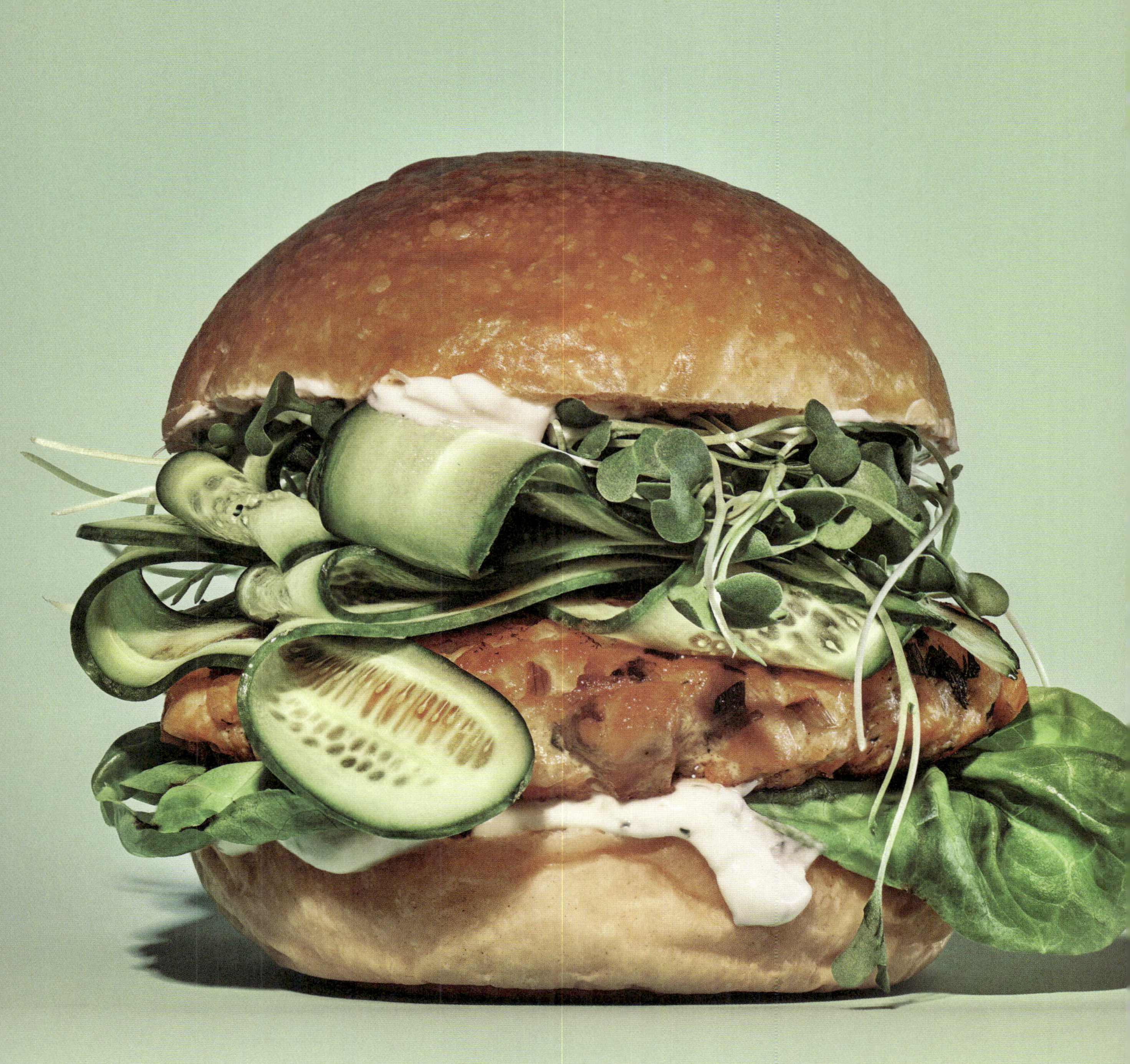

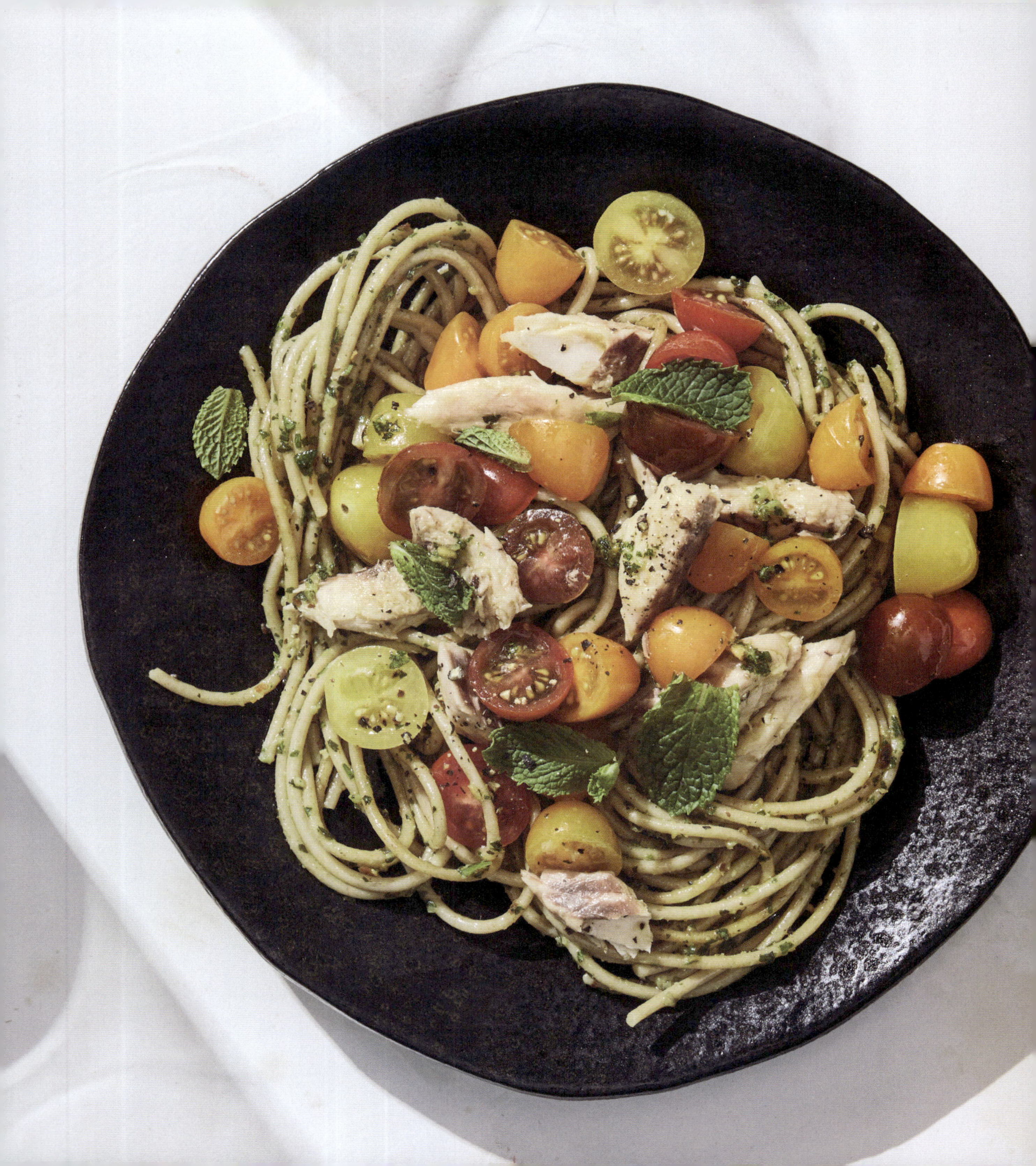

MACKEREL & TOMATO PASTA

ACTIVE 25 min. **TOTAL** 30 min. **SERVES** 4

10 oz whole-wheat spaghetti

3 4.4-oz cans boneless mackerel fillets in olive oil

12 oz mixed-color cherry tomatoes, halved (or quartered if large)

Kosher salt and pepper

2 cups mint leaves, plus more for serving

1 cup flat-leaf parsley leaves

1 large shallot, roughly chopped

4 fillets oil-packed anchovies, coarsely chopped

½ cup olive oil

⅔ cup roasted sliced almonds, divided

1. Cook pasta per package directions; drain and rinse under cold water to cool.
2. Meanwhile, drain mackerel, reserving 2 tablespoons oil; transfer mackerel to a medium bowl and break into bite-size pieces. Gently toss with tomatoes, reserved mackerel oil, and a pinch each of salt and pepper.
3. In a food processor, pulse mint, parsley, shallot, anchovies, and ¼ teaspoon each salt and pepper to finely chop. Add olive oil and ⅓ cup almonds and pulse until nuts are finely chopped.
4. In a large bowl, toss pasta with almond mint pesto. Spoon mackerel salad on top and scatter with remaining almonds and additional mint leaves, if desired.

PER SERVING *About 884 cal, 54.5 g fat (7.5 g sat), 33 mg chol, 541 mg sodium, 74 g carb, 15 g fiber, 4 g sugar (0 g added sugar) 33 g pro*

FIBER FIX

While the carb content is nearly the same, whole-wheat pasta typically has 2 to 3 times the fiber than regular white pasta, making for a more satisfying meal.

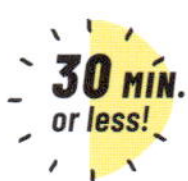

SEARED SALMON *with* LENTIL SALAD

ACTIVE 20 min. **TOTAL** 20 min. **SERVES** 4

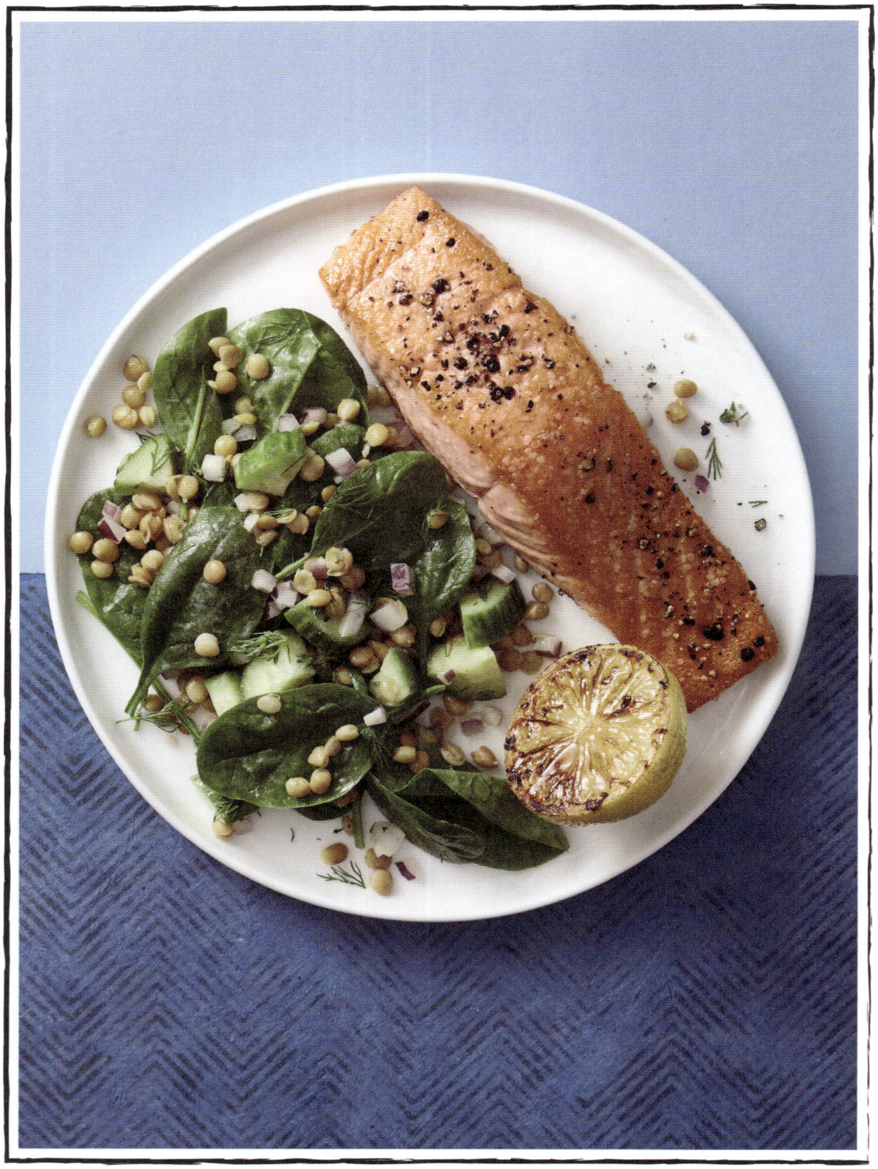

4 5-oz skinless salmon fillets
Kosher salt and pepper
2 Tbsp plus 2 tsp olive oil, divided
2 lemons, halved
2 tsp Dijon mustard
1 tsp fresh thyme
½ small red onion, finely chopped
1 15-oz can lentils, rinsed
1 small seedless cucumber, cut into pieces
4 cups baby spinach
¼ cup fresh dill, chopped

1. Heat a large skillet on medium. Season salmon with ¼ teaspoon each salt and pepper. Add 2 teaspoons oil to a skillet, then salmon and lemon halves, cut-sides down, and cook until salmon is opaque, 5 minutes per side.”

2. Into a bowl, squeeze 2 tablespoons lemon juice, then whisk in mustard, remaining 2 tablespoons oil, and ¼ teaspoon each salt and pepper; stir in thyme. Toss with onion and lentils then fold in cucumber, spinach, and dill. Serve with salmon.

PER SERVING *About 348 cal, 13.1 g fat (2.5 g sat), 66 mg chol, 488 mg sodium, 19 g carb, 9.5 g fiber, 3 g sugar (0 g added sugar), 37 g pro*

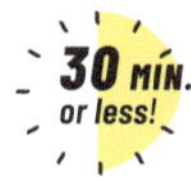

ROASTED GARLICKY SHRIMP *and* PITA

ACTIVE 10 min. **TOTAL** 20 min. **SERVES** 4

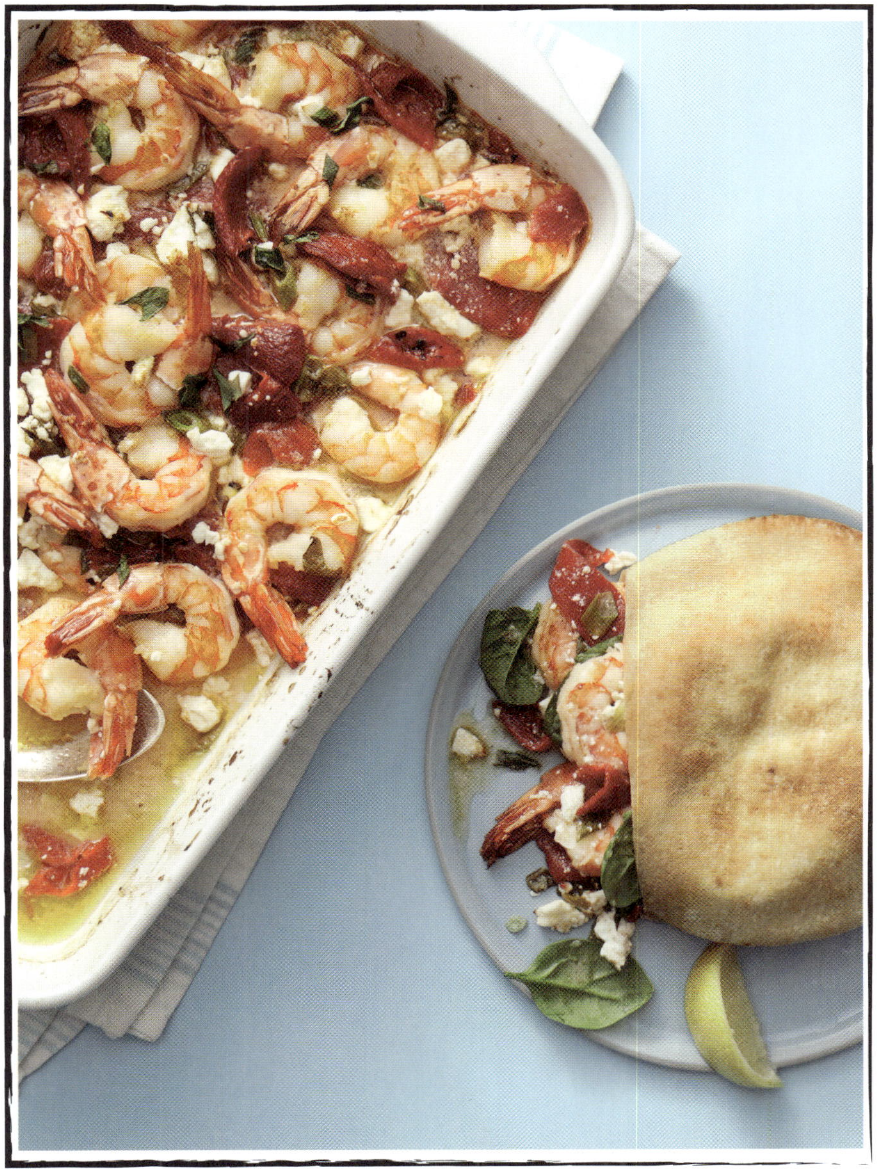

1½ lb large peeled and deveined shrimp
1 12-oz jar roasted red peppers, drained and cut into 1-in. pieces
4 scallions, sliced
2 cloves garlic, pressed
2 Tbsp dry white wine
1 Tbsp fresh lemon juice
Kosher salt and pepper
2 Tbsp olive oil
4 oz feta cheese, crumbled
Pitas and baby spinach, rice or couscous, or salad greens, for serving

1. Heat oven to 425°F. In a 1½-to 2-quart baking dish, combine shrimp, red peppers, scallions, garlic, wine, lemon juice, and ¼ teaspoon each salt and pepper.

2. Drizzle with olive oil and sprinkle with feta cheese. Bake until shrimp are opaque throughout, 12 to 15 minutes. Spoon into pitas along with baby spinach, serve over rice or couscous, or toss with your favorite salad greens.

PER SERVING *About 289 cal, 14.5 g fat (5.5 g sat), 240 mg chol, 1468 mg sodium, 10 g carb, 3 g fiber, 2 g sugar (0 g added sugar), 28 g pro*

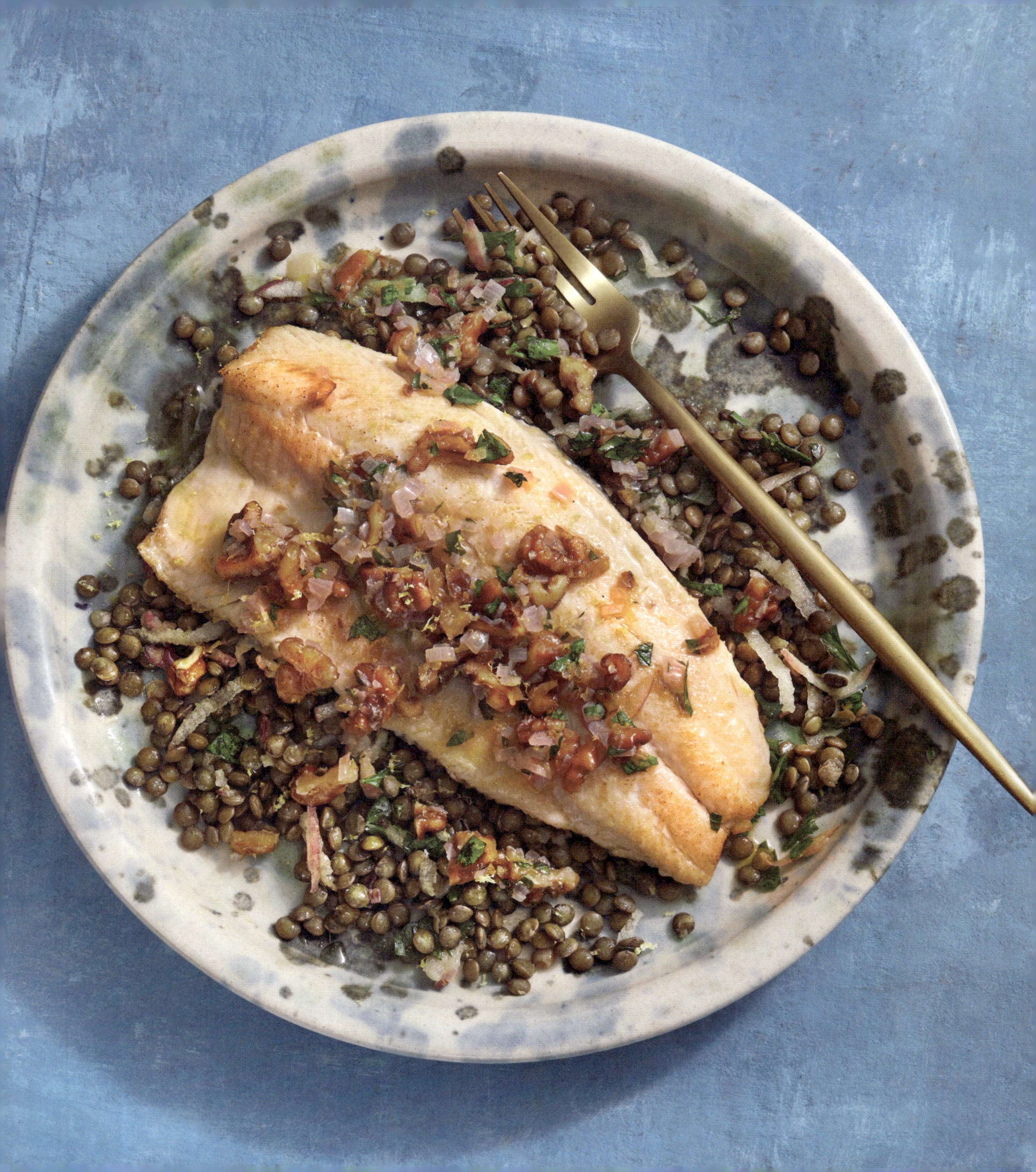

TROUT *with* LENTIL, APPLE & WALNUT SALAD

ACTIVE 40 min. **TOTAL** 40 min. **SERVES** 4

1 cup French green lentils, rinsed and picked over

½ cup flat-leaf parsley leaves, chopped, divided, stems reserved

2 sprigs thyme

¼ cup plus 1 Tbsp olive oil, divided

¼ cup raw walnut halves, chopped

1 small shallot, finely chopped

Kosher salt and pepper

2 tsp lemon zest plus 2 Tbsp lemon juice, divided

1 Honeycrisp apple

4 4-oz skin-on trout fillets

1. Cook lentils per package directions, adding parsley stems and thyme sprigs to cooking water. Drain, gently shaking out excess liquid; discard parsley stems and thyme sprigs.
2. Meanwhile, heat ¼ cup oil and walnuts in a large nonstick skillet on medium and cook, stirring occasionally, until nuts are fragrant and golden brown, 5 to 7 minutes. Add shallot and ¼ teaspoon salt and cook, stirring constantly, 1 minute. Transfer to a medium heatproof bowl and fold in 1 teaspoon lemon zest and half of chopped parsley; wipe out skillet and reserve.
3. Strain 1 tablespoon walnut oil into a large bowl, then stir in lemon juice and ½ teaspoon each salt and pepper; fold in lentils. Coarsely grate apple into lentils, add remaining chopped parsley, and toss to combine.
4. Heat ½ tablespoon olive oil in a reserved skillet on medium heat. Add 2 trout fillets and cook until golden brown and cooked through, 2 to 3 minutes per side; transfer to plates. Repeat with remaining ½ tablespoon olive oil and 2 fillets.
5. Serve trout topped with walnut mixture and remaining 1 teaspoon lemon zest alongside lentil salad.

PER SERVING *About 509 cal, 24.5 g fat (4 g sat), 60 mg chol, 414 mg sodium, 41 g carb, 8 g fiber, 6 g sugar (0 g added sugar), 33 g pro*

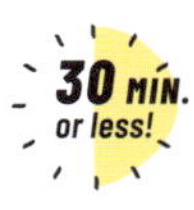

ROASTED SALMON, ARTICHOKES, *and* RED ONION

ACTIVE 10 min. **TOTAL** 30 min. **SERVES** 4

FOR SALMON
2 14-oz cans artichoke hearts, halved and patted dry

1 medium red onion, cut into 8 wedges

1 Tbsp olive oil

Kosher salt and pepper

2 small navel oranges

4 5-oz skinless salmon fillets

1 clove garlic, finely chopped

FOR PARSLEY OIL
1 cup flat-leaf parsley

½ cup olive oil

1 tsp fresh lemon juice

Kosher salt

1. Heat oven to 425°F. On a rimmed baking sheet, gently toss artichokes and onion with oil and ½ teaspoon each salt and pepper. Create 4 spaces for salmon to be added later. Roast veggies 15 minutes.

2. Cut 1 orange into wedges. Season salmon with garlic and ¼ teaspoon each salt and pepper and place in the spaces on the sheet; add orange wedges and continue roasting until salmon is opaque throughout, 12 to 15 minutes.

3. Meanwhile, prepare parsley oil: In a blender, puree parsley, oil, lemon juice, and ¼ teaspoon salt until smooth. Grate zest of remaining orange over vegetables and serve with parsley oil.

PER SERVING *About 540 cal, 36 g fat (5.5 g sat), 66 mg chol, 898 mg sodium, 21 g carb, 3 g fiber, 7.5 g sugar (0 g added sugar), 33 g pro*

LOVE YOUR LEFTOVERS
Only sauce what you plan to eat with the parsley oil. Refrigerate any leftover salmon and vegetables separately for up to three days.

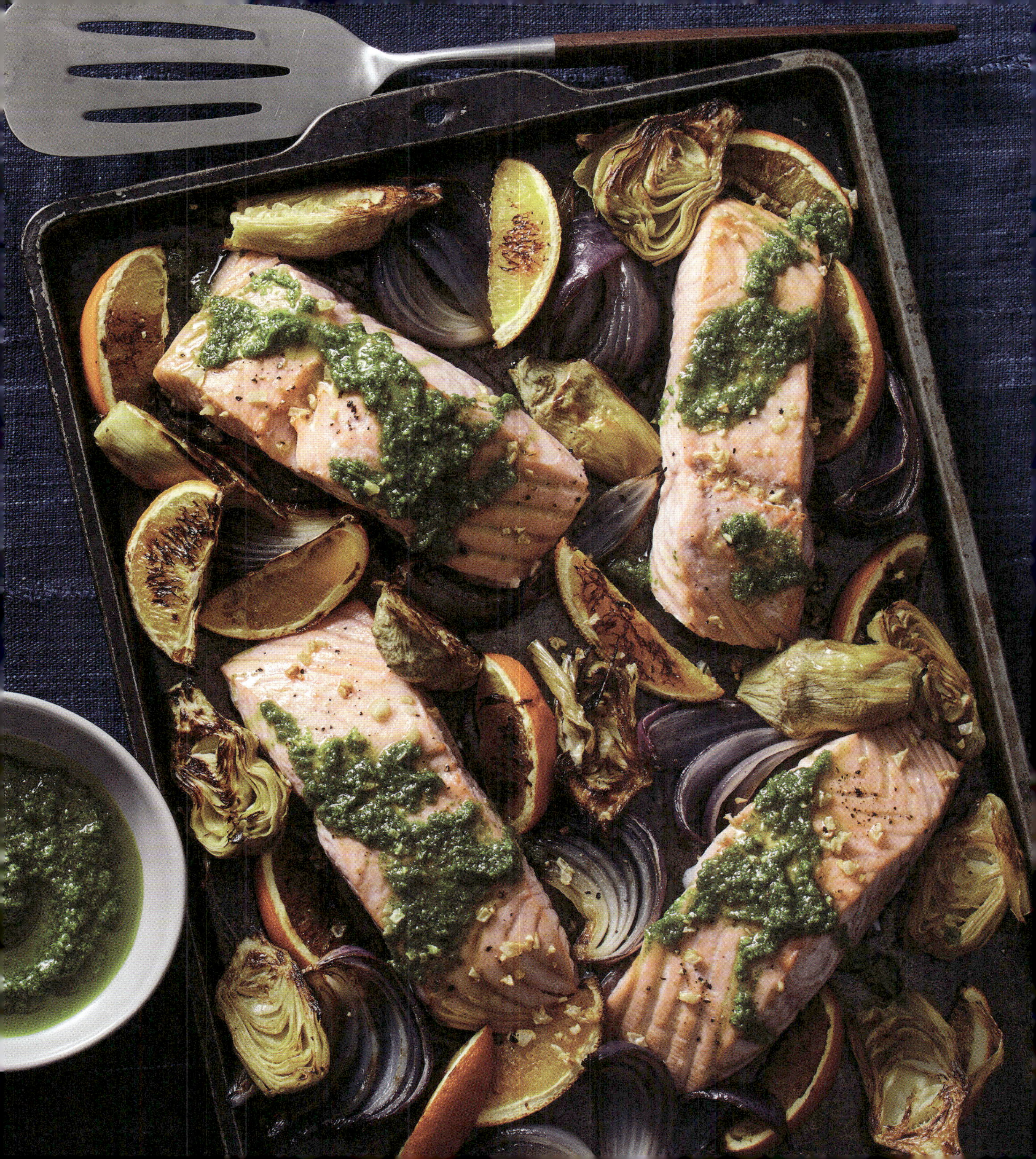

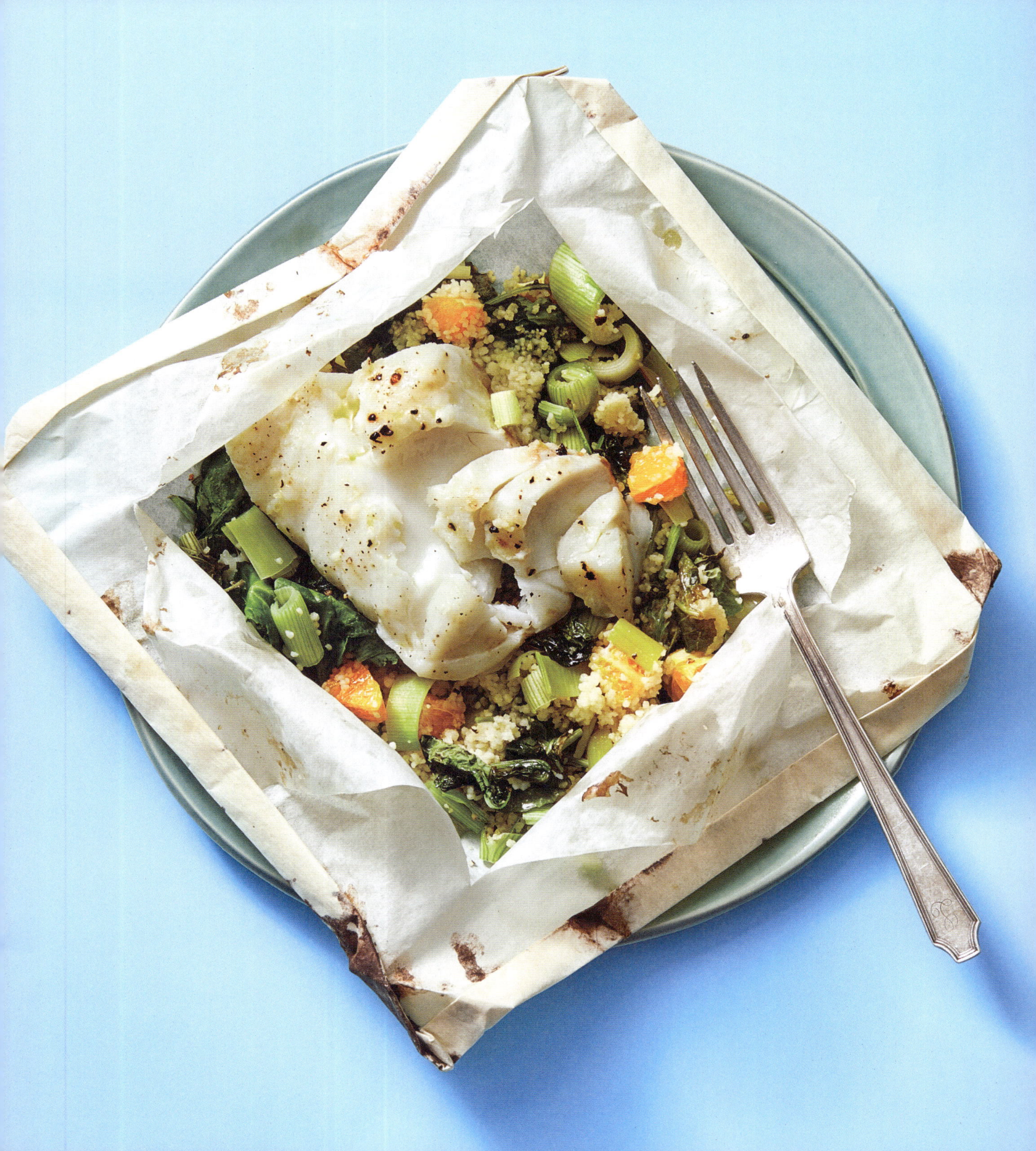

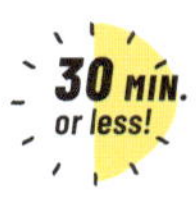

COD IN PARCHMENT *with* ORANGE LEEK COUSCOUS

ACTIVE 15 min. **TOTAL** 30 min. **SERVES** 4

1 cup couscous

1 orange

1 leek, white and light green parts only, cut in half lengthwise, then sliced ½-inch thick

3 cups baby kale

1¼ lb cod, cut into 4 portions

1 Tbsp olive oil

Kosher salt and pepper

1. Heat oven to 425°. Tear off four 12-in. squares of parchment paper and arrange on two baking sheets. In a bowl, combine couscous with ¾ cup water.
2. Cut orange in half, then peel one half and coarsely chop fruit. Fold orange into couscous along with leek and baby kale.
3. Divide couscous mixture among pieces of parchment and top each with a piece of cod. Drizzle with oil and sprinkle with ½ teaspoon salt and ¼ teaspoon pepper, then squeeze remaining orange half over tops.
4. Cover each with another piece of parchment and fold each edge up and under three times, tucking edges underneath. Roast 12 minutes.
5. Transfer each packet to a plate. Using scissors or a knife, cut an "X" in the center and fold back the triangles.

PER SERVING *About 338 cal, 4.8 g fat (0.5 g sat), 61 mg chol, 332 mg sodium, 40 g carb, 3.5 g fiber, 3.5 g sugar (0 g added sugar), 32 g pro*

KITCHEN TIP

This dish is cooked in single-serve portions, making it easy to halve or double the recipe based on how many people you're serving.

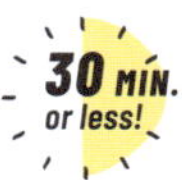

SALMON SALAD TARTINES

ACTIVE 15 min. **TOTAL** 15 min. **SERVES** 4

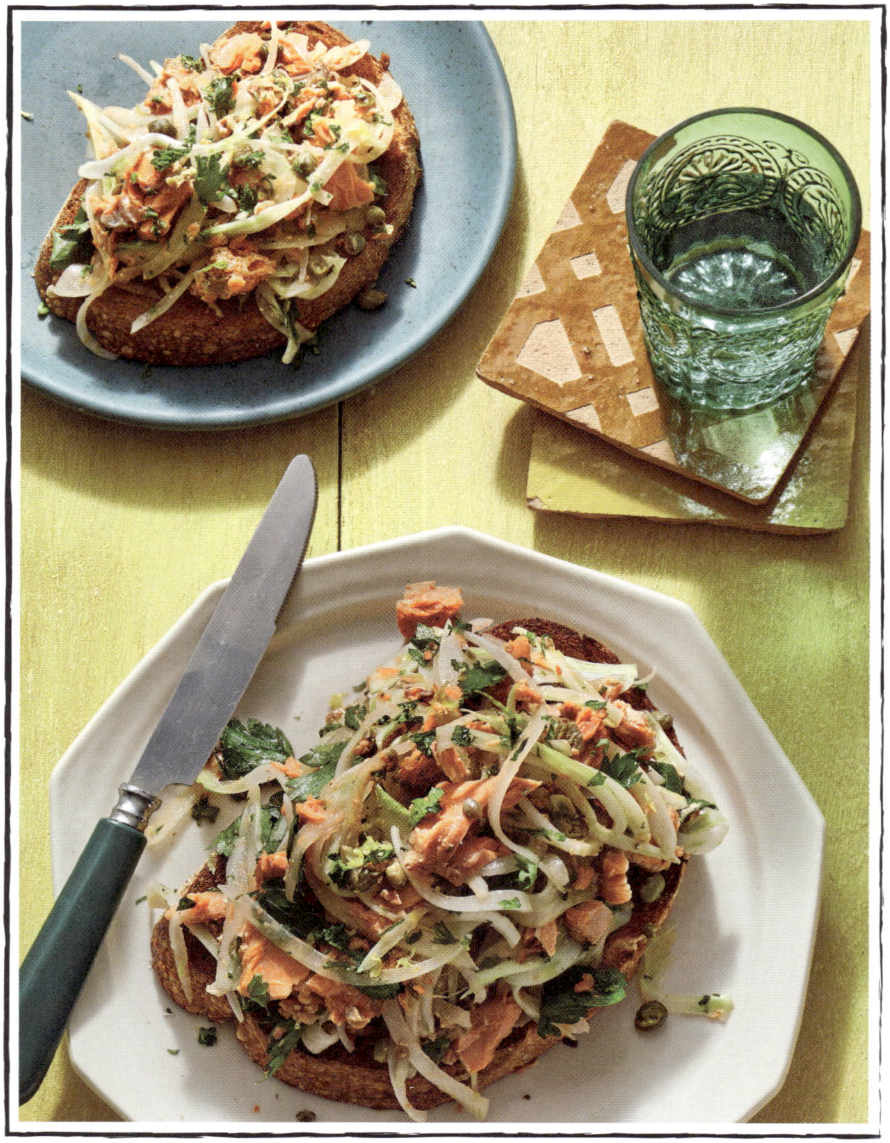

- ½ small Vidalia onion, thinly sliced on mandoline
- ½ bulb fennel
- ½ cup flat-leaf parsley leaves, chopped
- 2 Tbsp capers, drained and chopped
- 2 Tbsp olive oil
- 1 tsp lemon zest plus ½ Tbsp lemon juice
- Kosher salt and pepper
- 2 7.5-oz cans sockeye salmon, drained and gently broken apart
- 4 slices sourdough bread, toasted

1. In a small bowl, soak onion in ice water 10 minutes, then drain and squeeze dry.

2. Meanwhile, core fennel, then thinly slice on mandoline. Combine in a medium bowl with parsley, capers, oil, lemon zest and juice, and ¼ teaspoon each salt and pepper, then toss with squeezed onion. Fold in salmon and serve on toast.

PER SERVING *About 348 cal, 13 g fat (2.5 g sat), 56 mg chol, 860 mg sodium, 30 g carb, 3 g fiber, 5 g sugar (0 g added sugar), 29 g pro*

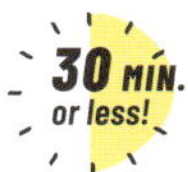

TUNA, ARTICHOKE & CHICKPEA TOASTS

ACTIVE 20 min. **TOTAL** 25 min. **SERVES** 4

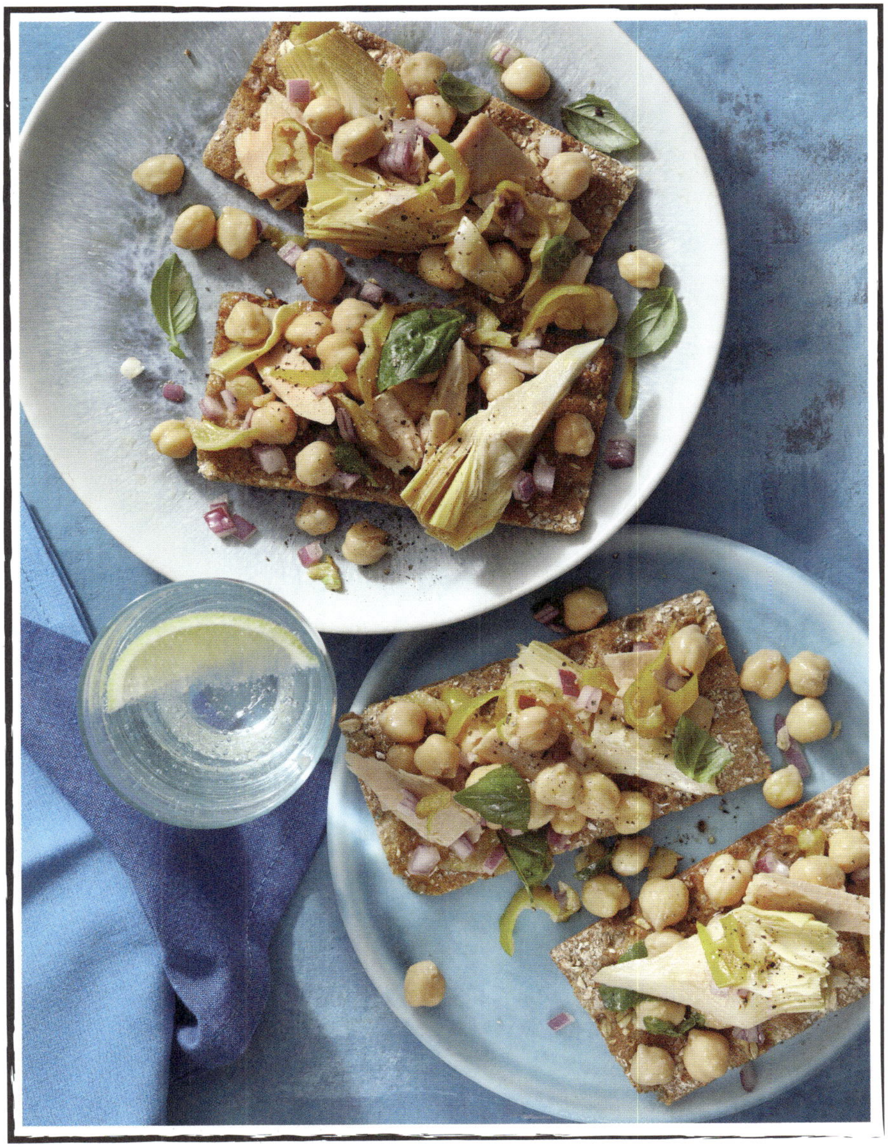

- 5 Tbsp olive oil
- ¼ cup red wine vinegar
- 1 tsp Dijon mustard
- Kosher salt and pepper
- 1 15.5-oz can low-sodium chickpeas, rinsed and roughly chopped
- 1 small red onion, finely chopped
- 6 jarred pepperoncini peppers, chopped
- 2 8-oz jars solid white tuna packed in olive oil, drained and flaked into pieces
- 1 14-oz can artichoke quarters, drained and halved lengthwise (halved again crosswise if large)
- ½ cup basil leaves, torn
- 8 pieces multigrain crispbread

1. In a large bowl, whisk together oil, vinegar, mustard, ½ teaspoon salt, and ¼ teaspoon pepper. Stir in chickpeas, red onion, and pepperoncini and let marinate at room temperature, 10 minutes.

2. Fold in tuna, artichokes, and basil. Serve with crispbread.

PER SERVING *About 507 cal, 25.5 g fat (4 g sat), 41 mg chol, 1,105 mg sodium, 39 g carb, 8 g fiber, 3.5 g sugar (0 g added sugar), 30 g pro*

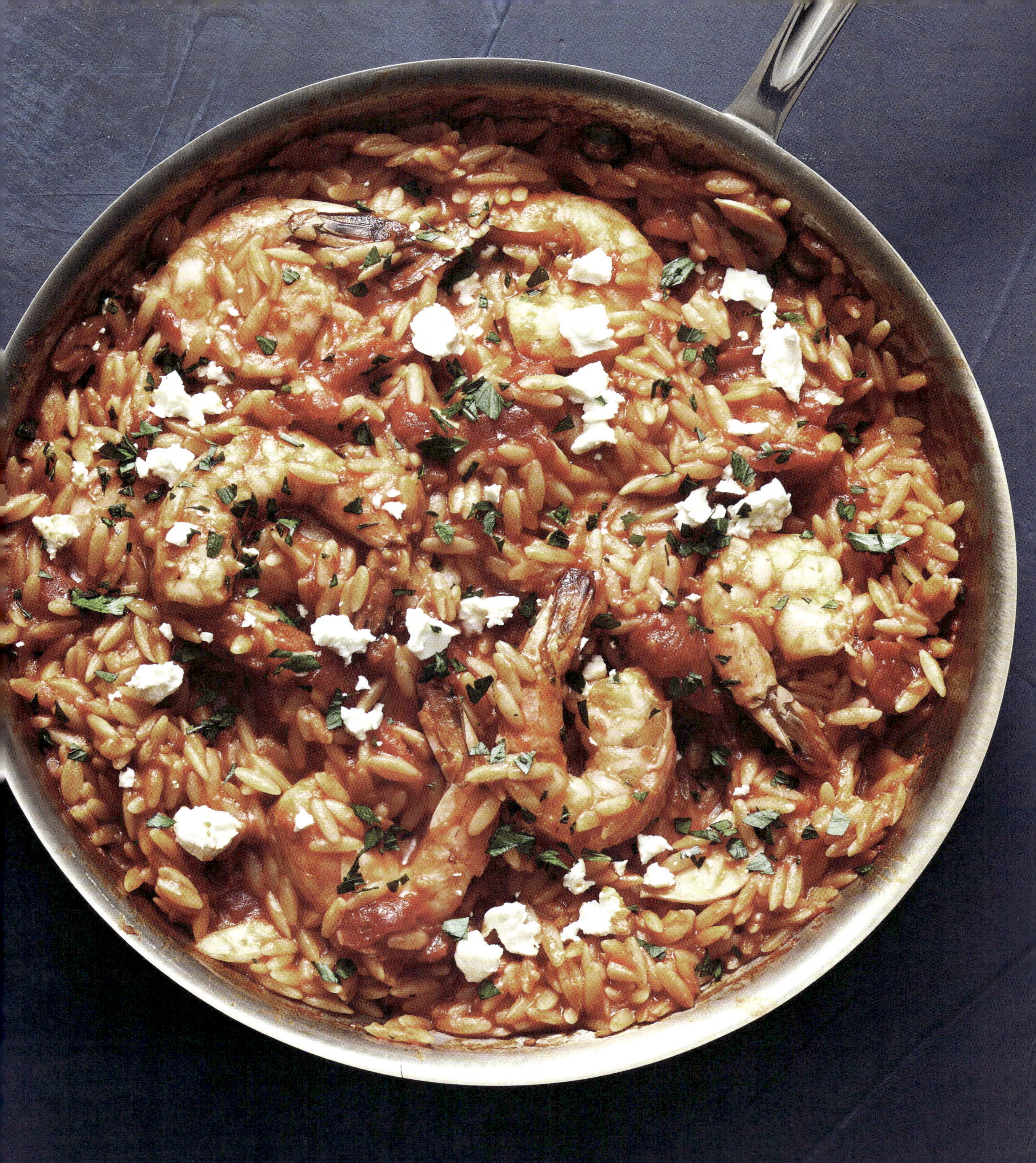

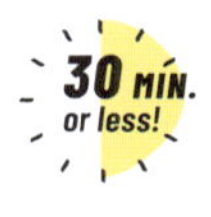

SKILLET SHRIMP *with* TOMATO-FETA ORZO

ACTIVE 30 min. **TOTAL** 30 min. **SERVES** 4

- 1 tsp lemon zest
- 2 large cloves garlic, grated, divided
- 3 Tbsp olive oil, divided
- Kosher salt
- 1 lb large peeled and deveined shrimp
- ½ tsp red pepper flakes
- ½ cup dry white wine
- 1 cup orzo
- 28-oz can whole peeled tomatoes
- ½ cup flat-leaf parsley, chopped
- 2 oz feta, crumbled

1. In a medium bowl, combine lemon zest, half of garlic, 1 tablespoon oil, and ½ teaspoon salt. Add shrimp and toss to coat; let marinate.
2. Meanwhile, in a large skillet, heat red pepper flakes, remaining garlic, and remaining 2 tablespoons oil on medium until sizzling. Stir in wine and simmer 1 minute. Stir in orzo to coat, then tomatoes and their juices, crushing with hands, and ½ cup water. Simmer, covered, stirring occasionally, until orzo is just barely tender, 8 to 10 minutes.
3. Add shrimp and cook, covered, until opaque throughout, 3 to 5 minutes. Sprinkle with parsley and feta.

PER SERVING *About 326 cal, 14 g fat (3.5 g sat), 195 mg chol, 804 mg sodium, 22 g carb, 3 g fiber, 6.5 g sugar (0 g added sugar), 28 g pro*

PROTEIN POWER
Shrimp are a fanatastic lean protein source, with roughly 22 to 25 grams of protein per 4 ounces.

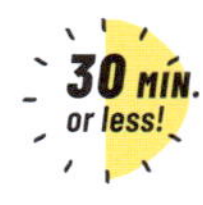

CAULIFLOWER COUSCOUS *with* PAPRIKA SHRIMP

ACTIVE 20 min. **TOTAL** 20 min. **SERVES** 4

- 1 medium head cauliflower (about 1¾ lb)
- 3 Tbsp olive oil, divided
- ½ cup dried apricots (or 3 fresh), roughly chopped
- Kosher salt and pepper
- 2 Tbsp fresh lemon juice
- 20 large shrimp, peeled and deveined
- 1 tsp paprika
- ½ seedless cucumber, cut into ½-in. pieces
- ¼ cup fresh mint leaves, roughly chopped

1. Remove and discard any leaves from the cauliflower. Thinly slice the head and place it in the bowl of a food processor. Roughly chop the thick stems and add them to the food processor. Pulse the cauliflower until it is finely chopped and resembles couscous (re-pulse any big pieces separately, if necessary).
2. Heat 1 tablespoon oil in a large skillet over medium heat. Add the cauliflower, apricots, and ½ teaspoon each salt and pepper and cook, covered, stirring occasionally, until the cauliflower is beginning to soften, 2 to 3 minutes. Transfer to a large bowl and toss with the lemon juice and 1 tablespoon oil.
3. Wipe out the skillet and heat the remaining tablespoon oil over medium heat. Season the shrimp with paprika and ¼ teaspoon salt. Working in batches, cook the shrimp until opaque throughout, 1 to 2 minutes per side.
4. Add the cucumber and mint to the cauliflower and toss to combine. Serve with the shrimp.

PER SERVING *About 274 cal, 10.5 g fat (1.8 g sat), 108 mg chol, 990 mg sodium, 20 g carb, 2.5 g fiber, 2 g sugar (0 g added sugar), 26 g pro*

KITCHEN TIP

Many grocery stores sell frozen pre-riced cauliflower, which can save you both time and cleanup. No need to thaw—you can cook it straight from frozen. Bump up the heat to medium-high and sauté for 5 to 7 minutes to keep it from getting soggy.

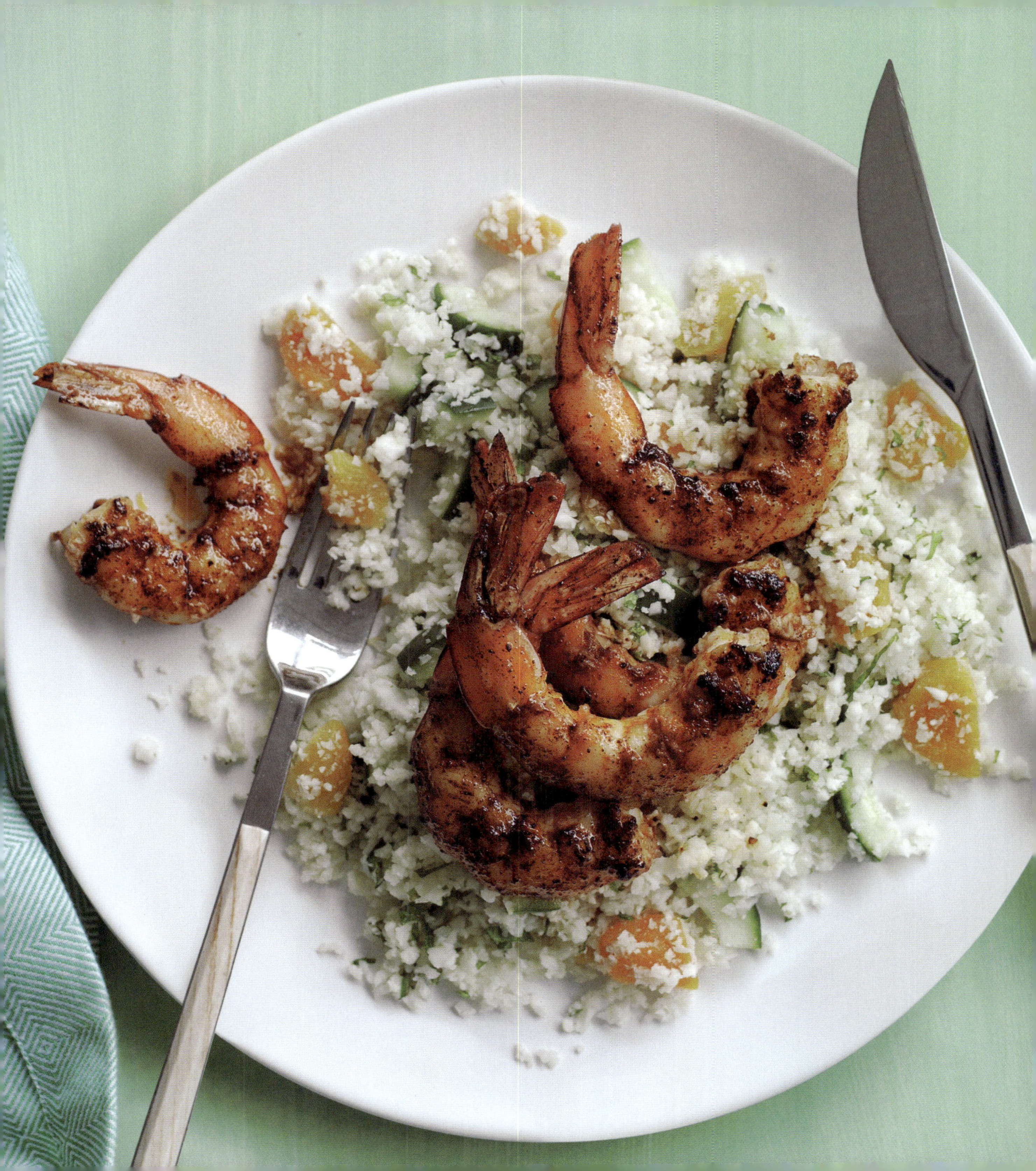

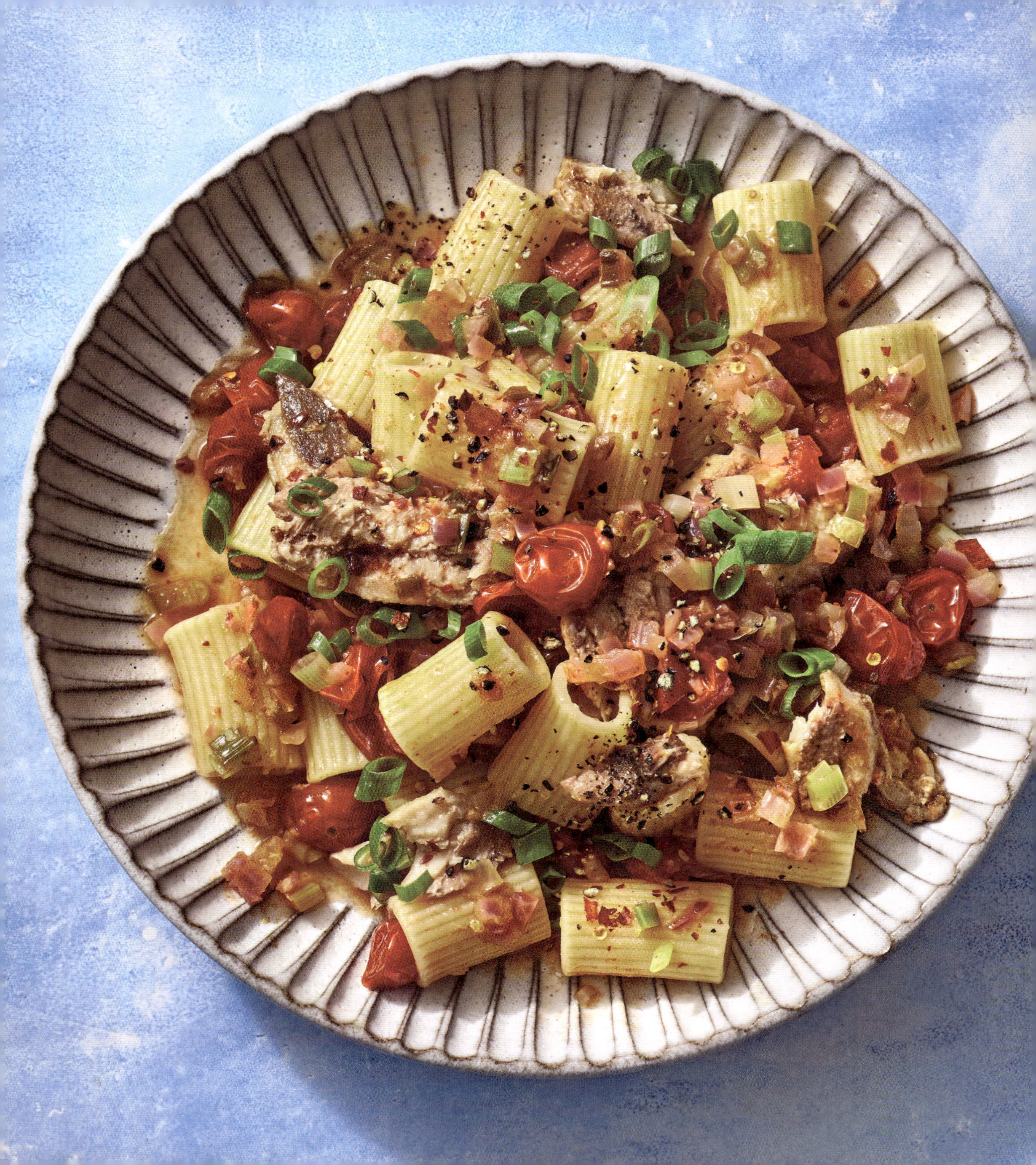

SARDINE PASTA *with* BURST TOMATOES

ACTIVE 30 min. **TOTAL** 30 min. **SERVES** 4

8 oz mezzi rigatoni

1 tsp lemon zest plus 2 Tbsp lemon juice

1 Tbsp olive oil

1 medium red onion, chopped

Kosher salt and pepper

2 cloves garlic, finely chopped

¼ tsp red pepper flakes

1 pint grape tomatoes, halved

1 bunch scallions, trimmed and thinly sliced, dark greens separated

2 4.25- to 4.5-oz cans skinless, boneless sardines packed in olive oil, drained

1. Cook pasta per package directions. Reserve 1 cup pasta cooking water; drain pasta and return to the pot. Add lemon juice and toss to combine.
2. While pasta cooks, heat oil in a large skillet on medium. Add onion and ¼ teaspoon each salt and pepper and cook, covered, stirring occasionally, 8 minutes. Stir in garlic and red pepper flakes and cook, stirring, 1 minute.
3. Add tomatoes and scallions, reserving ¼ cup dark scallion greens for topping, and cook, stirring occasionally, until onion and scallions are tender and tomatoes begin to break down, 8 to 10 minutes.
4. Add pasta to the skillet along with lemon zest and ¼ cup reserved pasta cooking water and toss to combine, adding more cooking water if pasta seems dry. Remove from heat and gently fold in sardines. Serve topped with reserved scallion greens and cracked black pepper if desired.

PER SERVING *About 410 cal, 13.5 g fat (4 g sat), 24 mg chol, 322 mg sodium, 54 g carb, 5 g fiber, 5 g sugar (0 g added sugar), 23 g pro*

KITCHEN TIP

Sardines are rich in heart healthy omega-3s, protein, calcium, and vitamin D—great for heart, bone, and brain health. Olive oil-packed varieties have richer flavor and a smoother texture than those in water. Use the oil for extra flavor in dressings or sautés.

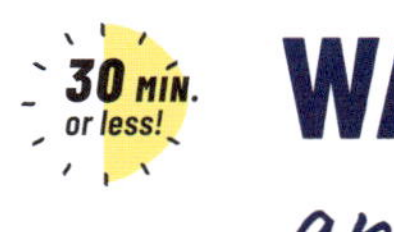

WARM LEMONY SALMON *and* BROWN RICE BOWLS

ACTIVE 25 min. **TOTAL** 25 min. **SERVES** 4

- 1 cup short-grain brown rice
- 4 cups baby spinach
- 3 6-oz cans boneless, skinless sockeye salmon in water
- ⅓ cup olive oil
- 5 cloves garlic, finely chopped
- 4 large pepperoncini, roughly chopped, plus 2 Tbsp pickling liquid
- 1 cup flat-leaf parsley leaves, chopped, plus more for serving
- 2 tsp lemon zest plus ¼ cup lemon juice
- Pepper

1. Cook rice per package directions. Fluff rice with fork and fold in spinach to wilt.
2. Meanwhile, drain salmon, reserving 2 tablespoons liquid. Break salmon into bite-size pieces. Heat oil in a large skillet on medium-low. Add garlic and cook, stirring, until fragrant and very pale golden, 1 to 2 minutes, adjusting heat if necessary.
3. Reduce heat to low and add pepperoncini and pickling liquid, salmon, and reserved packing liquid, and heat gently, shaking the pan occasionally, until salmon is just barely warmed through, 1 to 2 minutes. Gently fold in parsley and lemon zest and juice, keeping salmon intact as much as possible.
4. Divide rice mixture among plates and top with salmon mixture and any juices. Sprinkle with ¼ teaspoon coarsely ground pepper and scatter with additional parsley.

PER SERVING *About 497 cal, 25.5 g fat (4 g sat), 63 mg chol, 633 mg sodium, 41 g carb, 2 g fiber, 2 g sugar (0 g added sugar), 32 g pro*

KITCHEN TIP

Canned sockeye salmon is richer in flavor and color and higher in heart-healthy omega-3s and vitamin D than other varieties. For a more budget-friendly pick, sub in milder canned pink salmon.

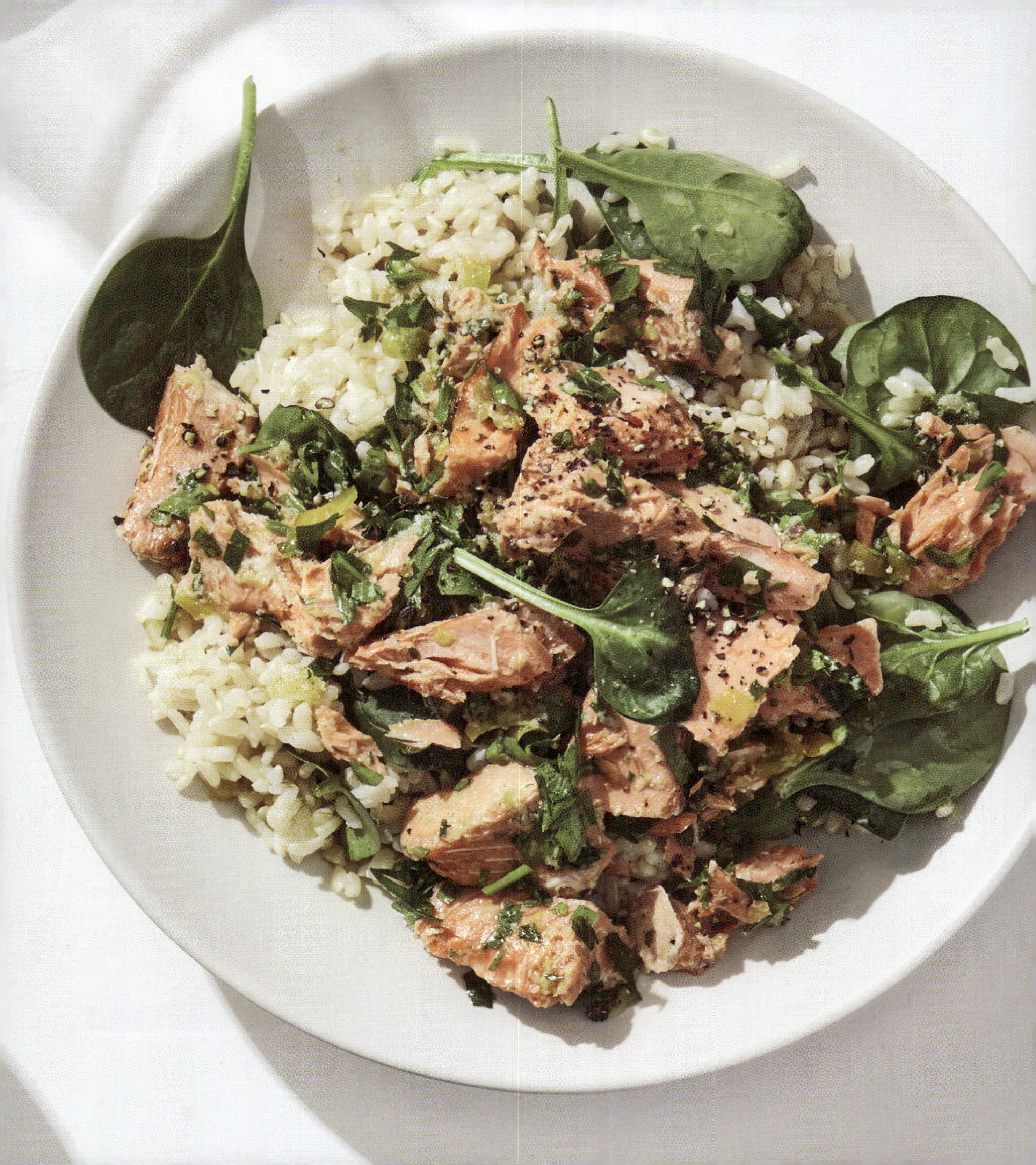

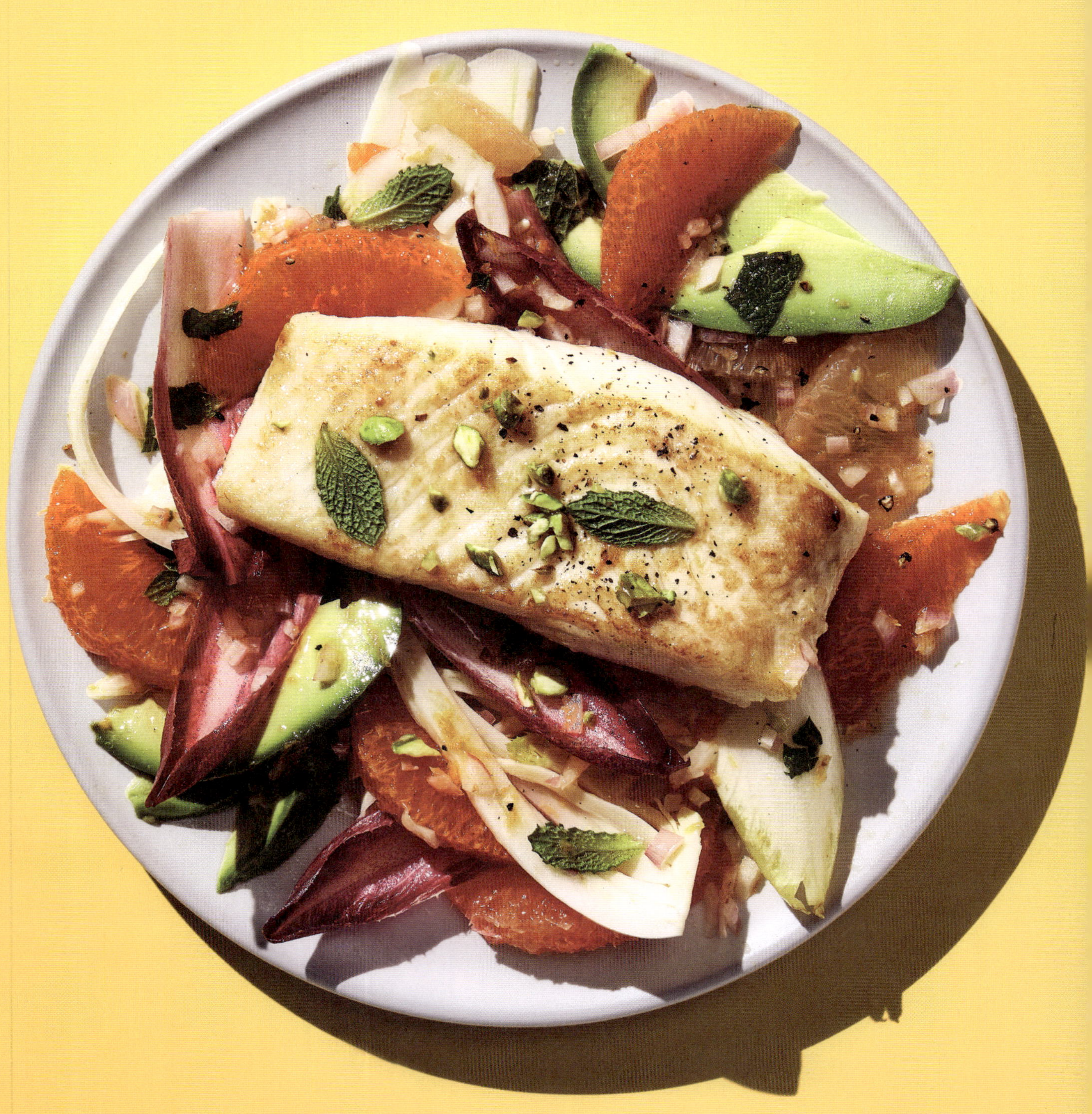

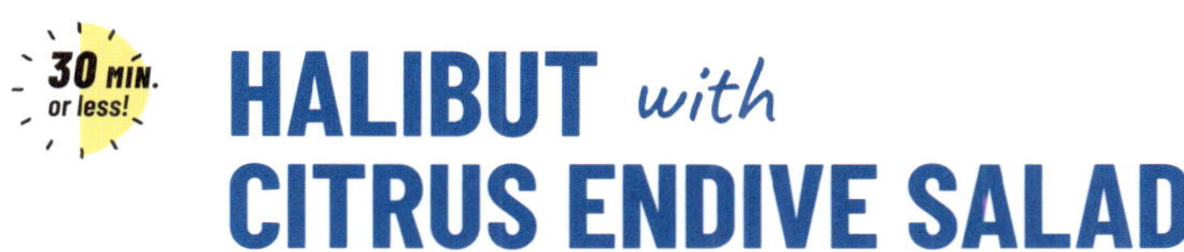

HALIBUT *with* CITRUS ENDIVE SALAD

ACTIVE 30 min. **TOTAL** 30 min. **SERVES** 4

- 1 medium grapefruit
- 1 Cara Cara orange
- 3 Tbsp white wine vinegar
- 2½ Tbsp olive oil, divided
- ½ tsp honey
- Kosher salt and pepper
- 2 medium shallots, finely chopped
- 4 5-oz skinless fillets halibut
- 3 small heads endive (combo of red and green), leaves separated
- 1 head fennel, cored and very thinly sliced
- ⅓ cup mint leaves, roughly chopped, plus whole mint leaves for serving
- 1 small avocado, sliced
- ¼ cup shelled, roasted pistachios, chopped

1. Grate 2 teaspoons zest from grapefruit into a large bowl. Cut tops and bottoms off grapefruit and orange, cut peel and pith away, then cut segments from between membranes and transfer to plate. Squeeze 1½ tablespoons juice from remaining membranes into bowl with zest; add vinegar, 1½ tablespoons oil, honey, and ½ teaspoon each salt and pepper and whisk to combine; stir in shallots and let sit 5 minutes.

2. Meanwhile, heat remaining 1 tablespoon oil in a large nonstick skillet on medium. Season fish with ¼ teaspoon each salt and pepper and cook, undisturbed, until golden brown on bottom, about 3 minutes. Flip and cook until opaque throughout, about 2 minutes more.

3. Add endive, fennel, and mint to shallot mixture and toss to combine. Gently fold in grapefruit and orange segments along with avocado. Serve with fish, topped with pistachios and additional mint leaves if desired.

PER SERVING *About 454 cal, 20.5 g fat (3 g sat), 77 mg chol, 566 mg sodium, 36 g carb, 17 g fiber, 15 g sugar (0.5 g added sugar), 37 g pro*

KITCHEN TIP
Cara Cara oranges are sweet, pink-fleshed navel oranges. Can't find any? Sub in a regular navel orange or a blood orange.

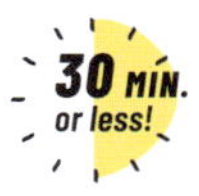

SHRIMP BOWLS with SCALLION VINAIGRETTE

ACTIVE 30 min. **TOTAL** 30 min. **SERVES** 4

1½ cups quinoa

1 lb broccoli, cut into small florets and stems cut into thin pieces

2 Tbsp olive oil, divided

Kosher salt and pepper

20 large peeled and deveined shrimp, tails removed

1 Tbsp rice vinegar

1 Tbsp finely grated fresh ginger

8 oz plum tomatoes, seeds removed and cut into ⅛-in. pieces

2 scallions, thinly sliced

1 avocado, cut into small pieces

1. Heat oven to 425°F. Heat a medium saucepan over medium, add quinoa, and cook, shaking pan occasionally, until lightly toasted, 5 minutes. Add 3 cups water and immediately cover (it will sputter). Simmer gently for 10 minutes. Remove from heat, remove lid, cover with a clean towel and let stand 10 minutes; fluff with a fork.

2. Meanwhile, on a rimmed baking sheet, toss broccoli with 1 tablespoon oil and ¼ teaspoon each salt and pepper. Spread in an even layer and roast 15 minutes. Season shrimp with a pinch each salt and pepper, toss with broccoli, and roast until opaque throughout, 6 to 8 minutes.

3. In a medium bowl, whisk together vinegar, ginger, and remaining tablespoon oil. Toss with tomatoes, then fold in scallions. Divide quinoa among 4 bowls, then top with shrimp, broccoli, and avocado. Spoon tomato-scallion vinaigrette over top.

PER SERVING *About 462 cal, 19 g fat (2.5 g sat), 58 mg chol, 458 mg sodium, 57 g carb, 12 g fiber, 6 g sugar (0 g added sugar), 20 g pro*

PROTEIN POWER

Quinoa might be small, but it's mighty. The tiny grain is one of the few plant-based foods that's a complete protein, packing all nine essential amino acids in one fluffy bite. Cook it in bone broth for a boost of protein and flavor.

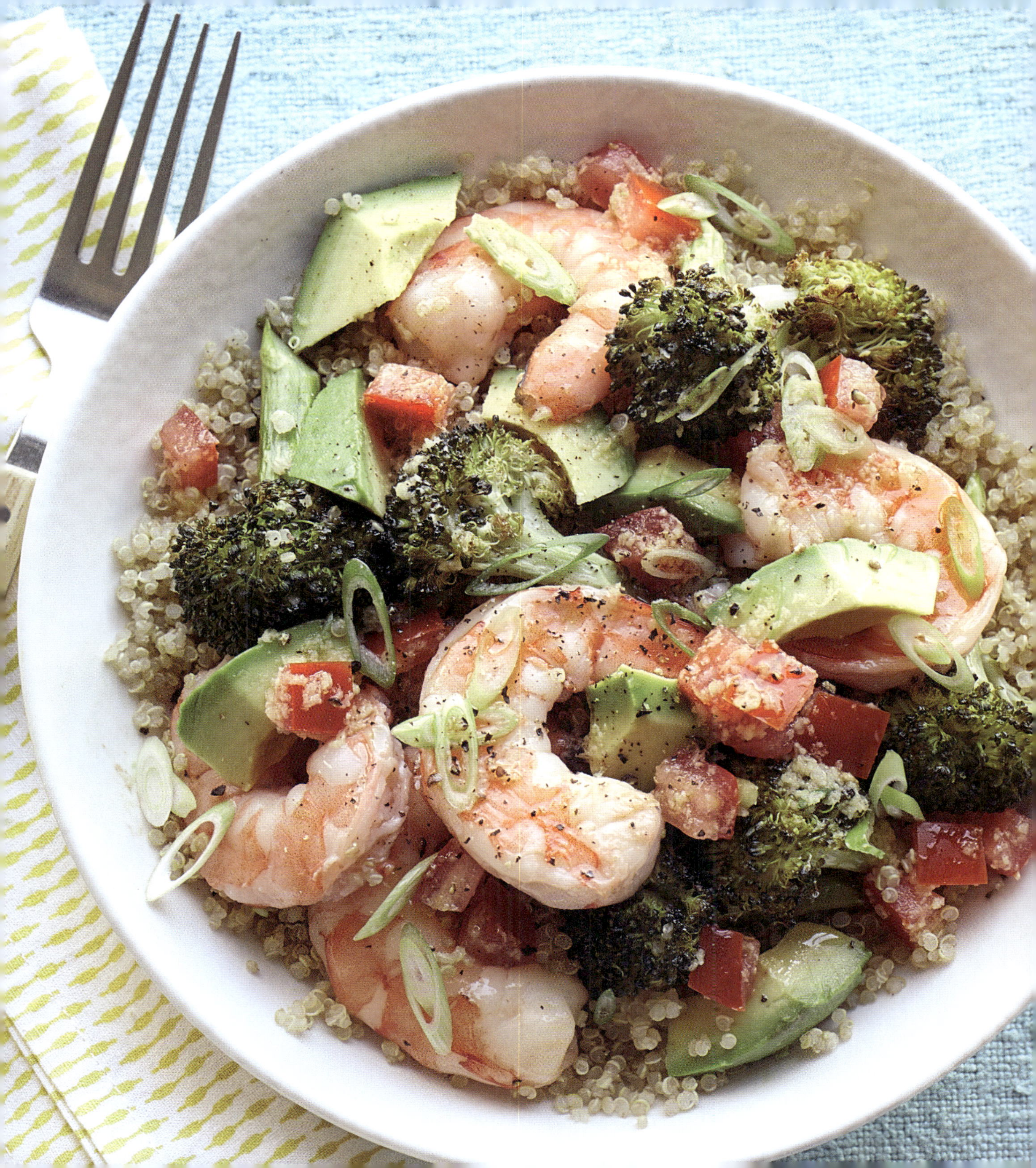

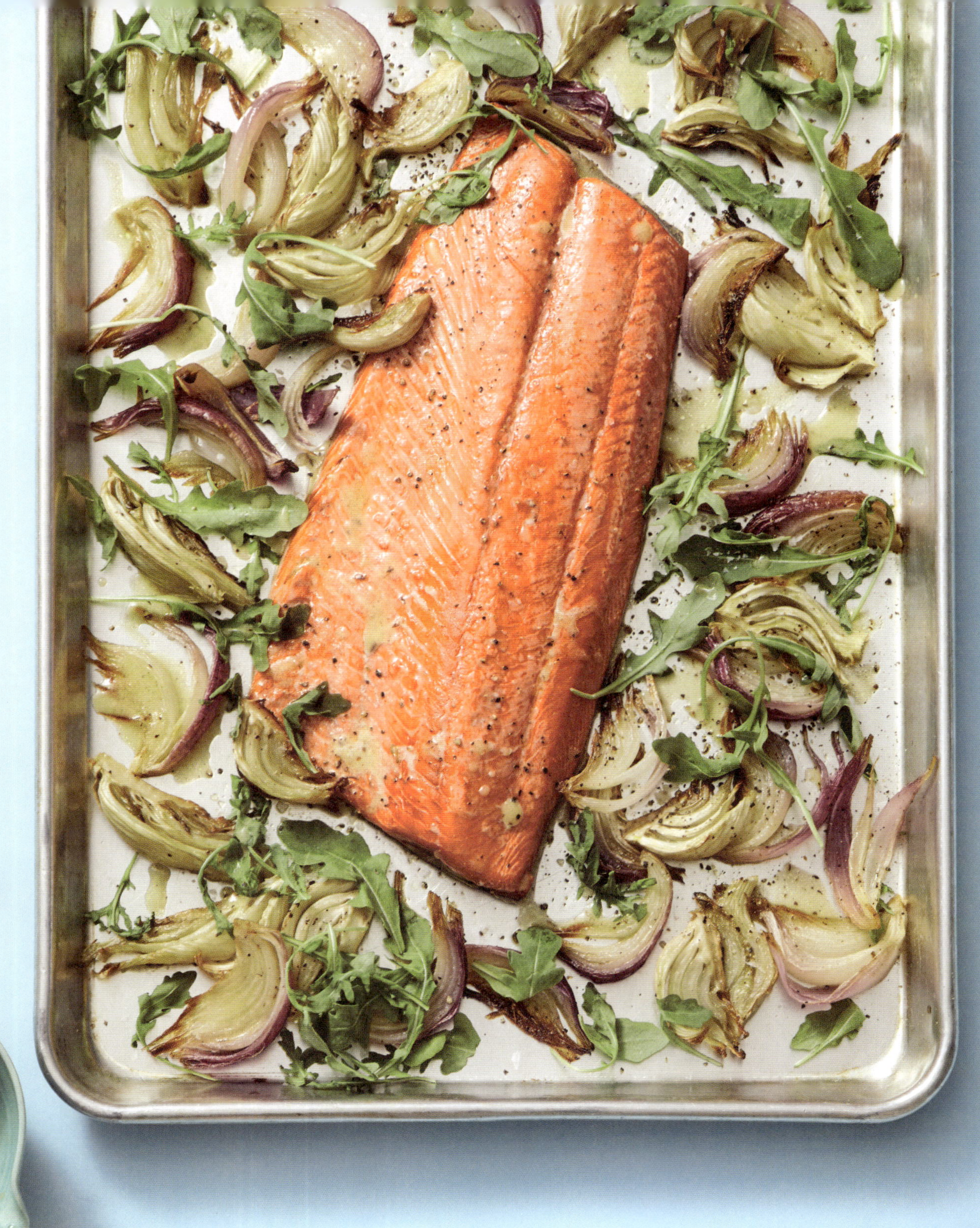

ROASTED SALMON *with* CHARRED LEMON VINAIGRETTE

ACTIVE 20 min. **TOTAL** 35 min. **SERVES** 4

- 1 lemon
- 2 bulb fennel, thinly sliced
- 2 small red onions, thinly sliced
- 2½ Tbsp olive oil, divided
- Kosher salt and pepper
- 1¼ lb skin-on salmon fillet
- 1 tsp stone-ground mustard
- 3 cups baby arugula

1. Heat broiler. Cut pointed ends off lemon, halve crosswise and place on a rimmed baking sheet, center cut sides up. Broil on top rack until charred, 5 minutes; transfer to a plate and set aside.
2. Reduce oven temperature to 400°F. On a rimmed baking sheet, toss fennel and onions with 1½ tablespoons oil and ¼ teaspoon each salt and pepper; arrange around edges of pan. Place salmon in center of pan and season with ¼ teaspoon each salt and pepper. Roast until vegetables are tender and salmon is opaque throughout, 17 to 20 minutes.
3. Juice charred lemon halves into a small bowl and whisk in mustard and remaining tablespoon oil. Remove baking sheet from oven and fold arugula into vegetables. Drizzle charred lemon vinaigrette over fish and vegetables and gently toss vegetables.

PER SERVING *About 305 cal, 13.9 g fat (2.5 g sat), 66 mg chol, 401 mg sodium, 14 g carb, 4.5 g fiber, 7 g sugar (0 g added sugar), 31 g pro*

LOVE YOUR LEFTOVERS

Refrigerate salmon and vegetables in separate airtight containers for up to three days, then add to a platter alongside boiled potatoes, eggs, and green beans for a twist on salmon Niçoise.

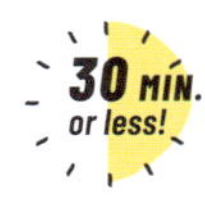

GRILLED HARISSA CHICKEN KEBABS *and* CHICKPEA SALAD

ACTIVE 20 min. **TOTAL** 20 min. **SERVES** 4

1 cup quick-cooking bulgur, cooked

¼ cup harissa pepper paste

2 Tbsp extra virgin olive oil

2 Tbsp honey

1¼ lb skinless, boneless chicken breasts, thinly sliced

15-oz can chickpeas, rinsed and drained

¾ cup finely chopped flat-leaf parsley

Kosher salt

1. Cook bulgur per package directions. Heat grill to medium-high.
2. In a large bowl, whisk together harissa pepper paste with oil and honey; transfer half to a small bowl and reserve for serving.
3. To remaining harissa mixture, add chicken breasts (cut into small pieces) and toss to coat, then thread onto skewers. Grill, turning once, until cooked through, 6 to 8 minutes.
4. Toss chickpeas with bulgur, flat-leaf parsley (finely chopped), and ½ teaspoon salt. Divide among plates and top with chicken skewers. Serve drizzled with reserved oil and honey mixture.

PER SERVING *About 497 cal, 13 g fat (2 g sat), 78 mg chol, 559 mg sodium, 57 g carb, 12 g fiber, 12.5 g sugar (8.5 g added sugar), 39 g pro*

LOVE YOUR LEFTOVERS

Refrigerate extra chickpea salad and chicken (removed from skewers) in separate airtight containers for up to three days. Try tossing the leftover chickpea mixture with arugula and squeezing on lemon juice for an easy salad. The chicken can be used for salads, sandwiches, or grain bowls.

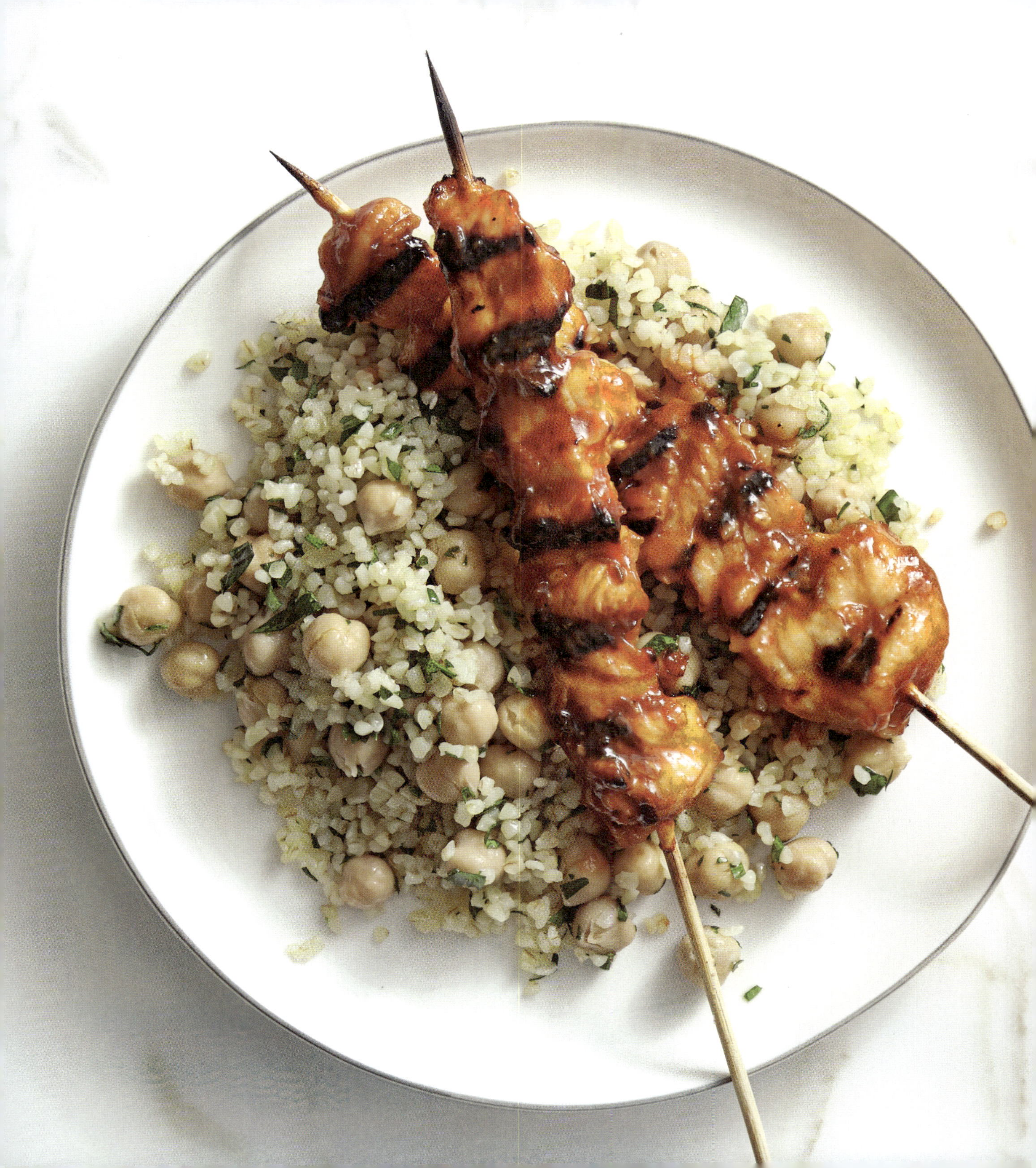

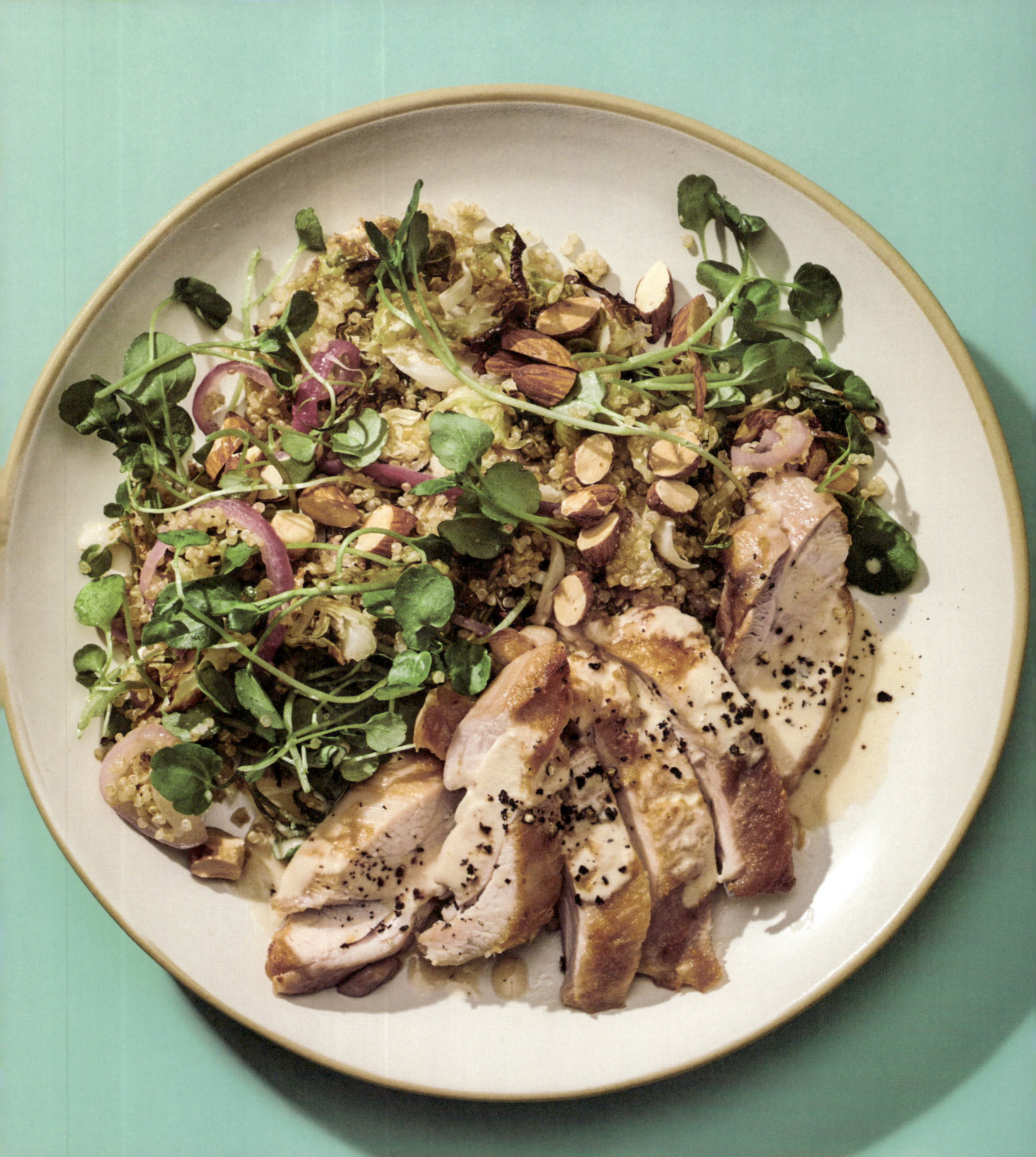

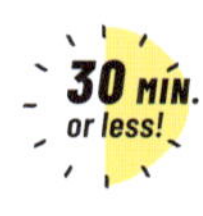

MUSTARDY CHICKEN *with* QUINOA-CRESS SALAD

ACTIVE 30 min. **TOTAL TIME** 30 min. **SERVES** 4

- 1 cup quinoa
- 8 oz Brussels sprouts, shaved (about 4 cups)
- 2 shallots, thinly sliced
- 4 Tbsp olive oil, divided
- Kosher salt and pepper
- 6 small boneless, skinless chicken thighs (about 1½ lb), trimmed
- 1½ Tbsp fresh lemon juice
- ¾ oz watercress (about 2 cups)
- ½ cup raw almonds, toasted and roughly chopped
- 3 Tbsp Dijon mustard
- 3 Tbsp whole-milk Greek yogurt

1. Heat oven to 450°F. Bring 1½ cups water to a boil in a medium saucepan. Stir in quinoa and return to a boil, then reduce heat and simmer, covered, 12 minutes. Remove from heat and let sit, covered, 5 minutes more. Fluff quinoa with a fork, transfer to a large bowl, and let cool.
2. While quinoa cooks, on a large rimmed baking sheet, toss Brussels sprouts and shallots with 2 tablespoons oil and ¼ teaspoon salt. Arrange in even layer and roast, stirring after 5 minutes, until tender and beginning to brown, 8 to 10 minutes total.
3. Heat 1 tablespoon oil in a large skillet over medium-high heat. Season chicken with ¼ teaspoon each salt and pepper and cook 6 minutes. Flip, reduce heat to medium, and cook until golden brown and just cooked through, 5 to 7 minutes more. Transfer to a cutting board and let rest 5 minutes before slicing (reserve skillet).
4. Add Brussels sprouts, lemon juice, and remaining 1 tablespoon oil to quinoa and toss to combine. Fold in watercress and almonds.
5. Return the skillet to medium heat, add mustard and ½ cup water, and cook, whisking often, until simmering, about 30 seconds. Remove from heat and whisk in yogurt and ¼ teaspoon pepper. Spoon sauce over chicken and serve with quinoa salad.

PER SERVING *About 633 cal, 32 g fat (5 g sat), 161 mg chol, 691 mg sodium, 40 g carb, 6 g fiber, 5 g sugar (0 g added sugar), 47 g pro*

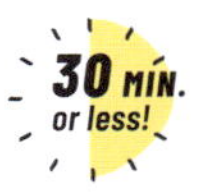

GREEK CHICKEN and FARRO SALAD

ACTIVE 20 min. **TOTAL** 20 min. **SERVES** 4

6 oz 10-minute farro (about 1¼ cups)

2 Tbsp olive oil, divided

½ small red onion, thinly sliced

4 Tbsp fresh lemon juice (from 1 juicy lemon)

Kosher salt and pepper

12 oz boneless skinless chicken breasts, sliced ½ in. thick

¼ cup fresh dill, chopped

8 oz grape tomatoes, halved

½ seedless cucumber, cut into ½-in. pieces

3 oz baby arugula (about 3 cups)

1 small avocado, diced

3 oz feta, crumbled

1. Bring a pot of water to a boil and cook farro according to package directions; drain, transfer to a large bowl and toss with 1 tablespoon oil.
2. Meanwhile, make pickled onions. In a small bowl, toss onion with 2 tablespoons lemon juice and a pinch of salt. Let sit, tossing twice, for at least 10 minutes.
3. Heat remaining 1 tablespoon oil in a large skillet over medium-high heat. Season chicken with ¼ teaspoon each salt and pepper and cook until golden brown and cooked through, 8 to 10 minutes.
4. Remove the pan from heat and add remaining 2 tablespoons lemon juice, scraping up any brown bits from the bottom of the pan.
5. Add chicken and any juices to farro along with dill, tomatoes, cucumber, and onions (and their juices) and toss to combine. Fold in the arugula, avocado, and feta.

PER SERVING *About 446 cal, 19 g fat (5 g sat), 68 mg chol, 414 mg sodium, 41 g carb, 9 g fiber, 4 g sugar (0 g added sugar), 30 g pro*

MAKE IT AHEAD

Assemble the farro salad without the dill, arugula, and avocado and refrigerate for up to two days. Fold in the remaining ingredients just before serving for maximum freshness.

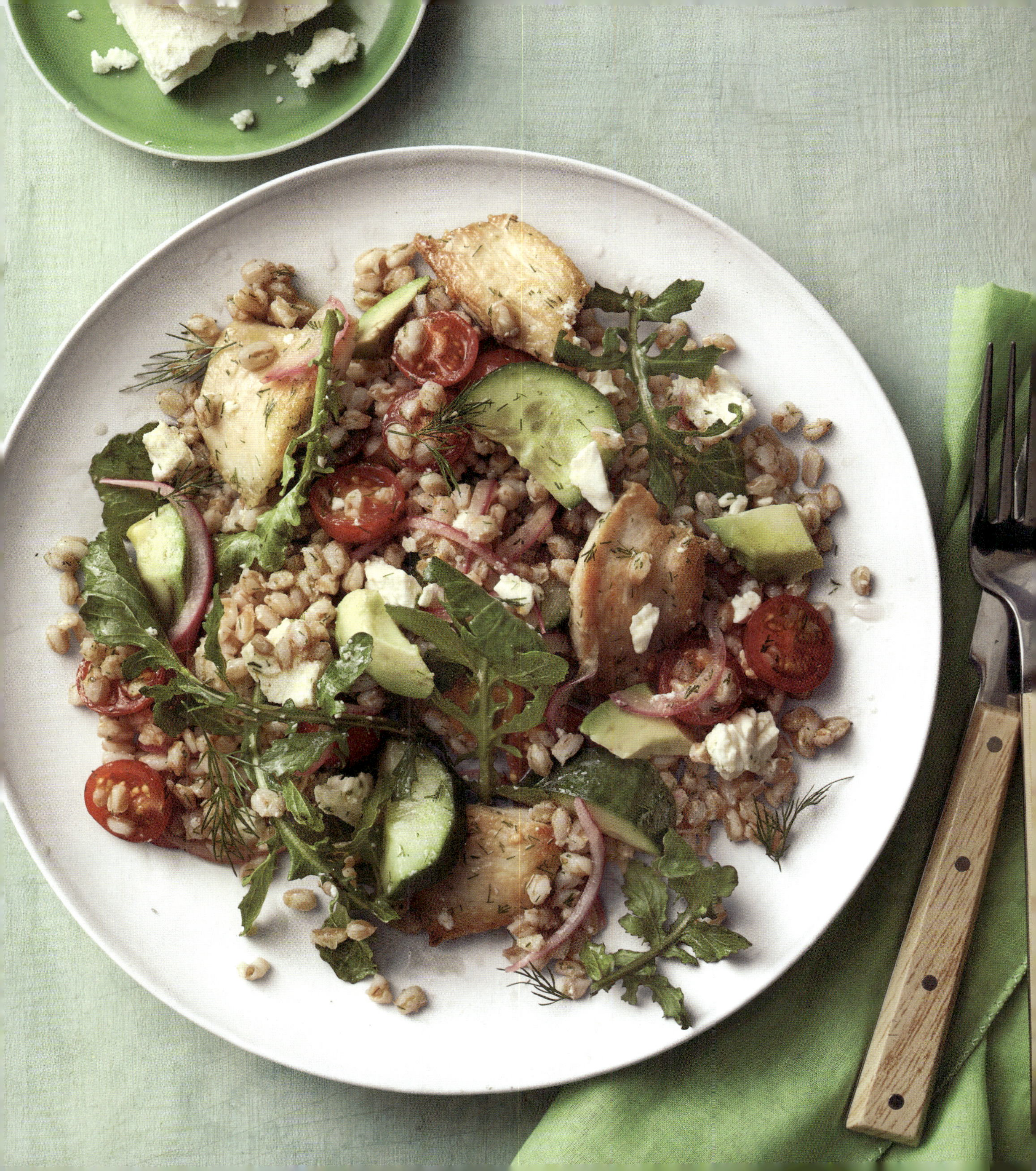

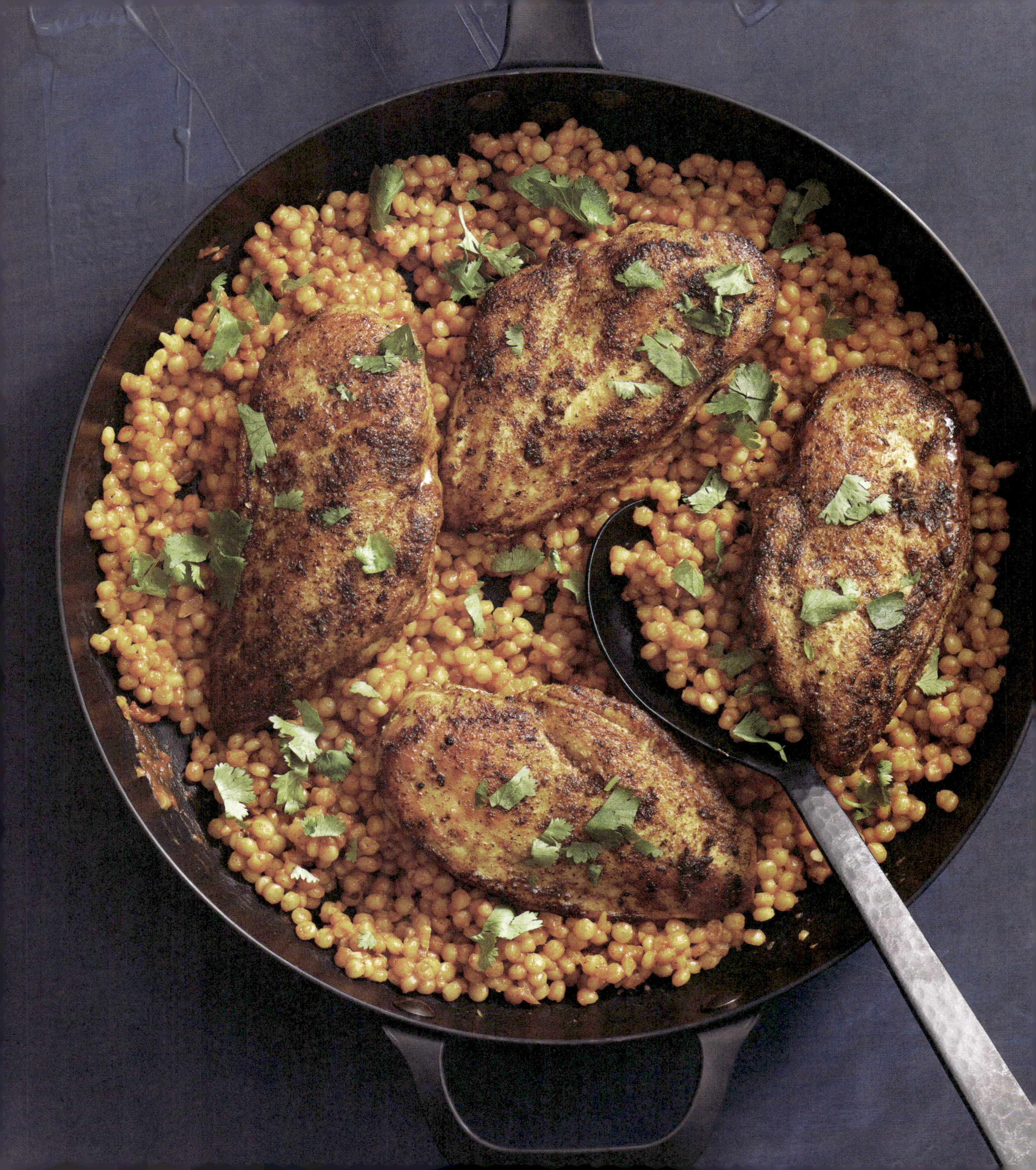

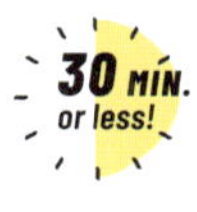

MOROCCAN-SPICED SKILLET CHICKEN

ACTIVE 30 min. **TOTAL** 30 min. **SERVES** 4

4 6-oz boneless, skinless chicken breasts

3 Tbsp olive oil, divided

1 Tbsp ras el hanout (see Tip)

Kosher salt and pepper

2 large cloves garlic, finely chopped

Rind from ¼ preserved lemon, pulp scraped and discarded, finely chopped (2 Tbsp)

2 Tbsp tomato paste

½ tsp smoked paprika

1 cup quick-cooking pearl couscous

1½ tsp chicken bouillon base, whisked into 1½ cups water

½ cup cilantro, chopped

1. Place chicken in a large bowl and toss with 1 tablespoon oil, then ras el hanout and ¼ teaspoon each salt and pepper to coat.
2. Heat 1 tablespoon oil in a large deep skillet or Dutch oven on medium. Add chicken and cook, undisturbed, until golden brown,7 to 8 minutes. Flip and cook until other side is golden brown, 2 to 3 minutes; transfer to plate (chicken will finish cooking later).
3. Add remaining tablespoon oil to the skillet along with garlic and preserved lemon rind; cook, stirring constantly, 15 to 30 seconds. Add tomato paste and smoked paprika; cook, stirring constantly, 1 minute.
4. Add couscous and stir to coat. Stir in bouillon mixture and bring to a boil. Nestle chicken, darker side up, in couscous and add any juices from plate. Cover, reduce heat, and simmer until couscous has absorbed most of liquid and chicken is cooked through, 14 to 15 minutes. Serve sprinkled with cilantro.

PER SERVING *About 476 cal, 15 g fat (2.5 g sat), 124 mg chol, 535 mg sodium, 38 g carb, 3 g fiber, 1.5 g sugar (0 g added sugar), 44 g pro*

KITCHEN TIP
Ras el hanout is a savory North African spice blend. Recipes can vary widely by region. If yours does not have cumin or cinnamon, add 1 teaspoon ground cumin and ¼ teaspoon cinnamon to the recipe when adding paprika.

FENNEL ROASTED CHICKEN & PEPPERS

ACTIVE 15 min. **TOTAL** 35 min. **SERVES** 4

1 Tbsp fennel seeds

1 Tbsp finely grated orange zest

3 bell peppers (red, yellow, and orange), cut into 1-in. chunks

6 cloves garlic, thinly sliced

2 Tbsp olive oil

Kosher salt and pepper

4 small chicken legs (about 2 lb)

4 cups baby spinach

2 oz feta cheese, crumbled

1. Heat oven to 425°F. In a small skillet, toast fennel seeds and orange zest until lightly browned and fragrant, 3 to 4 minutes. Transfer to spice grinder or blender and pulse to blend and grind. Set aside.
2. On a large rimmed baking sheet, toss bell peppers and garlic with 1 tablespoon oil and ½ teaspoon each salt and pepper. Rub chicken legs with remaining tablespoon oil, then with fennel-orange mixture. Nestle among vegetables on the baking sheet and roast until chicken is golden brown and cooked through and peppers are tender, 25 to 30 minutes.
3. Transfer chicken to plates, scatter spinach over peppers remaining on sheet, and toss until just beginning to wilt (pop back in oven, if necessary). Sprinkle with feta and serve with chicken.

PER SERVING *About 350 cal, 25 g fat (7 g sat), 167 mg chol, 350 mg sodium, 11 g carb, 3 g fiber, 2 g sugar (0 g added sugar), 25 g pro*

LOVE YOUR LEFTOVERS

Refrigerate chicken and vegetables in separate airtight containers for up to three days. Slice any leftover chicken and toss with the leftover vegetables in hot pasta or a grain bowl.

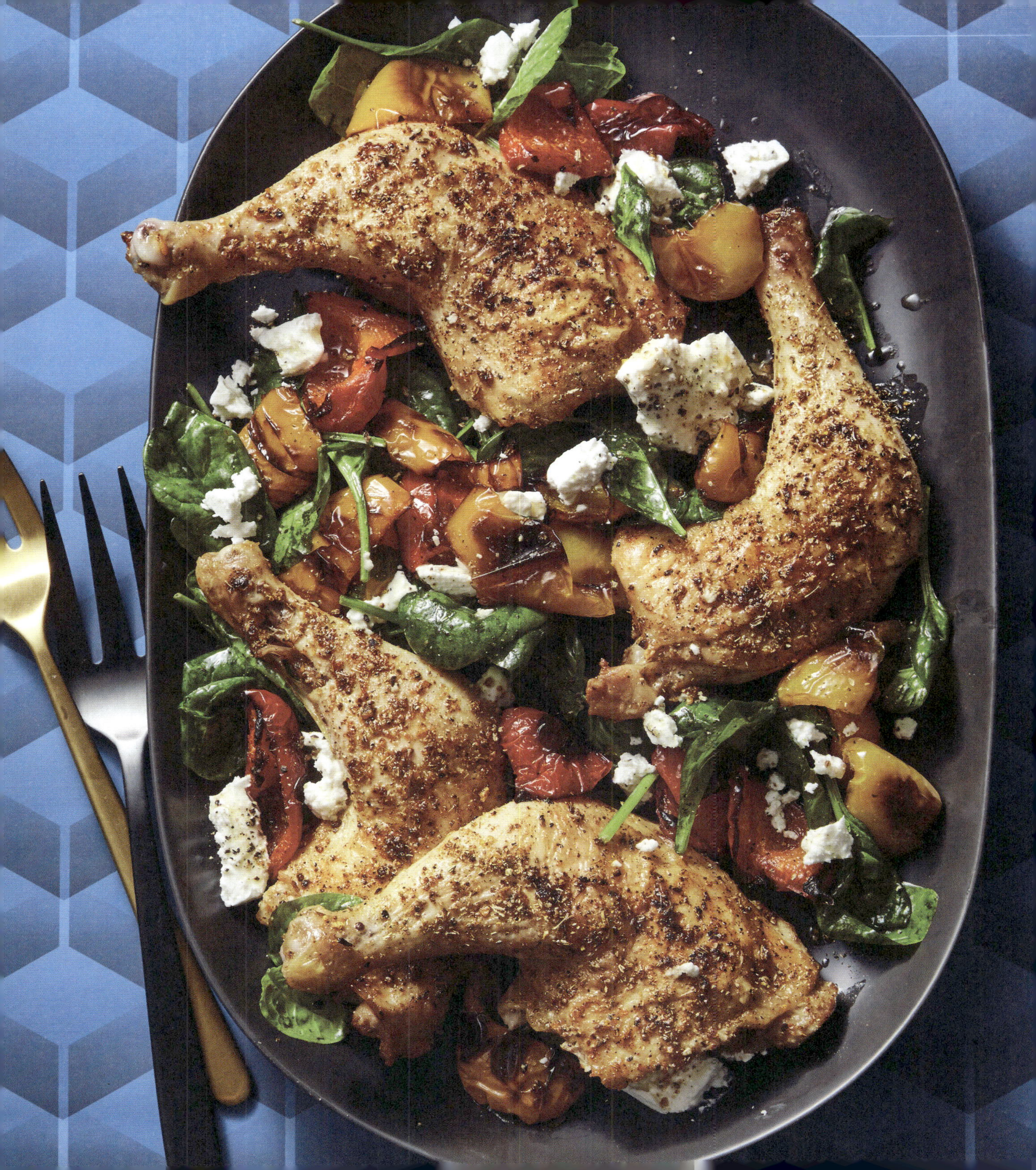

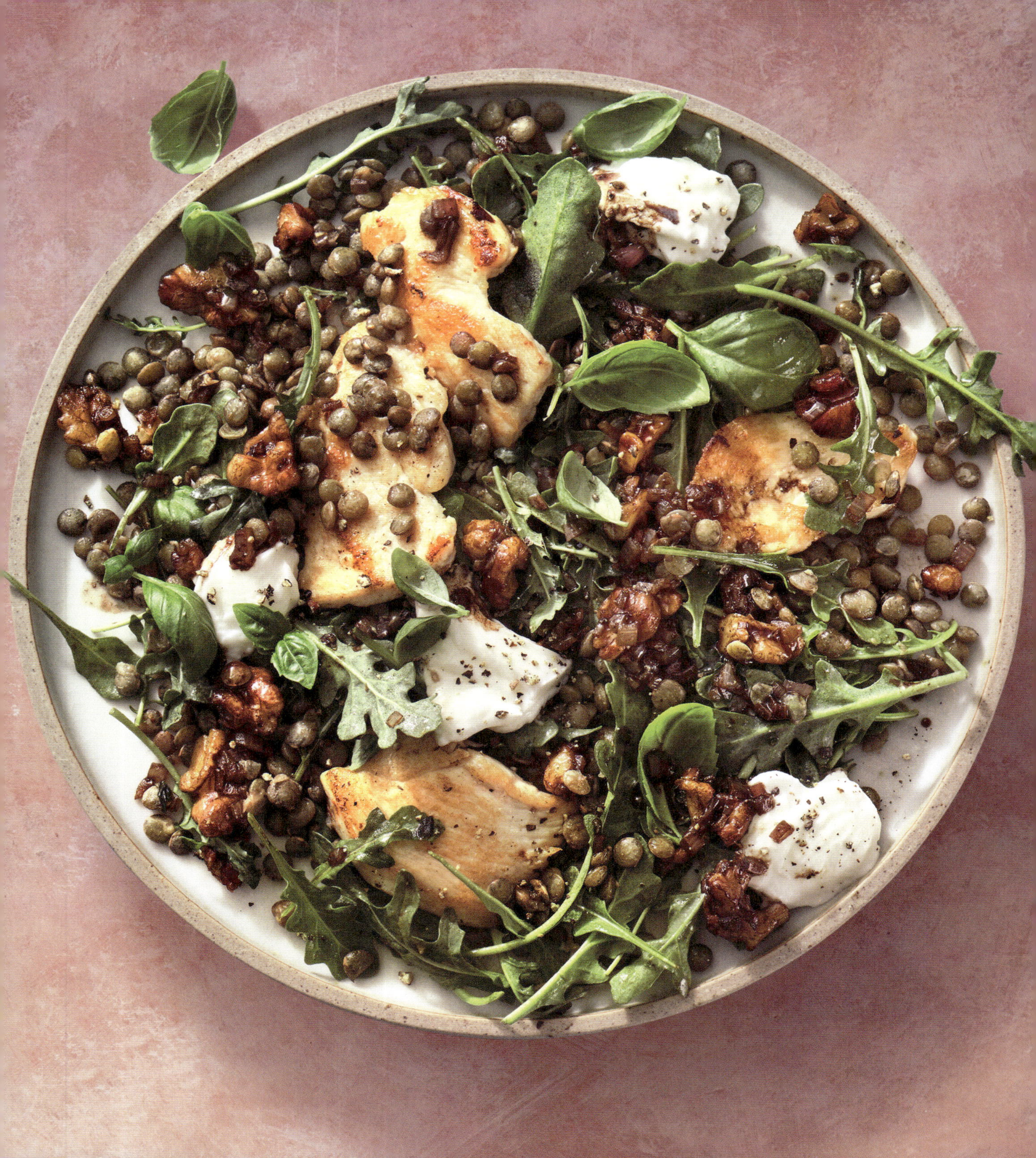

WARM LENTIL SALAD *with* CHICKEN *and* FRESH MOZZARELLA

ACTIVE 25 min. **TOTAL** 35 min. **SERVES** 4

1 cup French green lentils, rinsed and picked over

¼ cup plus 1 Tbsp olive oil, divided

1 lb boneless, skinless chicken breasts, sliced crosswise ¼ in. thick

Kosher salt and pepper

¼ cup raw walnut halves, chopped

1 clove garlic, smashed

2 thyme sprigs

1 medium shallot, finely chopped

2½ Tbsp balsamic vinegar

2 cups baby arugula

1 cup basil leaves, roughly chopped

4 oz small fresh mozzarella balls, torn

1. Cook lentils per package directions. Drain and rinse under cool water.
2. Meanwhile, heat 1 tablespoon oil in a large skillet over medium-high heat. Season chicken with ¼ teaspoon each salt and pepper; cook, turning occasionally, until golden brown all over, 3 to 4 minutes Transfer to plate.
3. Reduce heat to medium-low and add remaining ¼ cup oil (seeing brown bits in skillet is OK). Add walnuts, garlic, and thyme and cook, stirring occasionally, until nuts are fragrant and golden brown, 2 to 3 minutes. Add shallot and cook, stirring constantly, 2 to 3 minutes.
4. Remove from heat and discard garlic and thyme sprigs. Whisk in vinegar, ½ teaspoon salt, and ¼ teaspoon pepper. Fold in lentils, then arugula, basil, and chicken. Transfer to a platter and top with mozzarella.

PER SERVING *About 601 cal, 30.5 g fat (7.5 g sat), 106 mg chol, 438 mg sodium, 37 g carb, 8 g fiber, 4 g sugar (0 g added sugar), 44 g pro*

PROTEIN POWER

Lentils pull double duty—they're loaded with plant-based protein and fiber, making them a powerhouse for energy, satiety, and gut health all in one tiny package.

PAN-FRIED CHICKEN *with* LEMONY ROASTED BROCCOLI

ACTIVE 25 min. **TOTAL** 35 min. **SERVES** 4

- 1½ lb broccoli, cut into florets
- 2 cloves garlic, thinly sliced
- 3 Tbsp olive oil, divided
- Kosher salt and pepper
- 4 6-oz boneless, skinless chicken breasts
- 1 cup all-purpose flour
- 1 lemon, cut into ½-inch pieces
- 2 Tbsp lemon juice

1. Heat oven to 425°F. On a rimmed baking sheet, toss broccoli and garlic with 1 tablespoon oil and ¼ teaspoon each salt and pepper; roast 10 minutes.
2. Meanwhile, pound chicken breasts to even thickness, season with ¼ teaspoon each salt and pepper then coat in flour. Heat 1 tablespoon oil in a large skillet over medium-high heat and cook chicken until golden brown, 3 to 5 minutes per side. Nestle chicken amidst broccoli and roast until chicken is cooked through and broccoli is golden brown and tender, about 6 minutes.
3. Return the skillet to medium heat; add remaining tablespoon oil, then lemon pieces, and cook, stirring, until beginning to brown, 3 minutes. Add lemon juice and ⅓ cup water and cook, stirring and scraping up any browned bits. Spoon over chicken and serve with broccoli.

PER SERVING *About 367 cal, 15.5 g fat (2.5 g sat), 124 mg chol, 375 mg sodium, 15 g carb, 5 g fiber, 3.36 g sugar (0 g added sugar), 44 g pro*

LOVE YOUR LEFTOVERS

Refrigerate broccoli and chicken in separate airtight containers for up to three days. The broccoli is great on grain bowls, tossed in salads, or chopped as a relish to jazz up your favorite sandwich. You can slice and use leftover chicken on the same sandwich or use for another dish.

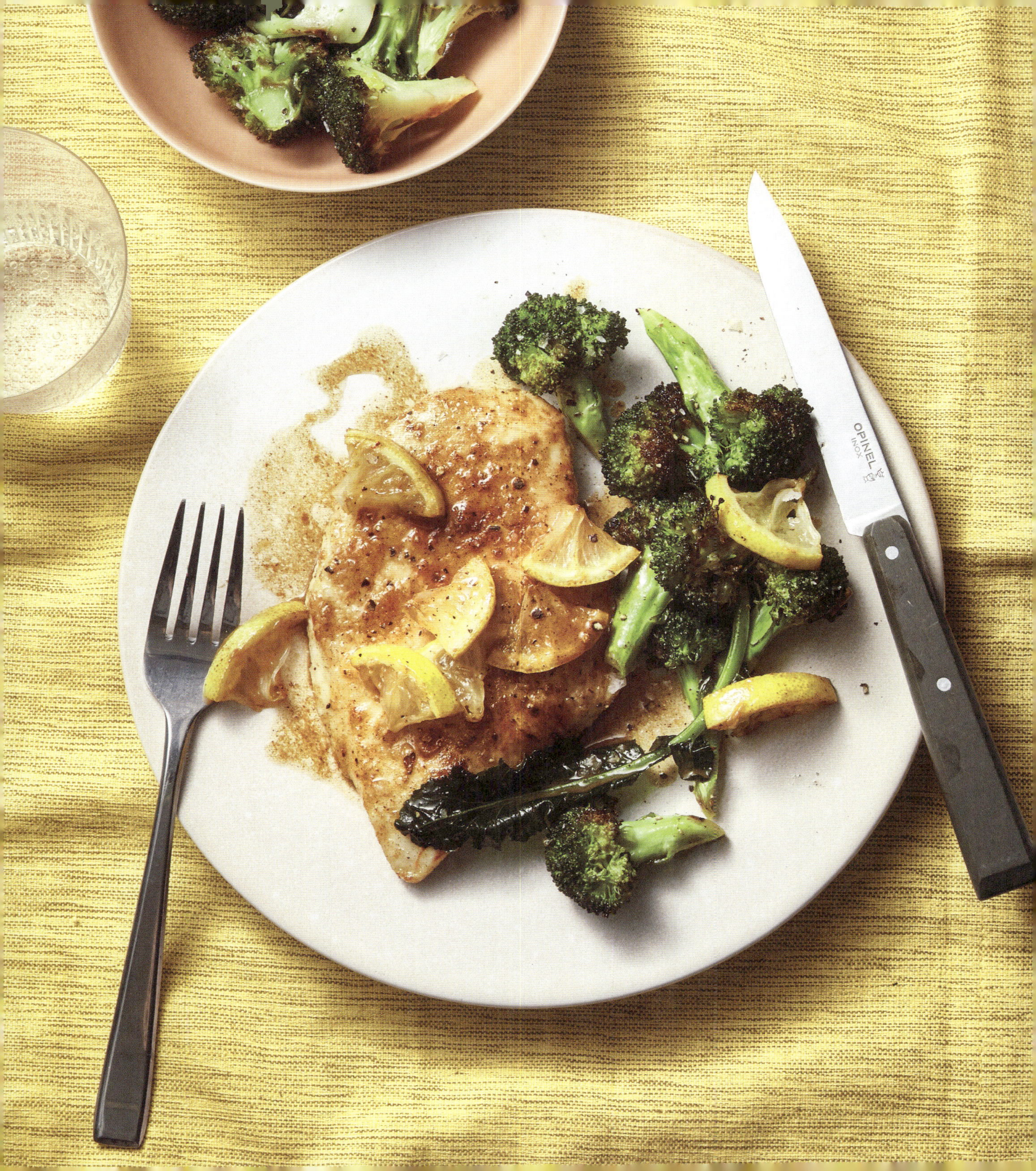
OPINEL
INOX

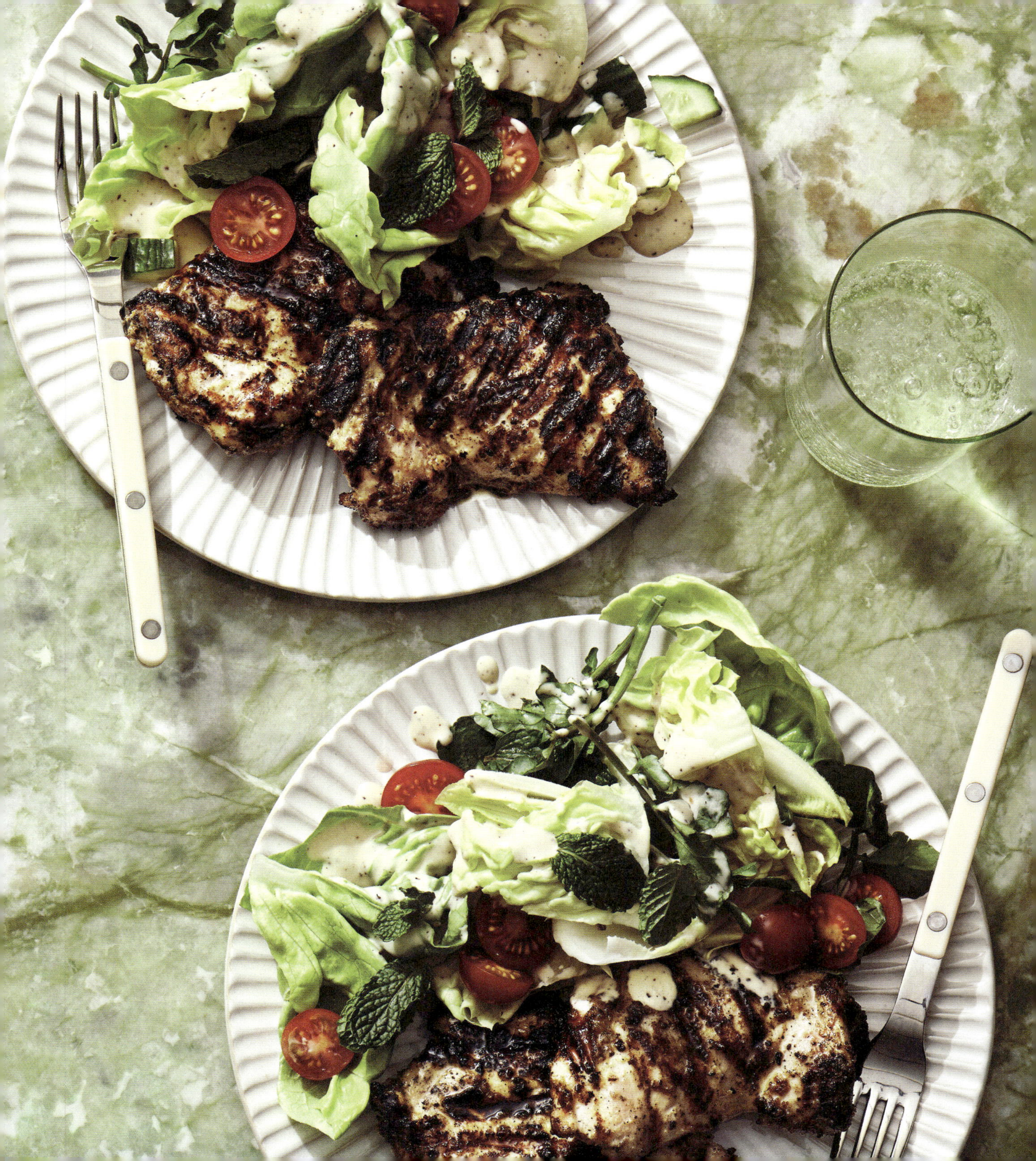

LEMON TAHINI-MARINATED CHICKEN

ACTIVE 15 min. **TOTAL** 25 min. (plus marinating) **SERVES** 4

1 cup tahini

2 tsp finely grated lemon zest plus 1½ Tbsp lemon juice

2 tsp honey

1 tsp sumac

2 cloves garlic, grated

Kosher salt and pepper

8 small boneless, skinless chicken thighs (about 2 lb)

1 Tbsp olive oil, divided, plus more for brushing grill

6 cups salad greens

2 Persian cucumbers, quartered and chopped

1 pint grape tomatoes, halved

¼ cup mint leaves, torn

1. In a large bowl, whisk tahini, lemon zest, honey, sumac, garlic, ½ teaspoon salt, and ¼ teaspoon pepper until smooth. Remove ¼ cup and set aside.
2. Add chicken to remaining tahini mixture and turn chicken to coat completely. Let marinate at least 1 hour or transfer to a resealable plastic bag and refrigerate overnight.
3. Heat the grill to medium and brush grates with oil. Grill chicken until instant-read thermometer registers 165°F, 7 to 8 minutes per side (discard marinade from bag).
4. Meanwhile, in a large bowl, whisk together reserved tahini mixture, lemon juice, 2 tablespoons water, and remaining 1 tablespoon oil.
5. Arrange salad greens, cucumbers, tomatoes, and chicken on a platter. Drizzle with tahini dressing and sprinkle with mint.

PER SERVING *About 625 cal, 40.5 g fat (7.5 g sat), 208 mg chol, 378 mg sodium, 24 g carb, 8 g fiber, 4.5 g sugar (1.5 g added sugar), 49 g pro*

KITCHEN TIP

Tahini is a creamy paste made from ground sesame seeds that's rich in healthy fats, plant-based protein, and minerals like calcium and iron—making it as nourishing as it is delicious.

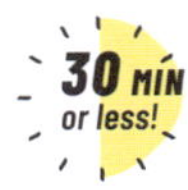

SHAWARMA-SPICED CHICKEN *with* CUCUMBER SALAD

ACTIVE 30 min. **TOTAL** 30 min. **SERVES** 4

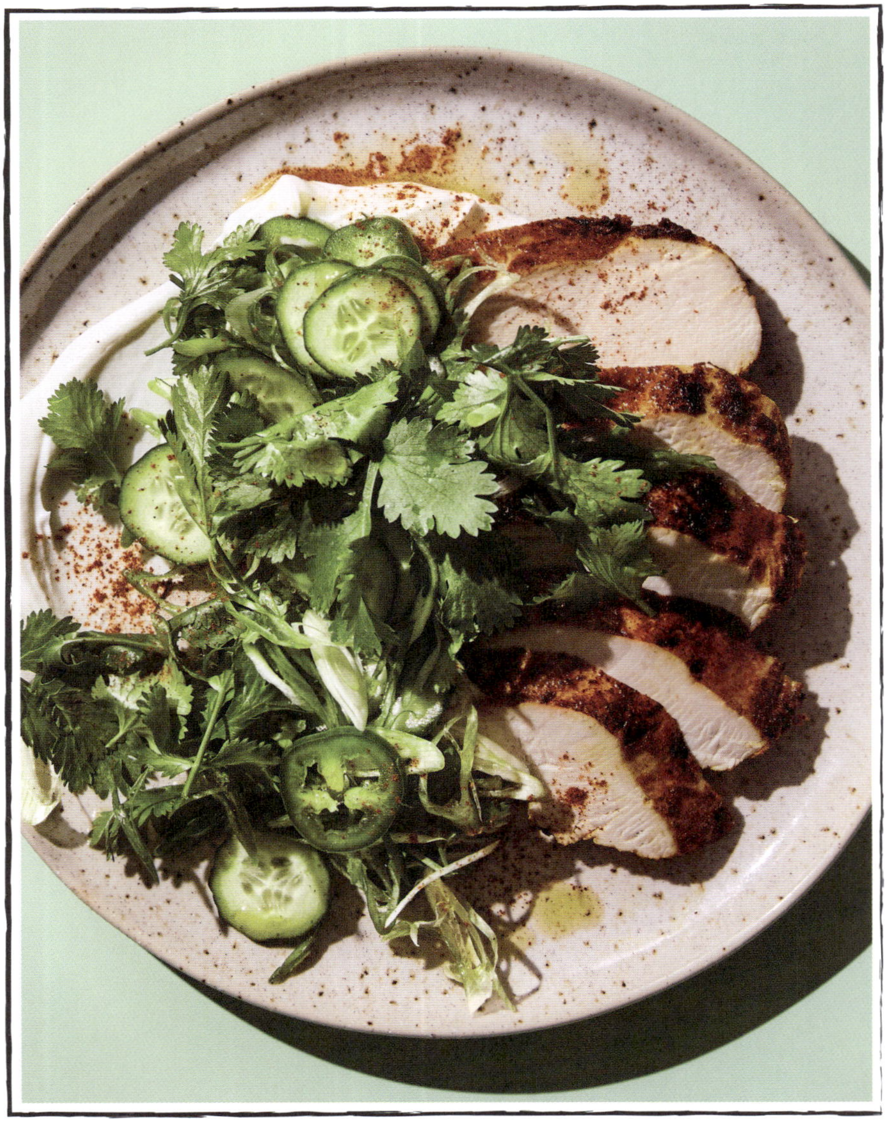

1. In a medium bowl, combine ½ cup plain **Greek yogurt** with 2 Tbsp fresh **lemon juice**, then 2 tablespoons **shawarma seasoning**, 1 large clove **garlic**, grated, and ½ teaspoon **kosher salt**. Add 4 6-ounce **boneless, skinless chicken breasts** and coat thoroughly. Let marinate 5 minutes.

2. Remove chicken from marinade, pat dry, and season with ¼ teaspoon salt. Heat 1 tablespoon **olive oil** in a large cast-iron skillet over medium heat and cook chicken, adjusting heat as needed to prevent burning, until deep golden brown and cooked through, 6 to 7 minutes per side. Transferto a cutting board and let rest at least 3 minutes before slicing.

3. Meanwhile, in another bowl, toss 2 **Persian cucumbers**, thinly sliced; 4 **scallions**, thinly sliced; 1 **jalapeño**, thinly sliced; and 1 cup **cilantro** leaves. Divide ¾ cup yogurt among plates. Top with chicken and salad. Drizzle with additional oil.

PER SERVING *About 276 cal, 10 g fat (3 g sat), 100 mg chol, 273 mg sodium, 6 g carb, 1 g fiber, 3 g sugar (0 g added sugar), 39 g pro*

30 MIN. or less!

OPEN-FACE CHICKEN & WHITE BEAN SALAD SANDWICHES

ACTIVE 20 min. **TOTAL** 20 min. **SERVES** 4

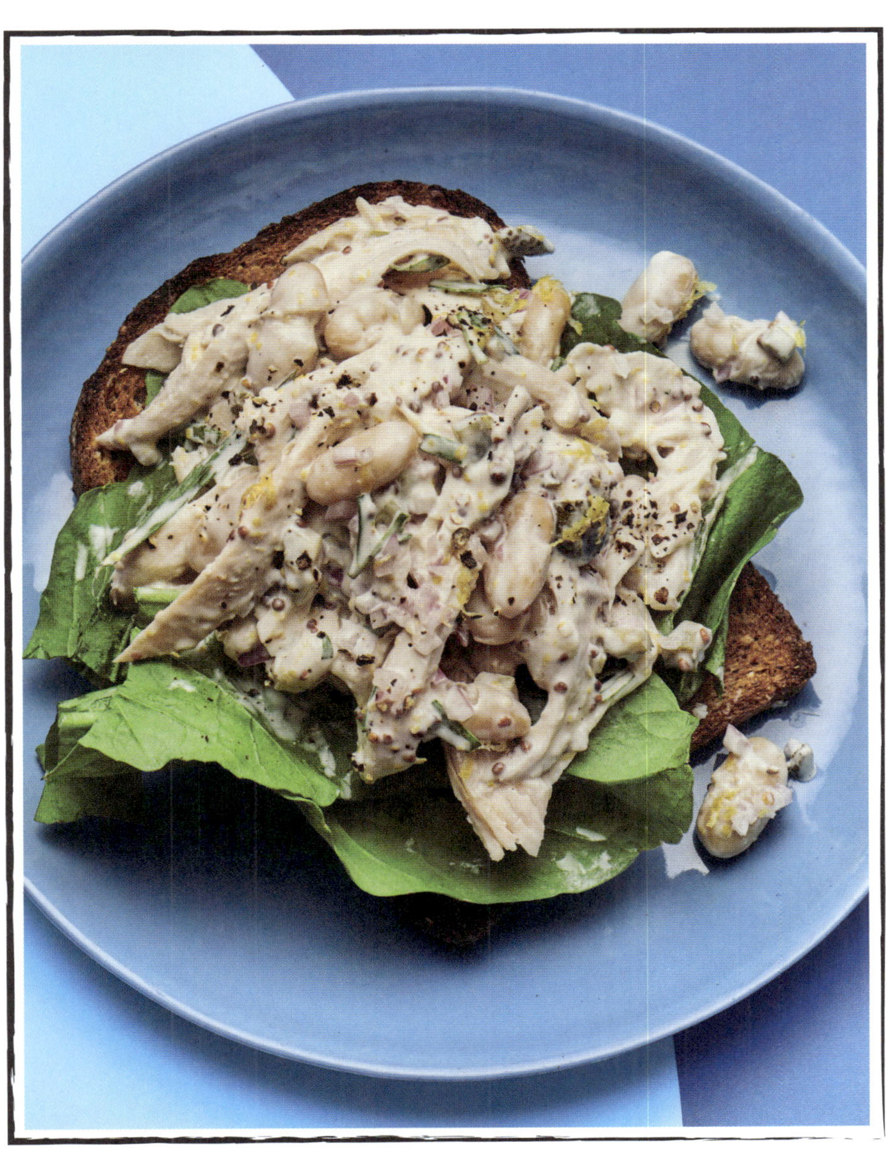

1. In a large bowl, stir together 2 tablespoons whole milk plain **Greek yogurt**, 2 tablespoons **mayonnaise**, 1 tablespoon country-style **Dijon mustard**, ½ teaspoon **lemon zest** and 1 tablespoon **lemon juice**, ¼ teaspoon **kosher salt**, and ½ teaspoon **pepper**; stir in 6 **cornichons** chopped (¼ cup), 2 tablespoons finely chopped **shallots**, and 2 tablespoons **tarragon,** chopped.

2. Fold in 1½- to 2-pounds **rotisserie chicken**, skin discarded, meat shredded (about 4 cups; 12 ounces) and 1 cup canned no-salt **cannellini beans**, rinsed. Divide 2 cups **arugula** among 4 slices **Ezekiel 4:9 bread**, toasted and top with chicken salad.

PER SERVING *About 347 cal, 20.5 g fat (5 g sat), 56 mg chol, 890 mg sodium, 28 g carb, 6 g fiber, 2 g sugar (0 g added sugar), 26 g pro*

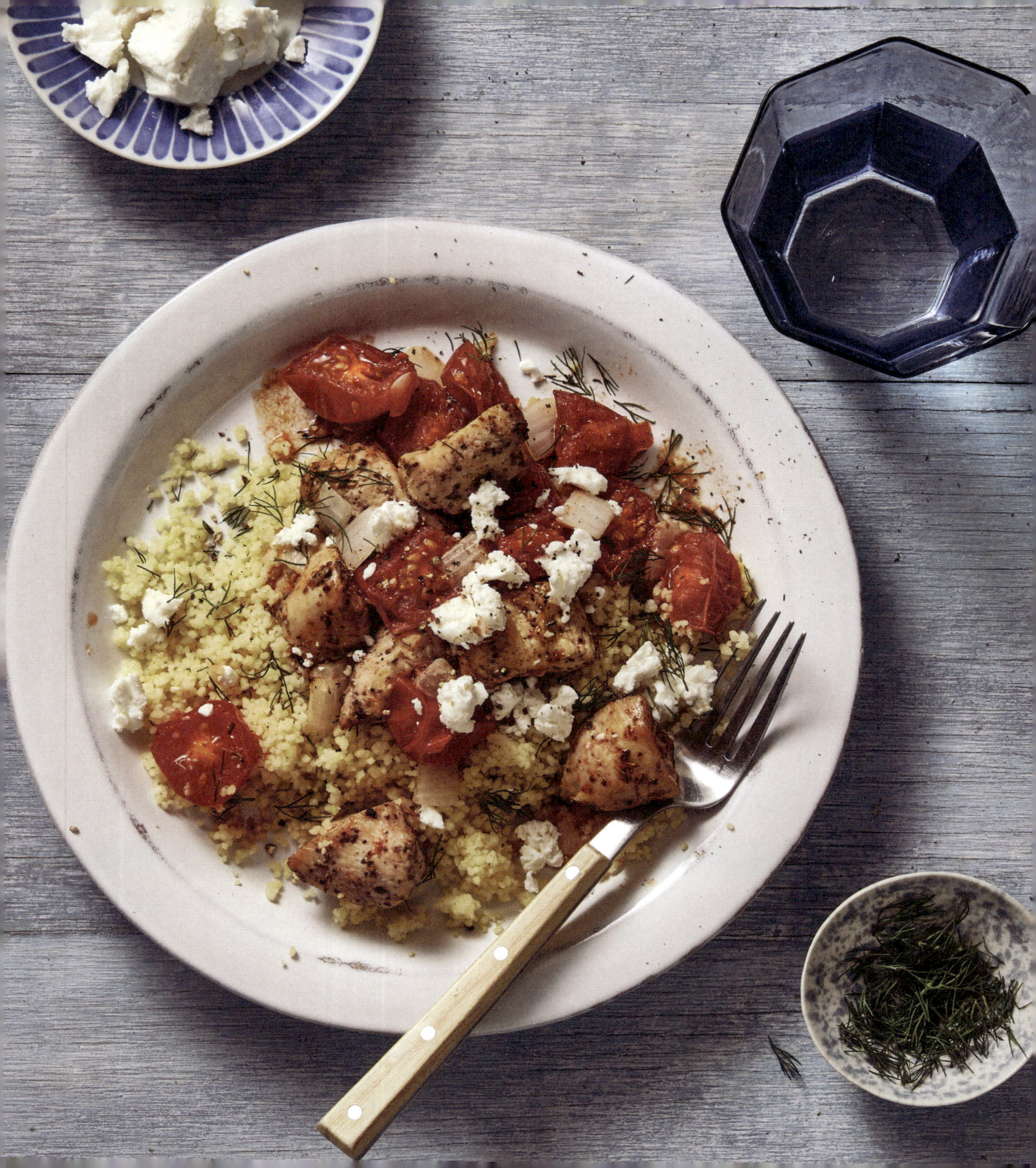

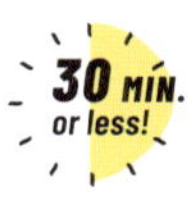

MEDITERRANEAN CHICKEN BOWLS

ACTIVE 15 min. **TOTAL** 30 min. **SERVES** 2 to 4

1 lb boneless, skinless chicken breasts, cut into 1½-inch pieces

1 Tbsp olive oil

1 tsp dried oregano

1 tsp ground sumac

Kosher salt and pepper

1 pint grape or cherry tomatoes

1 medium onion, roughly chopped

1 cup couscous

1 tsp grated lemon zest plus 1 Tbsp lemon juice, plus lemon wedges for serving

¼ cup fresh dill, divided

Crumbled feta, for serving

1. In a large bowl, toss chicken with oil, then oregano, sumac, and ½ teaspoon each salt and pepper. Add tomatoes and onion and toss to combine.
2. Arrange in even layer in an air fryer basket and air-fry at 400°F, shaking basket occasionally, until chicken is golden brown and cooked through, 15 to 20 minutes.
3. Meanwhile, toss couscous with lemon zest and prepare per package directions. Fluff with fork and fold in lemon juice and 2 tablespoons dill.
4. Serve chicken and vegetables over couscous, spooning any juices collected at bottom of the air fryer over top. Sprinkle with remaining dill and feta and serve with lemon wedges if desired.

PER SERVING *About 475 cal, 9.5 g fat (1.5 g sat), 110 mg chol, 425 mg sodium, 53 g carb, 5 g fiber, 5 g sugar (0g added sugar), 43 g pro*

KITCHEN TIP

Sumac is a tangy Middle Eastern spice with a lemony kick—great for brightening dishes. Don't have any? Sub in a sprinkle of lemon zest or a splash of vinegar.

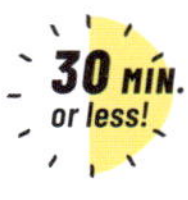

BALSAMIC CHICKEN & ONION SALAD

ACTIVE 25 min. **TOTAL** 25 min. **SERVES** 4

- 4 medium red onions, cut into 1-in.-thick wedges
- 4 Tbsp olive oil, divided
- 2 sprigs fresh thyme, plus more for sprinkling
- Kosher salt and pepper
- 3 Tbsp balsamic vinegar, divided
- 4 5-oz boneless, skinless chicken breasts
- 1 head Gem lettuce, leaves separated
- 1 bunch arugula, thick stems discarded
- 1 Tbsp fresh lemon juice
- ½ cup flat-leaf parsley leaves

1. Heat oven to 400°F. On a large rimmed baking sheet, toss onions with 2 tablespoons oil, thyme sprigs, and ¼ teaspoon each salt and pepper and roast 10 minutes.
2. Toss onions with 1 tablespoon vinegar and continue roasting until golden brown and tender, 10 to 15 minutes more. Transfer to a shallow bowl and sprinkle with additional thyme if desired.
3. Meanwhile, heat 1 tablespoon oil in a large skillet over medium heat. Season chicken with ½ teaspoon each salt and pepper and cook until golden brown and cooked through, 7 to 10 minutes per side. Remove the skillet from heat, add remaining 2 tablespoons vinegar, and turn chicken to coat. Transfer to a cutting board, drizzle with any remaining vinegar in the pan, and let rest 5 minutes before slicing.
4. In a large bowl, toss lettuce and arugula with lemon juice, remaining tablespoon oil, and ¼ teaspoon each salt and pepper. Toss with parsley and onions. Serve with chicken.

PER SERVING *About 360 cal, 17.5 g fat (2.5 g sat), 104 mg chol, 584 mg sodium, 16 g carb, 3 g fiber, 7.5 g sugar (0 g added sugar), 34 g pro*

MAKE IT AHEAD

Prep the chicken and onions and refrigerate in separate airtight containers for up to three days. Just before serving, toss the lettuce, arugula, and parsley with the lemon juice, oil, and salt and pepper, then top with the chicken and onions.

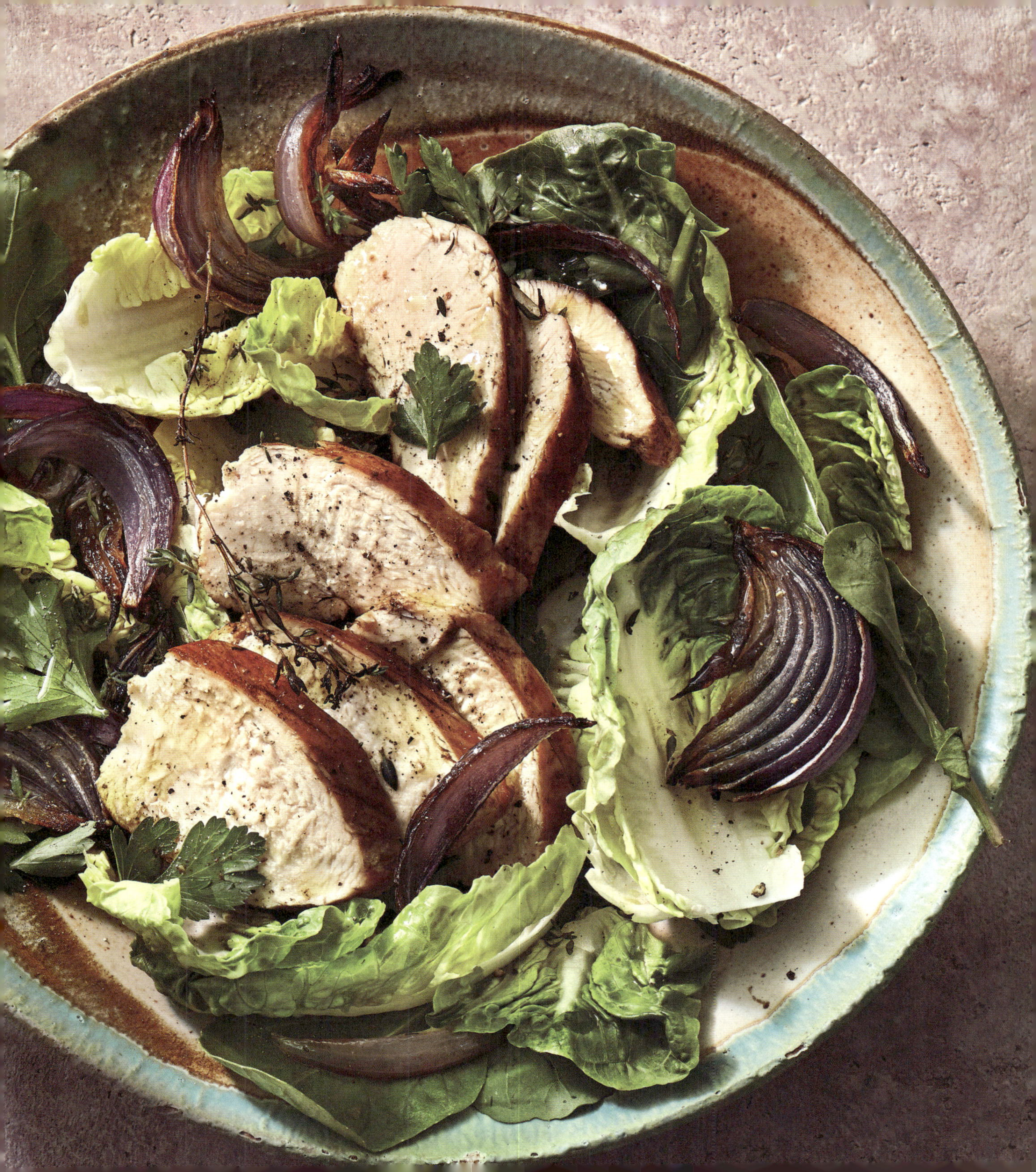

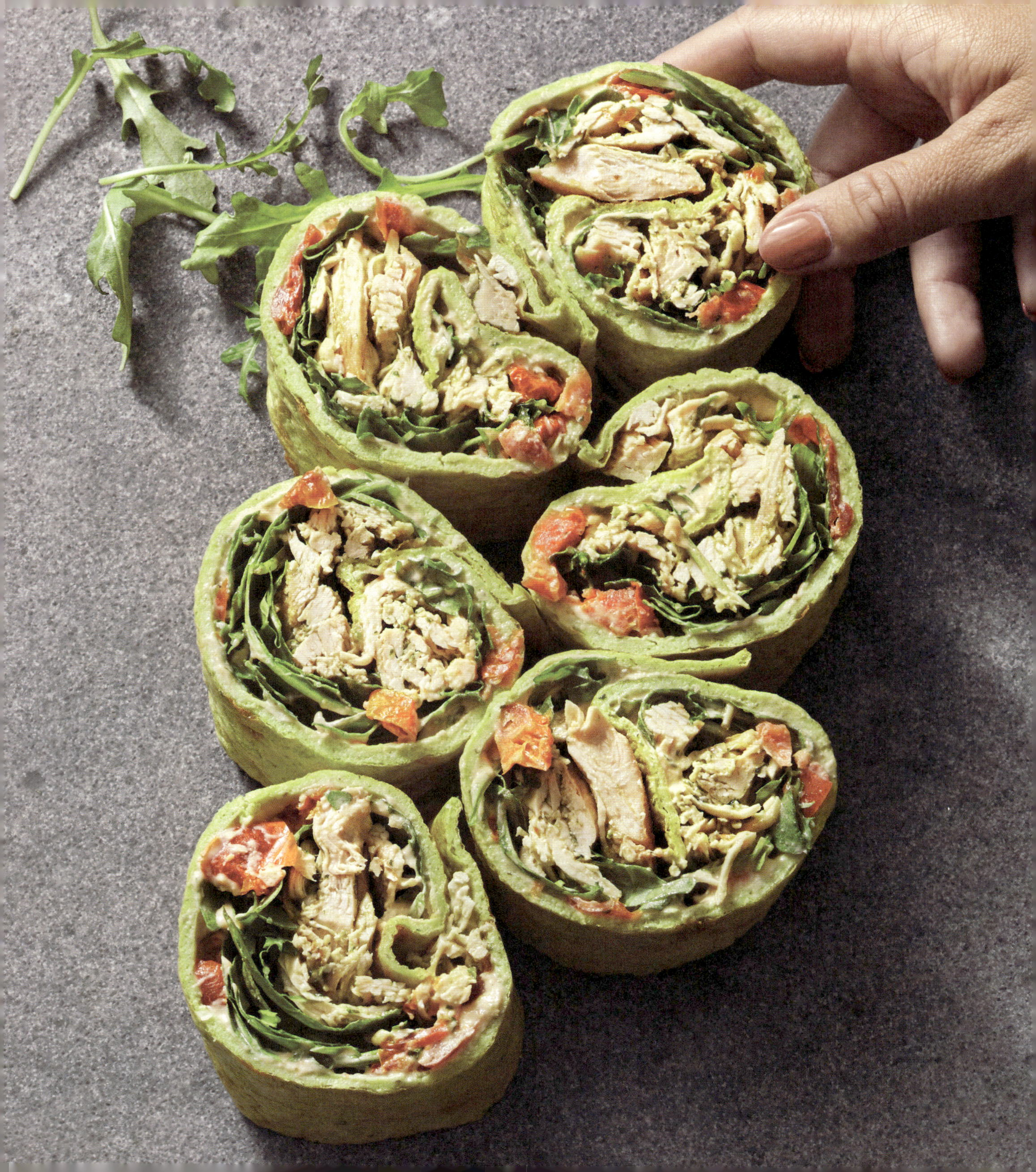

COTTAGE CHEESE WRAP PINWHEELS

ACTIVE 35 min. **TOTAL** 55 min. (plus cooling) **SERVES** 4

1 Tbsp olive oil

2 8-oz boneless, skinless chicken breasts

1½ cups low-fat cottage cheese, drained if necessary

3 large eggs, beaten

¼ cup sliced chives

¼ cup flat-leaf parsley leaves, chopped

2 Tbsp pesto

½ cup hummus

Half of 5-oz pkg. baby arugula

⅔ cup roasted tomatoes, chopped (homemade or store bought)

1. Heat oven to 350°F. Heat oil in a large skillet over medium heat. Add chicken and cook until lightly golden on bottom, 4 to 5 minutes. Reduce heat to medium-low. Flip chicken, cover, and cook until internal temp reaches 165°F, 8 to 10 minutes more. Remove from heat and let sit, covered, 5 minutes. Transfer to a cutting board and let sit until cool enough to handle. Using 2 forks, shred; set aside.

2. Meanwhile, line a large rimmed baking sheet with parchment paper. In blender on high, puree cottage cheese and eggs until smooth. Add chives and parsley and blend until just combined. Pour onto prepared the baking sheet, spread in even layer (about 14 by 10 inches) and bake, rotating the pan halfway through, until lightly browned in spots and set, 27 to 30 minutes. Let cool 10 minutes on the baking sheet.

3. Meanwhile, in a medium bowl, toss shredded chicken with pesto. Refrigerate until ready to use.

4. Invert flatbread onto a cutting board, then peel off parchment. Spread hummus evenly on top and scatter with arugula, pesto chicken, and tomatoes. Starting from long end closest to you, roll flatbread into log. Cut log into 8 pinwheels and serve.

PER SERVING *About 405 cal, 21.5 g fat (4.5 g sat), 214 mg chol, 653 mg sodium, 11 g carb, 2 g fiber, 5 g sugar (0 g added sugar), 41 g pro*

MAKE IT AHEAD

This gluten-free flatbread is perfect for meal prep. Make the wrap up to three days ahead, then let cool completely and refrigerate in an airtight container with parchment between layers to prevent sticking. Enjoy it warm or cold as a high-protein wrap base filled with your favorite fixings.

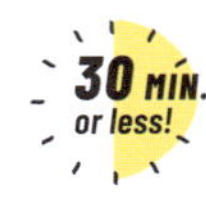

CHICKEN & ASPARAGUS RIBBONS *with* MEYER LEMON VINAIGRETTE

ACTIVE 15 min. **TOTAL** 25 min. **SERVES** 4

- 1 lb thick asparagus, trimmed
- Kosher salt and pepper
- 1½ lb boneless, skinless chicken breasts, cut into 1½-in. pieces
- 2 Tbsp olive oil, divided
- 1 Meyer lemon
- 1 tsp Dijon mustard
- ¼ cup grated pecorino cheese
- 5 oz mixed greens
- ¼ cup roasted almonds, chopped

1. Bring a medium pot of water to a boil. Reserve 4 thick spears asparagus, then cut others into 2-inch pieces. Add 1 teaspoon salt to water, then add asparagus pieces and cook until bright green, about 2 minutes; immediately transfer to bowl of ice water to cool. Drain and pat dry.
2. Season chicken with ½ teaspoon each salt and pepper. Heat 1 tablespoon olive oil in a large skillet over medium-high heat, add chicken and cook, tossing occasionally, until golden brown on all sides and just cooked through, about 12 minutes.
3. Into a large bowl, grate zest from lemon and squeeze in juice. Whisk in mustard and remaining tablespoon oil, then stir in pecorino.
4. With vegetable peeler, pressing down firmly, create long strips from reserved asparagus. Add to a bowl of dressing along with cooked asparagus and toss to coat; fold in chicken, mixed greens, and almonds.

PER SERVING *About 350 cal, 18 g fat (4 g sat), 104 mg chol, 555 mg sodium, 6 g carb, 3 g fiber, 2 g sugar (0 g added sugar), 41 g pro*

KITCHEN TIP

Meyer lemons are a sweet, floral cross between a lemon and a mandarin orange. Can't find any? Sub in lemon juice with a splash of orange juice.

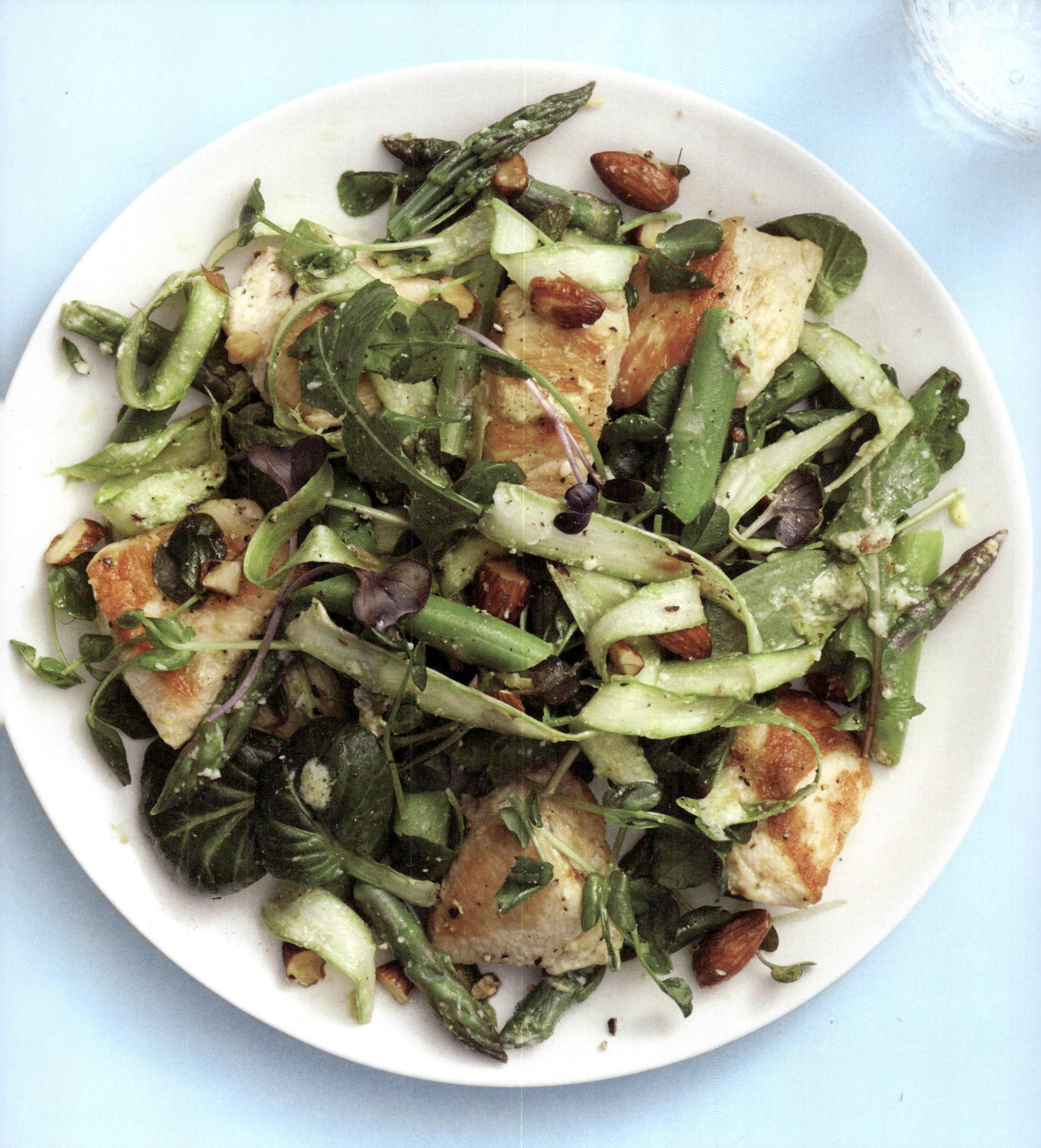

CHICKEN & BROCCOLI PARCHMENT

ACTIVE 35 min. **TOTAL** 45 min. **SERVES** 4

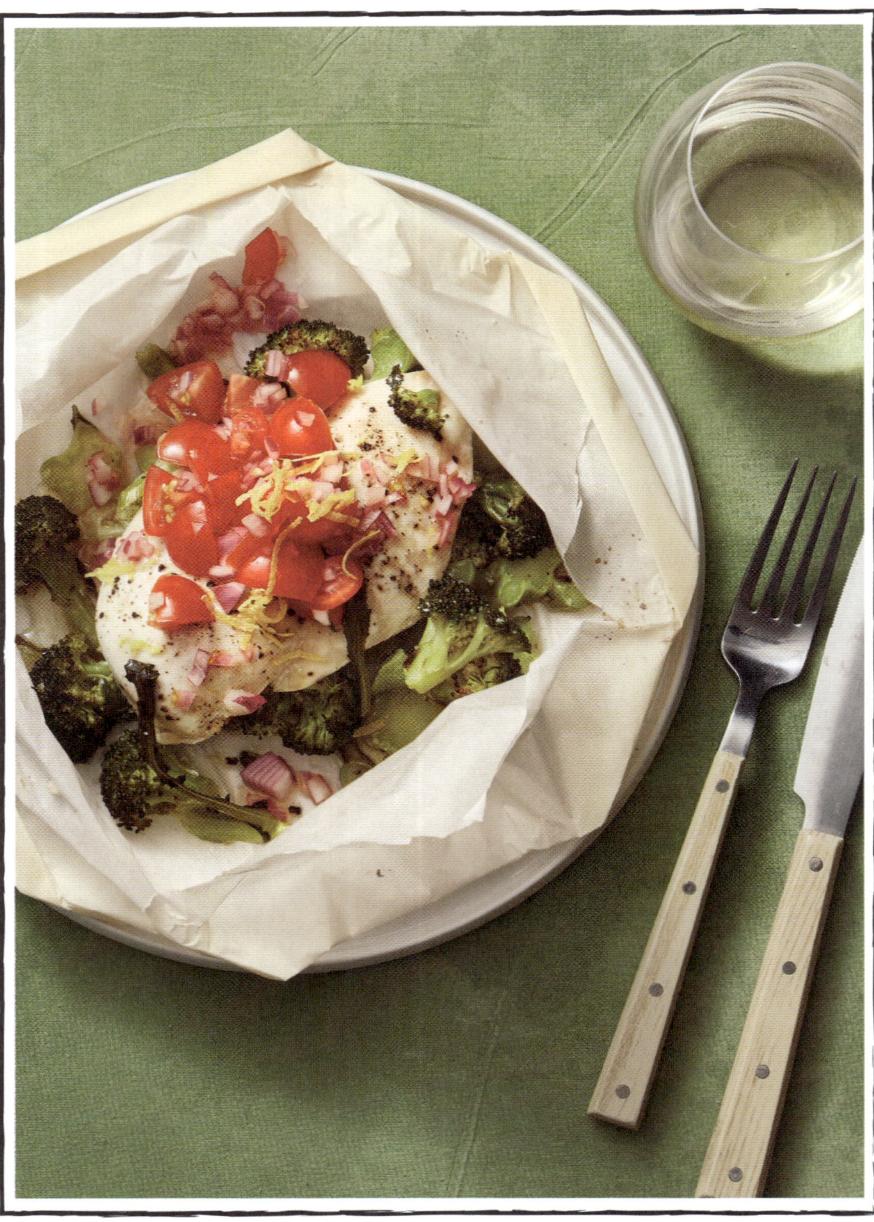

- 1¼ lb broccoli, cut into small florets
- 2 cloves garlic, pressed
- 2 Tbsp olive oil, divided
- Kosher salt and pepper
- 4 6-oz boneless, skinless chicken breasts
- ½ small red onion, finely chopped
- 1 lemon
- 8 oz tomatoes, chopped

1. Heat oven to 400°F. Toss broccoli, garlic, 1 tablespoon oil, and ¼ teaspoon each salt and pepper. Divide among four 12-inch squares of parchment.

2. Season chicken with ¼ teaspoon each salt and pepper and place on top of broccoli. Cover with parchment and seal. Place the packets on 2 rimmed baking sheets and roast 15 minutes.

3. Meanwhile, finely grate zest of lemon and squeeze 2 tablespoons juice. In medium bowl, combine onion, lemon juice, remaining tablespoon oil, and ¼ teaspoon each salt and pepper. Let sit 4 minutes, then toss with tomatoes. Cut open packets; top with vinaigrette and lemon zest.

PER SERVING *About 330 cal, 12 g fat (2 g sat), 124 mg chol, 485 mg sodium, 14 g carb, 5 g fiber, 4.5 g sugar (0 g added sugar), 43 g pro*

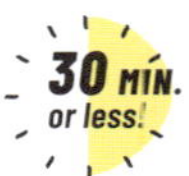

CHICKEN CUTLET SANDWICHES

ACTIVE 20 min. **TOTAL** 20 min. **SERVES** 4

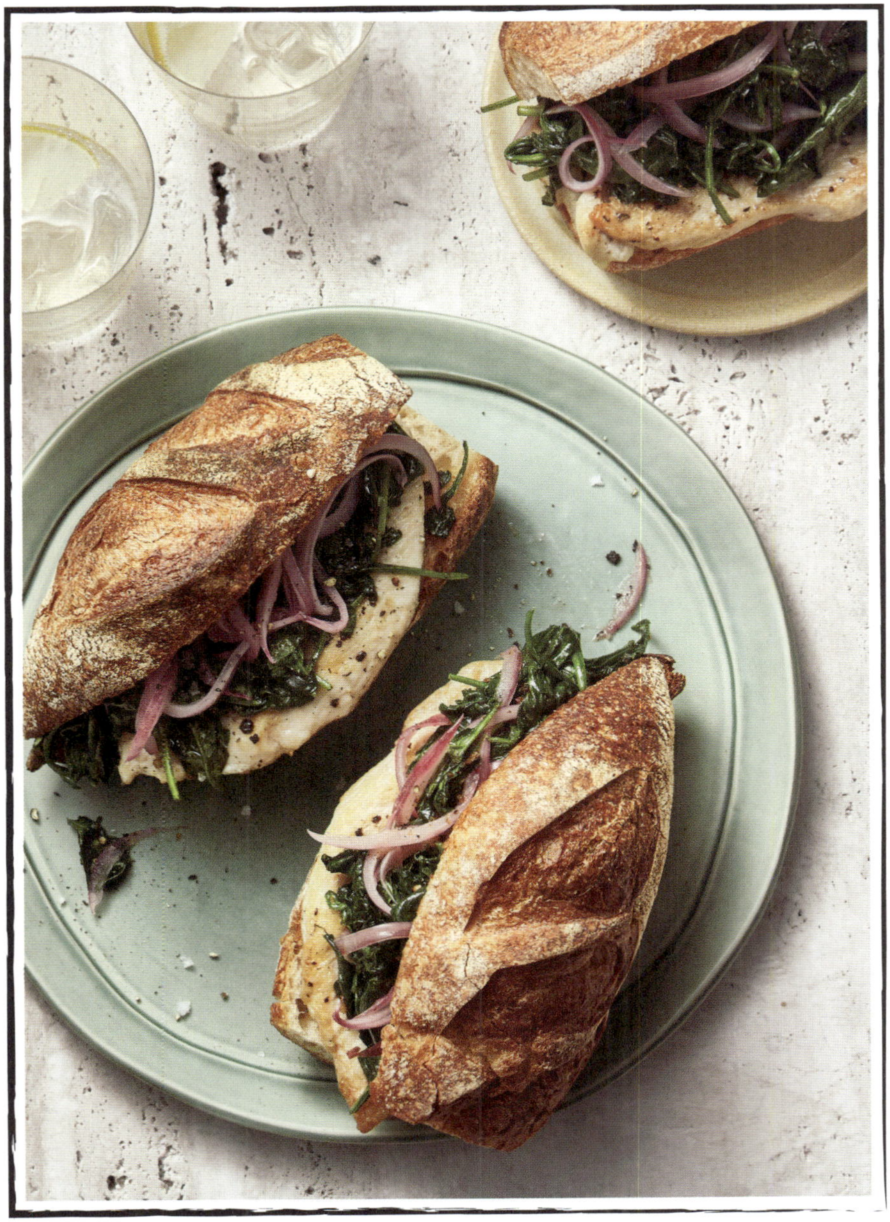

1. Toss ½ small **red onion**, thinly sliced with 1 tablespoon **red wine vinegar** and ⅛ teaspoon each **kosher salt** and **pepper**; let sit.

2. Cut 1 lb **boneless, skinless chicken breasts** into 6 thin cutlets. Heat 1 tablespoon **olive oil** in a large skillet over medium-high heat. Season chicken with ½ teaspoon Kosher each salt and pepper and cook until browned and cooked through, 2 minutes per side; transfer to a cutting board.

3. Add 6 cups **baby spinach** to a skillet, season with salt and pepper and cook until just beginning to wilt.

4. Slice chicken and sandwich between 4 5-inch pieces **baguette**, split and toasted, halves with spinach and onions.

PER SERVING *About 330 cal, 7 g fat (1 g sat), 83 mg chol, 705 mg sodium, 32 g carb, 3 g fiber, 1.5 g sugar (0 g added sugar), 33 g pro*

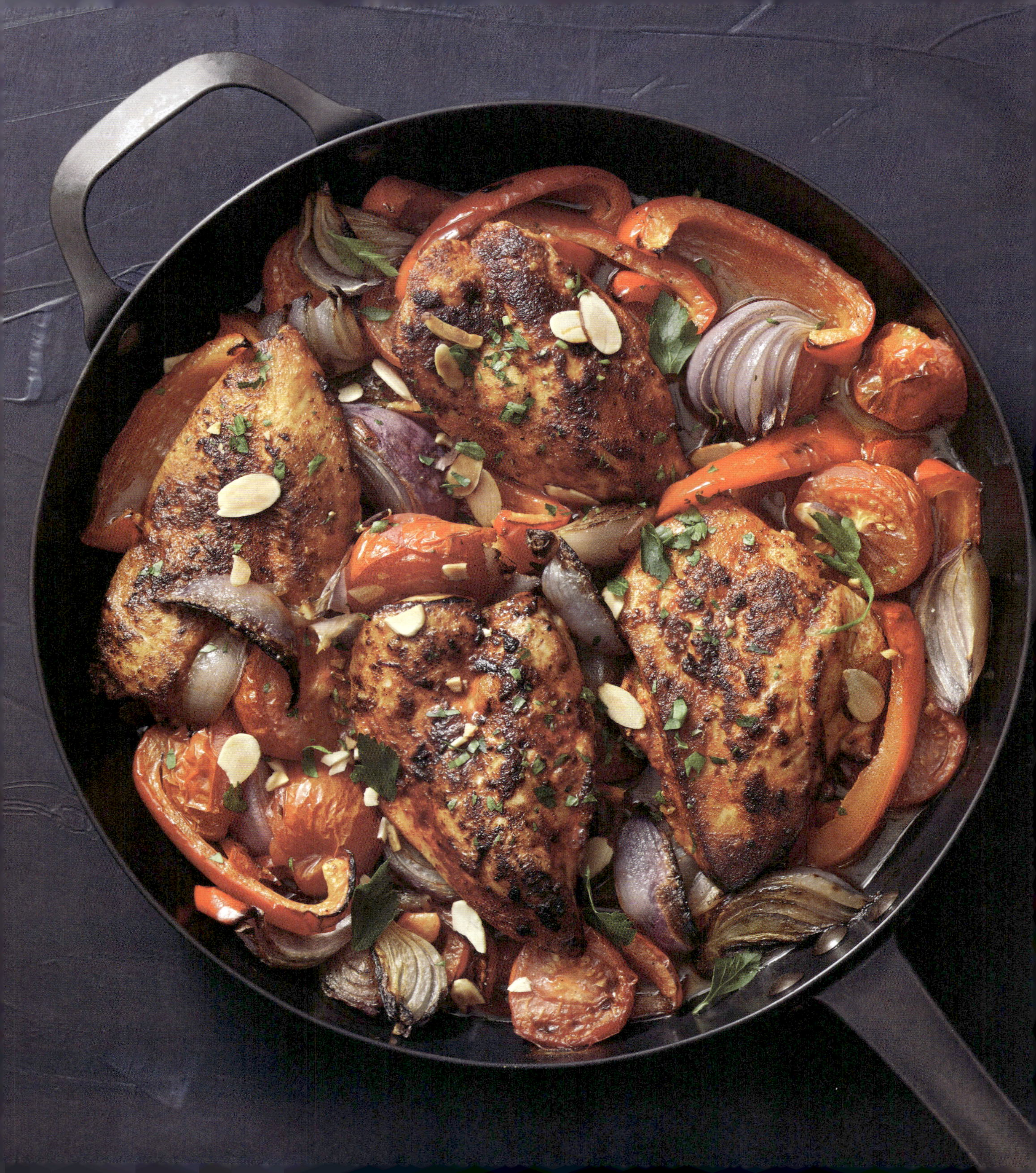

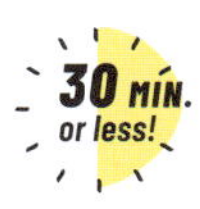

CHICKEN *with* STEWED PEPPERS *and* TOMATOES

ACTIVE 10 min. **TOTAL** 25 min. **SERVES** 4

4 6-oz boneless, skinless chicken breasts

1 Tbsp smoked paprika

Kosher salt and pepper

1 Tbsp olive oil

2 small red onions, cut into ½-in.-thick wedges

2 red peppers, quartered and sliced crosswise ½ in. thick

½ lb Campari or large cherry tomatoes, halved

2 cloves garlic, thinly sliced

Chopped flat-leaf parsley leaves and sliced almonds, for serving

1. Heat oven to 450°F. Pat chicken dry with paper towels, then rub with paprika and ½ teaspoon each salt and pepper.
2. Heat oil in a large ovenproof skillet over medium heat and cook chicken until browned on one side, 4 to 5 minutes. Flip chicken. Add onions, peppers, tomatoes, and garlic and season with ½ teaspoon each salt and pepper.
3. Transfer the skillet to oven and roast, stirring vegetables once, until chicken is cooked through and vegetables are tender, 14 to 16 minutes. Serve sprinkled with chopped parsley leaves and almonds if desired.

PER SERVING *About 325 cal, 12 g fat (2 g sat), 124 mg chol, 566 mg sodium, 13 g carb, 4 g fiber, 6.5 g sugar (0 g added sugar), 40 g pro*

LOVE YOUR LEFTOVERS

For an easy lunch, warm ½ cup cooked brown rice in a small bowl and top with leftover vegetables, 1 cup mixed greens, and a drizzle of red wine vinegar. Slice any leftover chicken and arrange on top. Scatter with crispy chickpeas.

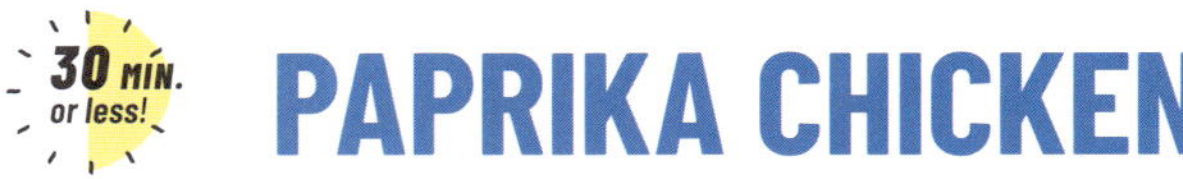

PAPRIKA CHICKEN

ACTIVE 15 min. **TOTAL** 20 min. **SERVES** 4

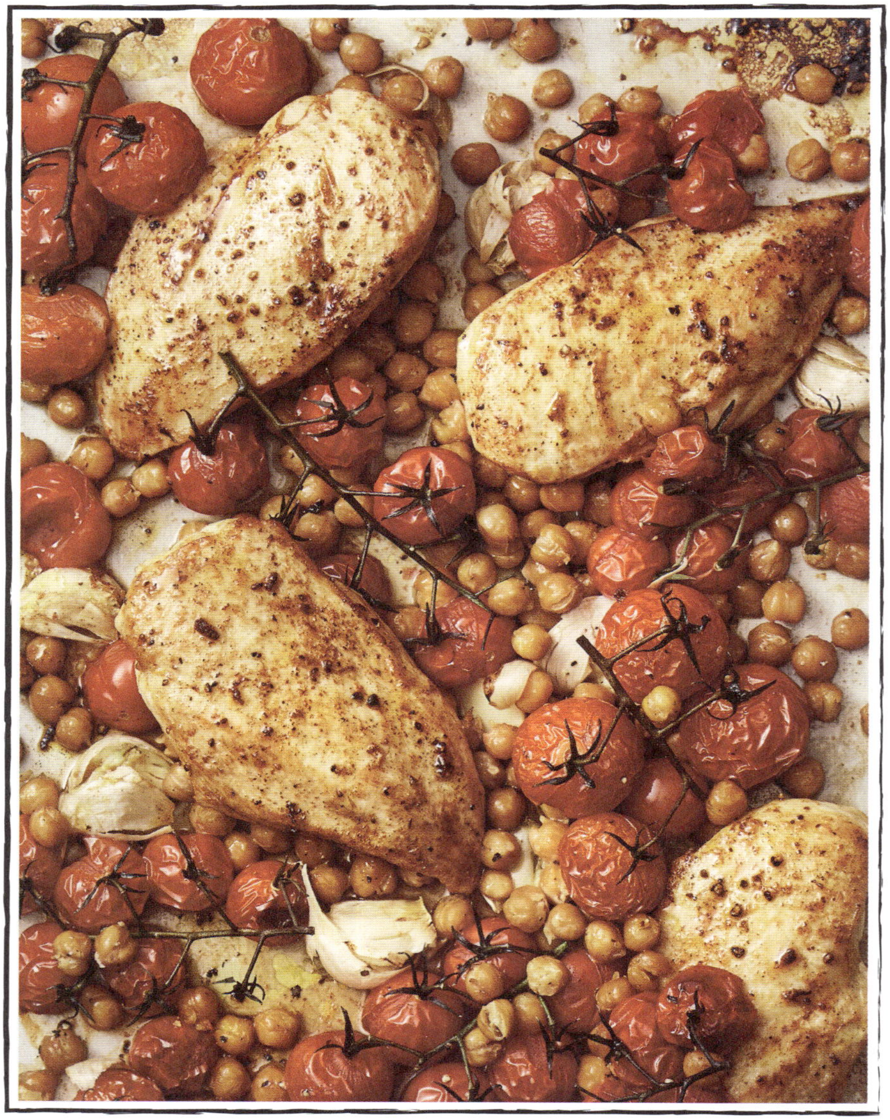

1. Heat oven to 425°F. On a rimmed baking sheet, toss 12 ounces **tomatoes**, 8 cloves **garlic**, smashed, in their skins, and 1 15-ounce can **chickpeas**, rinsed, with 2 tablespoons **olive oil** and ¼ teaspoon each **kosher salt** and **pepper**.

2. Roast 10 minutes. Heat 1 tablespoon olive oil in a large skillet over medium heat. Season 4 6-ounce boneless, skinless **chicken breasts** with 2 teaspoons **paprika** and ½ teaspoon each salt and pepper and cook until golden brown on one side, 5 to 6 minutes. Flip and cook 1 minute more.

3. Transfer to a baking sheet with tomatoes and chickpeas and roast until cooked through, 6 minutes more. Before serving, discard garlic skins.

PER SERVING *About 301 cal, 6 g fat (1.5 g sat), 94 mg chol, 589 mg sodium, 21 g carb, 6 g fiber, 5 g sugar (0 g added sugar), 40 g pro*

LEMONY CHICKEN SOUP

ACTIVE 25 min. **TOTAL** 1 hr. **SERVES** 4

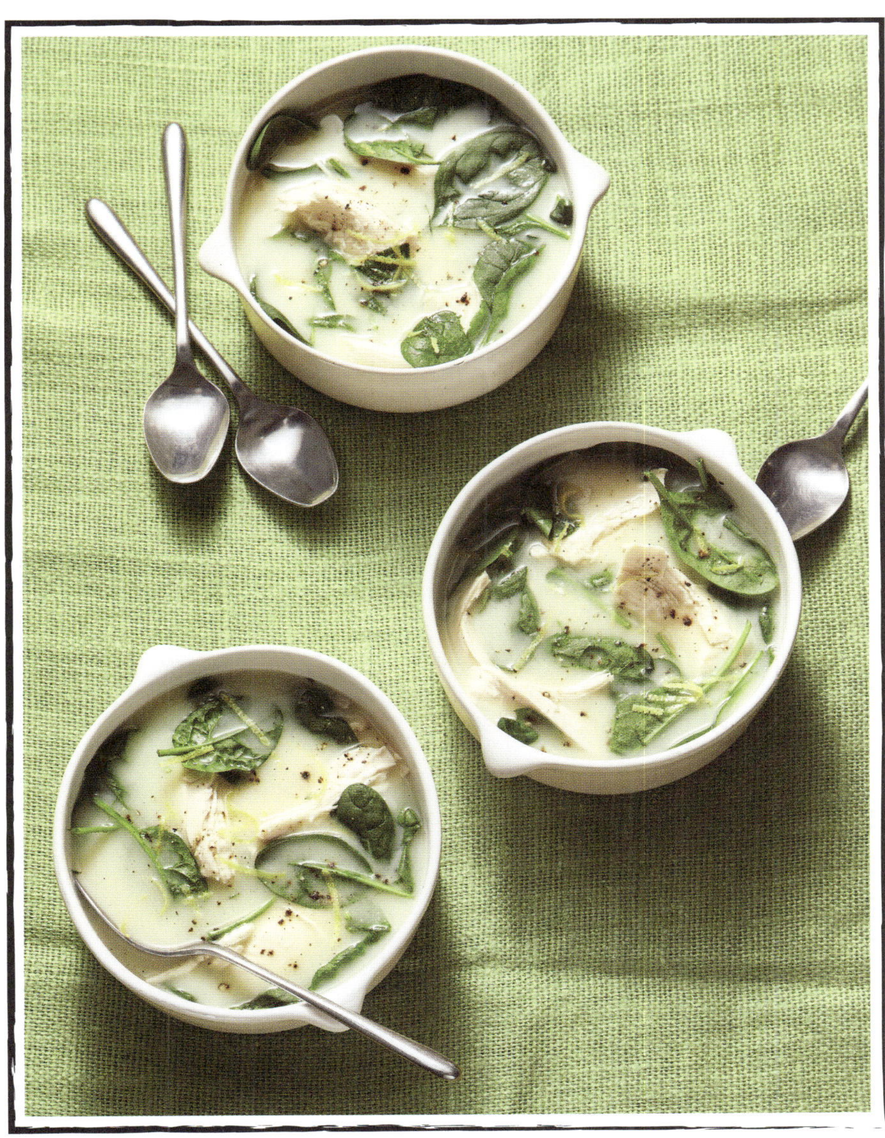

1. In a large pot, simmer 2 halved **yellow onions**, 1 halved head of **garlic**, and 1 **Parmesan rind** in 12 cups **water** for 25 minutes. Strain over a bowl, discard solids, and return liquid to the pot. Season with ½ teaspoon each **kosher salt** and **black pepper**, then return to a simmer. Add 3 small **boneless, skinless chicken breasts** (about 1¼ pounds) and poach until cooked through, 11 to 13 minutes. Transfer chicken to a bowl, let cool slightly, and shred.

2. Meanwhile, whisk 2 large **eggs** with 6 tablespoons fresh **lemon juice** until foamy. Slowly whisk in 1 cup hot broth, 1 tablespoon at a time. Next: whisk broth in the pot constantly, gradually pour in the egg mixture. Reduce heat to medium-low and cook until slightly thickened and velvety, about 5 minutes. Remove from heat, stir in shredded chicken and 6 cups **baby spinach**. Let sit 5 minutes before serving.

PER SERVING *About 270 cal, 6.5 g fat (1.5 g sat), 197 mg chol, 410 mg sodium, 14 g carb, 4 g fiber, 4 g sugar (0 g added sugar), 38 g pro*

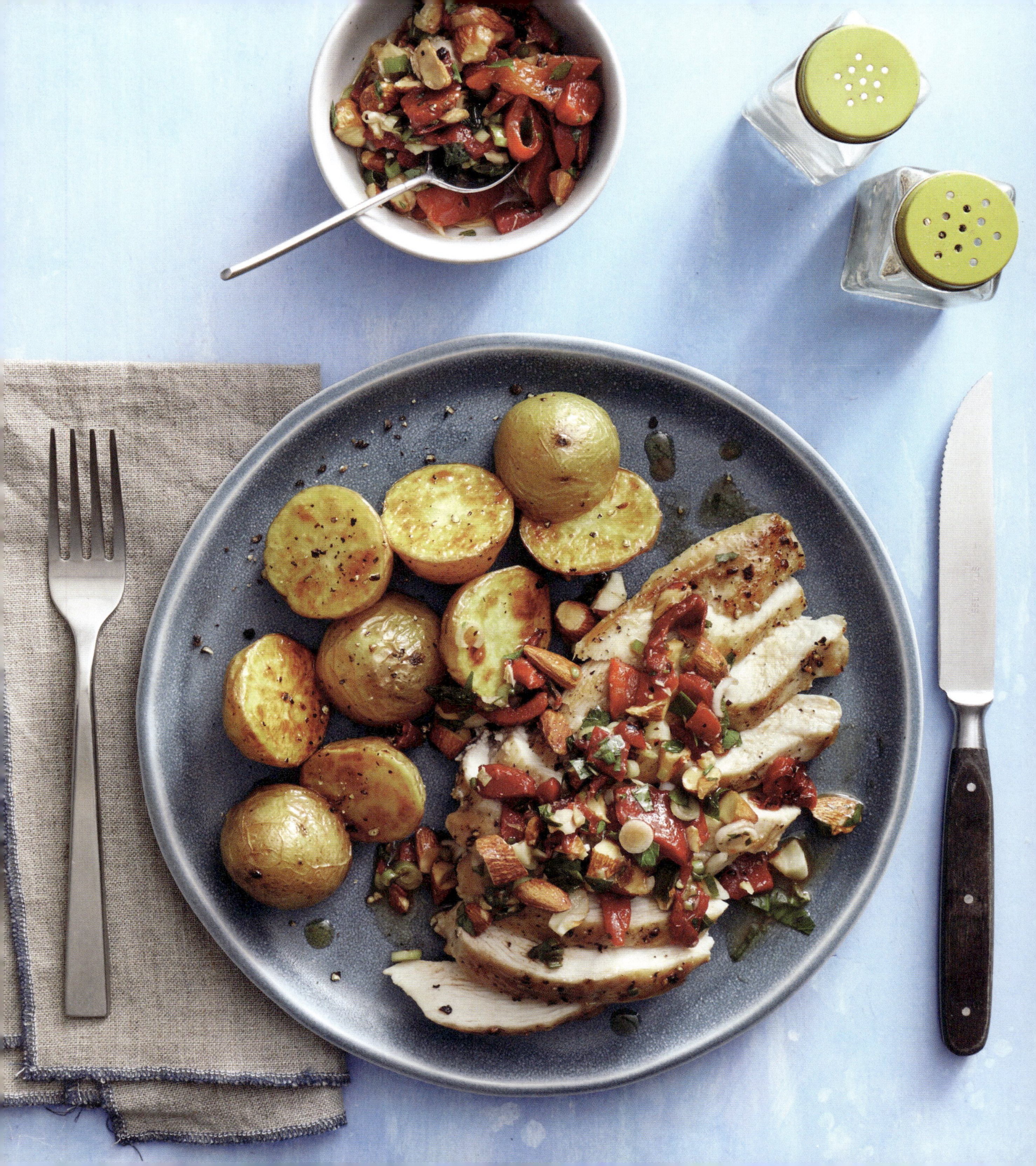

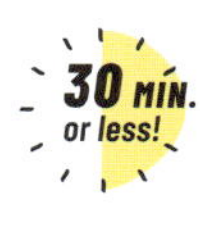

ROASTED CHICKEN *and* GARLIC POTATOES *with* RED PEPPER RELISH

ACTIVE 30 min. **TOTAL** 30 min. **SERVES** 4

1½ lb golden new potatoes (about 24), halved

4 Tbsp olive oil

4 cloves garlic (2 cloves smashed)

Kosher salt and pepper

4 6-oz boneless, skinless chicken breasts

¾ cup roasted red peppers, drained and cut into ⅛-in. pieces

2 scallions, finely chopped

⅓ cup roasted almonds, chopped

1 Tbsp sherry vinegar

2 Tbsp chopped flat-leaf parsley

1. Heat oven to 425°F. On a large rimmed baking sheet, toss potatoes with 2 tablespoons oil. Press 2 cloves garlic over top, sprinkle with ¼ teaspoon salt, and toss to combine. Roast 15 minutes.
2. Meanwhile, heat a large skillet over medium-high heat. Season chicken with ¼ teaspoon each salt and pepper. Add 1 tablespoon oil to skillet, then add chicken and cook until browned, about 4 minutes.
3. Turn chicken over, add smashed garlic to skillet and cook 1 minute more. Transfer skillet to oven along with potatoes and roast until chicken is cooked through and potatoes are golden brown and tender, 6 to 8 minutes more; transfer chicken and garlic to a cutting board.
4. While chicken cooks, in a bowl, combine peppers, scallions, almonds, vinegar, remaining tablespoon oil, and ¼ teaspoon salt. Chop smashed garlic, add to pepper mixture along with parsley and mix to combine. Serve with chicken and potatoes.

PER SERVING *About 520 cal, 23.5 g fat (3.5 g sat), 94 mg chol, 590 mg sodium, 38 g carb, 6 g fiber, 1 g sugar (0 g added sugar), 40 g pro*

LOVE YOUR LEFTOVERS

This relish is inspired by romesco, a tangy red pepper and nuts sauce. Make a double batch and refrigerate it in an airtight container for up to a week—it's perfect for adding a burst of flavor to roasted veggies, meats, or fish, or even spooned over grain bowls or eggs.

HERB-MARINATED CHICKEN

ACTIVE 25 min. **TOTAL** 40 min. (plus marinating and resting) **SERVES** 4

3 Tbsp white wine vinegar

2 Tbsp red wine vinegar

2 cloves garlic

2 tsp Dijon mustard

1 tsp agave or honey

6 fresh basil leaves

½ Tbsp fresh thyme leaves

Kosher salt and pepper

⅔ cup olive oil

½ tsp red pepper flakes

¼ tsp dried oregano

4 6-oz boneless, skinless chicken breasts

2 peppers (one red, one orange), thinly sliced

1 cup grape or cherry tomatoes, halved

½ small red onion, thinly sliced

12 cups (about 6 oz) mixed salad greens, torn into bite-size pieces

1 oz Parmesan, shaved

1. In a blender, combine vinegars, garlic, mustard, agave, basil, thyme, and ½ teaspoon each salt and pepper; blend until smooth. Add oil and blend on low until just incorporated but not emulsified, about 10 seconds. Stir in red pepper flakes and oregano.
2. In a small baking dish, coat chicken with ⅓ cup dressing and marinate at least 10 minutes at room temperature or up to overnight in refrigerator.
3. Meanwhile, transfer 3 tablespoons remaining dressing to a large bowl. Add peppers, tomatoes, and onion and toss to coat.
4. Heat large skillet over medium heat and cook chicken until golden brown and cooked through, 5 to 7 minutes per side. Transfer to a cutting board and let rest 5 minutes before slicing.
5. Add greens to peppers and toss to coat. Top with Parmesan and serve with chicken.

PER SERVING *About 424 cal, 24.5 g fat (5 g sat), 100 mg chol, 526 mg sodium, 14 g carb, 3 g fiber, 4g sugar (1.33 g added sugar), 39 g pro*

AIR FRYING INSTRUCTIONS

Heat air fryer to 400°F. Add marinated chicken and cook for 4 minutes. Using tongs, flip and cook until golden brown and cooked through, 8-9 minutes more.

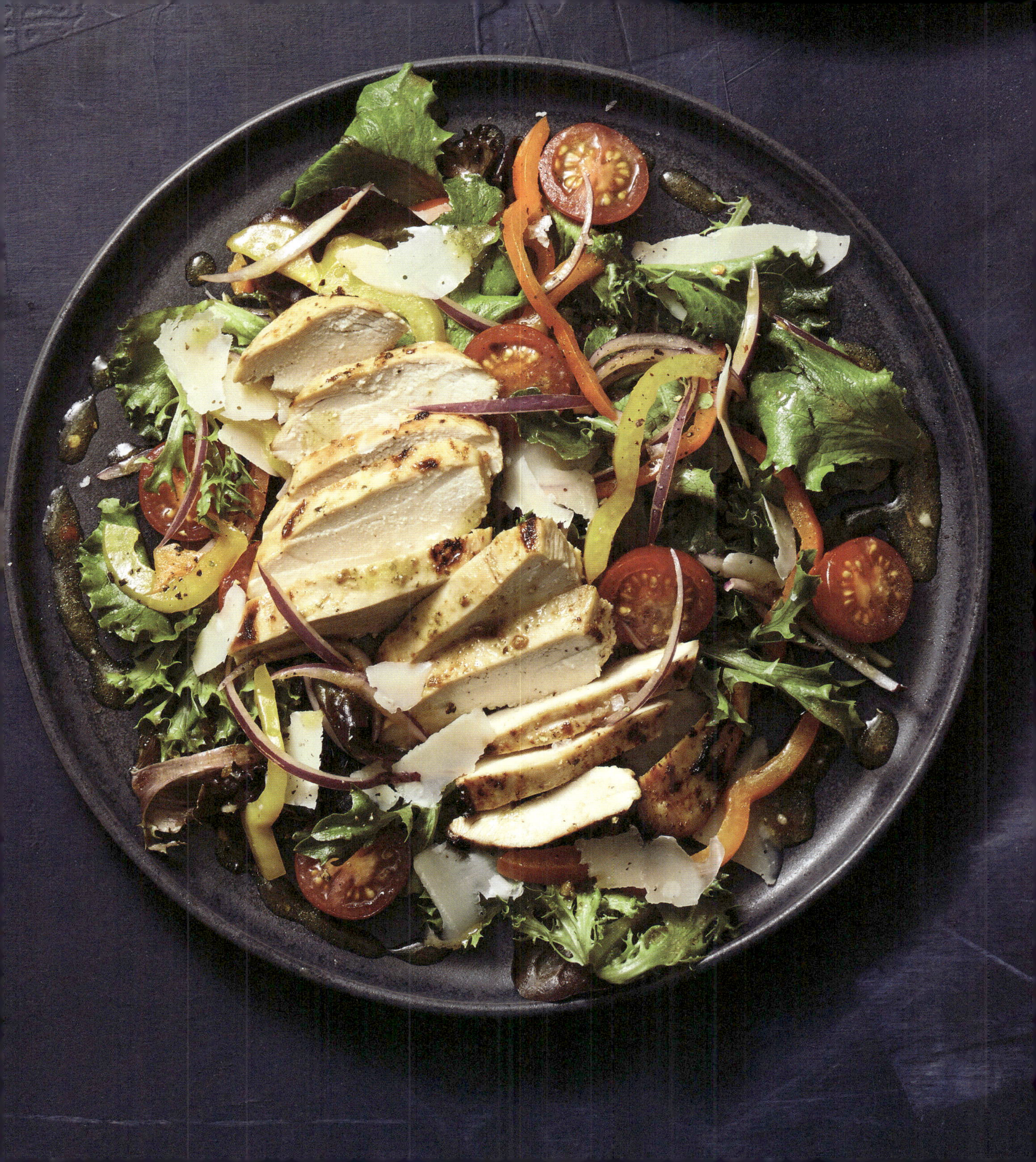

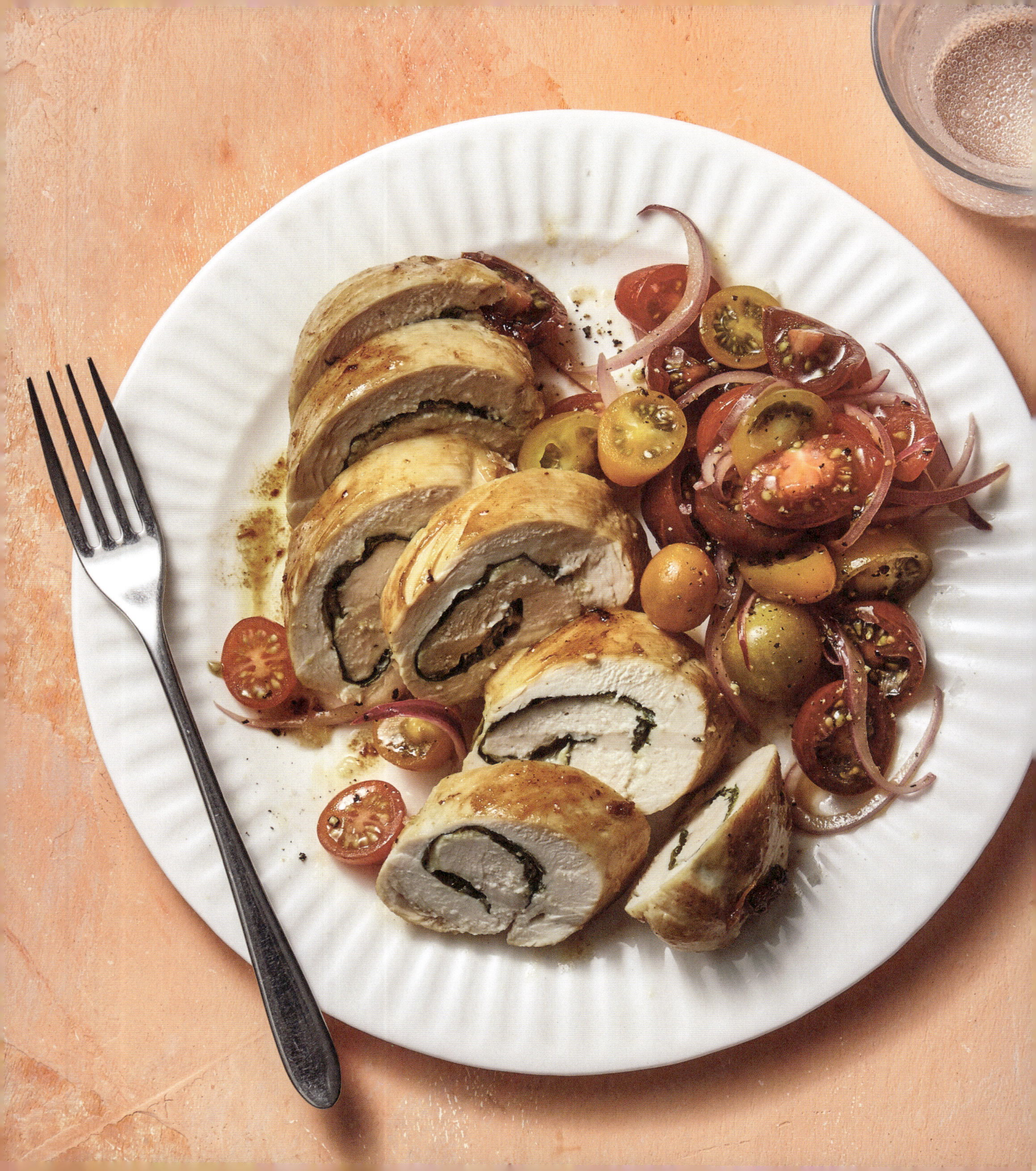

CHICKEN ROULADES *with* MARINATED TOMATOES

ACTIVE 35 min. **TOTAL** 35 min. **SERVES** 4

4 boneless, skinless chicken breasts

2 cloves garlic, finely grated

2 Tbsp lemon zest plus 2 Tbsp lemon juice

½ cup finely grated Parmesan

32 baby spinach leaves

Kosher salt and pepper

3 Tbsp olive oil, divided

2 pints grape or cherry tomatoes, sliced

¼ small red onion, thinly sliced

2 Tbsp red wine vinegar

1. Heat oven to 450ºF. Pound chicken breasts into thin cutlets. In a small bowl, combine garlic, lemon zest, and Parmesan. Lay 8 spinach leaves on each chicken cutlet, then sprinkle garlic mixture on top. Roll chicken up and secure with a toothpick (place toothpick in parallel to seam to make turning roulades easier). Season chicken with ½ teaspoon each salt and pepper.

2. Heat 1 tablespoon oil in a large ovenproof skillet over medium-high heat. Carefully add roulades, seam-side down, and cook, turning until browned on all sides, 6 to 7 minutes. Transfer to oven and bake until cooked through, 8 to 9 minutes more. Drizzle lemon juice on roulades.

3. While chicken roasts, toss together tomatoes, onion, vinegar, remaining 2 tablespoons oil, and ½ teaspoon each salt and pepper. Serve with chicken.

PER SERVING *About 310 cal, 16.5 g fat (4 g sat), 82 mg chol, 735 mg sodium, 10 g carb, 3 g fiber, 4.5 g sugar (0 g added sugar), 31 g pro*

MAKE IT AHEAD

The chicken roulades can be rolled up and refrigerated raw for up to two days. Once cooked, the roulades can be refrigerated for up to two days. They can be sliced cold and added to sandwiches and salads. The marinated tomatoes are best made the day you plan on serving them.

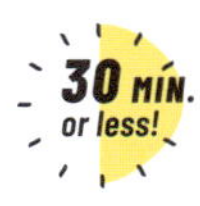

ROASTED CHICKPEA, TOMATO *and* CHICKEN BOWL

ACTIVE 20 min. **TOTAL** 30 min. **SERVES** 4

- ½ Tbsp coriander seeds
- 1 tsp cumin seeds
- ¼ tsp red pepper flakes
- ½ tsp ground sumac, divided
- Kosher salt and pepper
- 1 pint grape tomatoes
- 4 cloves garlic, smashed
- 2 Tbsp plus 1 tsp olive oil, divided
- 8-oz boneless, skinless chicken breast
- 15-oz can chickpeas, rinsed
- 1 cup cooked farro
- 1 scallion, thinly sliced
- 1½ Tbsp white wine vinegar
- Kosher salt and pepper
- 4 cups baby greens (spinach, kale, arugula, or a combination)

1. Heat oven to 425°F. With a mortar and pestle, coarsely crush coriander and cumin seeds. Stir in red pepper flakes, ¼ teaspoon sumac, and a pinch of salt.
2. On a rimmed baking sheet, toss tomatoes and garlic with 1 tablespoon oil and spices. Roast 12 minutes.
3. Meanwhile, heat 1 teaspoon oil in a small skillet over medium heat. Season chicken with ¼ teaspoon each salt and pepper and cook until golden brown, 5 to 6 minutes. Turn and cook 1 minute.
4. Toss tomato mixture with chickpeas, nestle chicken among tomatoes, and continue roasting until chicken is cooked through, 6 to 8 minutes more. Transfer chicken to a cutting board and let rest 5 minutes before slicing.
5. In bowl, toss farro, scallion, vinegar, remaining 1 tablespoon oil, and a pinch each of salt and pepper. Fold in chickpea-tomato mixture and chicken, then greens.

PER SERVING *About 309 cal, 11.5 g fat (1.5 g sat), 31 mg chol, 375 mg sodium, 37 g carb, 9 g fiber, 4 g sugar (0 g added sugar), 21 g pro*

KITCHEN TIP

Dark leafy greens like spinach, kale, and arugula are packed with vitamins and antioxidants—and are more nutrient-dense than lighter lettuces like iceberg. Mix and match a combination for optimal crunch and nutrition.

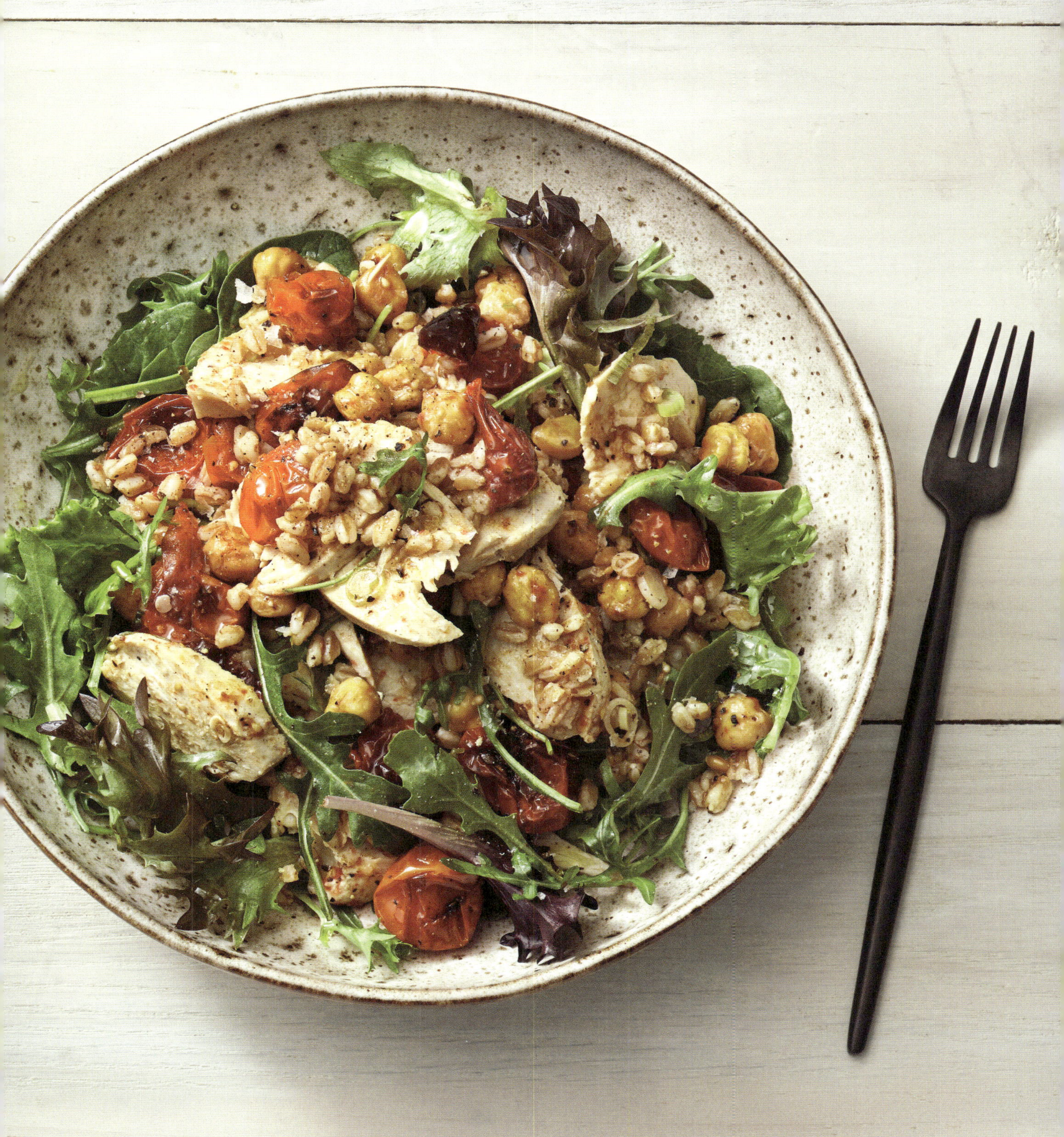

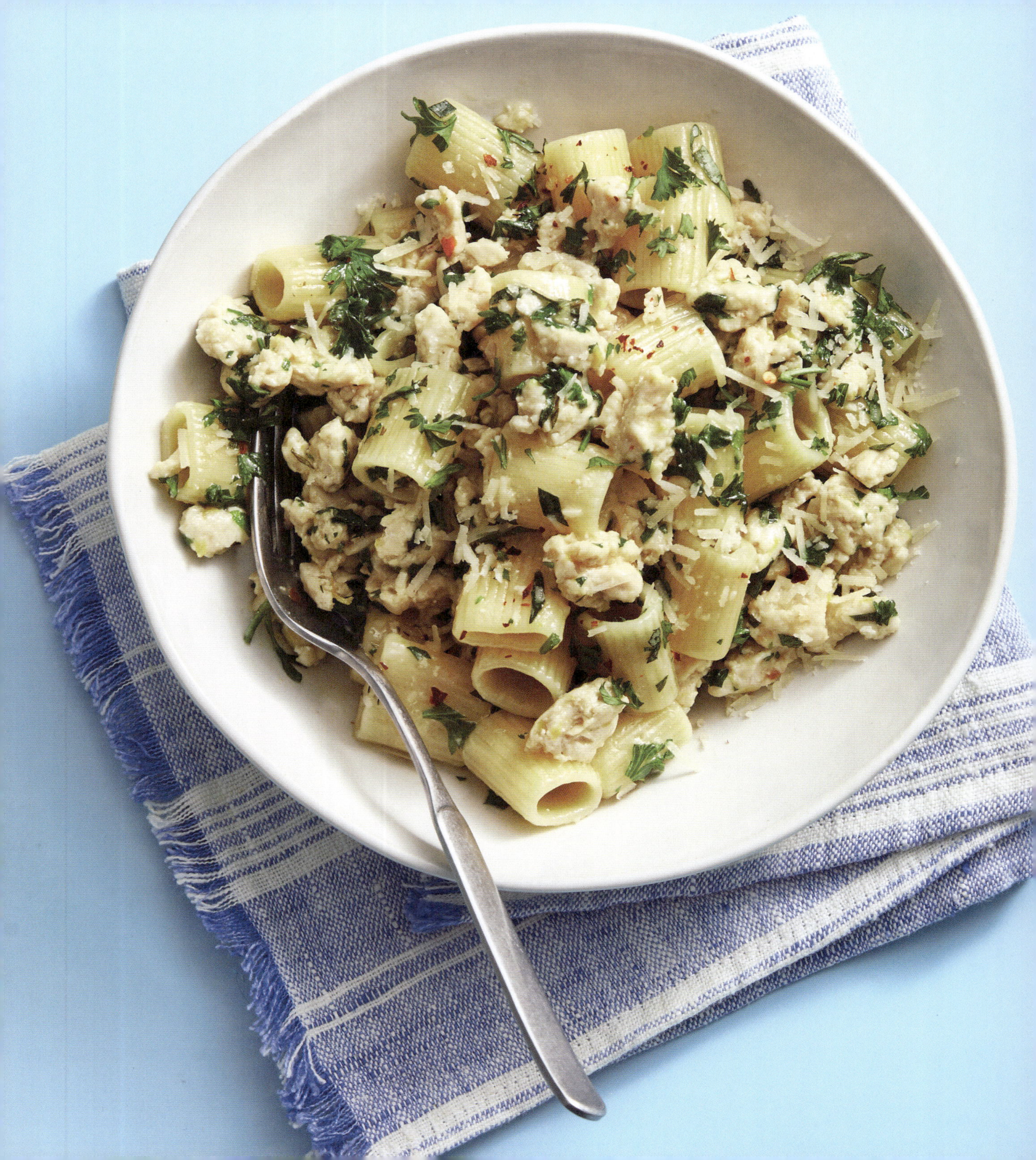

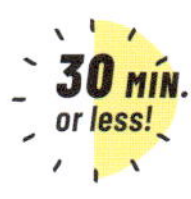

CHICKEN BOLOGNESE

ACTIVE 15 min. **TOTAL** 20 min. **SERVES** 4

- 12 oz mezze rigatoni
- 1 Tbsp olive oil
- 2 cloves garlic, pressed
- 1 lb ground chicken
- ½ tsp red pepper flakes
- Kosher salt and pepper
- ½ cup dry white wine
- ½ cup low-sodium chicken broth
- 1 Tbsp finely grated lemon zest
- ½ cup finely grated Parmesan, plus more for serving
- ¾ cup flat-leaf parsley, chopped
- 1 Tbsp tarragon, chopped
- ¼ cup chopped chives
- 2 Tbsp cold unsalted butter (optional)

1. Cook pasta per package directions. Reserve 1 cup cooking liquid, then drain pasta and return to pot.
2. Meanwhile, heat oil in large skillet over medium heat. Add garlic and cook, stirring, until it starts to sizzle, about 1 minute.
3. Add chicken, season with red pepper flakes and ½ teaspoon each salt and pepper, and cook, breaking up into tiny pieces, until nearly cooked through, 4 to 5 minutes. Add wine and simmer until nearly evaporated, about 2 minutes.
4. Add broth and toss to combine, then bring to a simmer. Fold in lemon zest, Parmesan, and herbs. Remove from heat and add butter if using, stirring and tossing until melted.
5. Toss with rigatoni and ½ cup reserved cooking liquid, adding more if pasta seems dry. Top with additional Parmesan if desired.

PER SERVING *About 563 cal, 17 g fat (5 g sat), 35 mg chol, 510 mg sodium, 68 g carb, 3 g fiber, 4 g sugar (0 g added sugar), 35 g pro*

MAKE IT AHEAD

Refrigerate the bolognese and pasta in separate airtight containers for up to four days. When ready to serve, bring a pot of water to a boil and reheat the pasta. Warm the bolognese in a skillet over medium heat. You can also freeze the bolognese in an airtight container for up to three months. Thaw in the refrigerator overnight

CHICKEN *and* RICE *with* FETA VINAIGRETTE

ACTIVE 15 min. **TOTAL** 1 hr. **SERVES** 4

- 1 lemon, plus lemon wedges for serving
- 3 cloves garlic, smashed
- 2 rice cooker cups (1½ cups) basmati rice, rinsed
- Kosher salt and pepper
- 2 8- to 9-oz boneless, skinless chicken breasts
- ½ tsp honey
- 1 scallion, finely chopped
- 4 Tbsp olive oil
- ¼ cup fresh mint, chopped
- 4 cups baby greens
- 1 oz feta, cut into chunks

1. Using vegetable peeler, remove 2 strips lemon zest and add to a rice cooker along with garlic, rice, and ¼ teaspoon salt. Fill with water to second line on cooker and stir.
2. Season chicken with ½ teaspoon salt and ¼ teaspoon pepper and place on steam rack, then transfer to the rice cooker. Cook on white rice setting until program is complete and chicken is cooked through, 30 to 60 minutes.
3. Meanwhile, squeeze 1½ tablespoons lemon juice into a small bowl and whisk in honey and ¼ teaspoon each salt and pepper. Stir in scallion and oil, then mint.
4. Once rice and chicken are ready, transfer chicken and steam rack to a cutting board. Discard lemon zest and garlic cloves. Fluff rice, add greens, close lid and let sit 5 minutes, then fold into rice.
5. Slice chicken and serve with rice, dressing, feta, and lemon wedges.

PER SERVING *About 523 cal, 19 g fat (3.5 g sat), 94 mg chol, 634 mg sodium, 53 g carb, 3 g fiber, 1.5 g sugar (0.5 g added sugar), 33 g pro*

FIBER FIX

Sub in brown rice for more fiber, vitamins, and minerals, plus an overall more filling plate. If your rice cooker has a brown rice setting, use that for best results. If not, extend the cook time to 45 to 60 minutes.

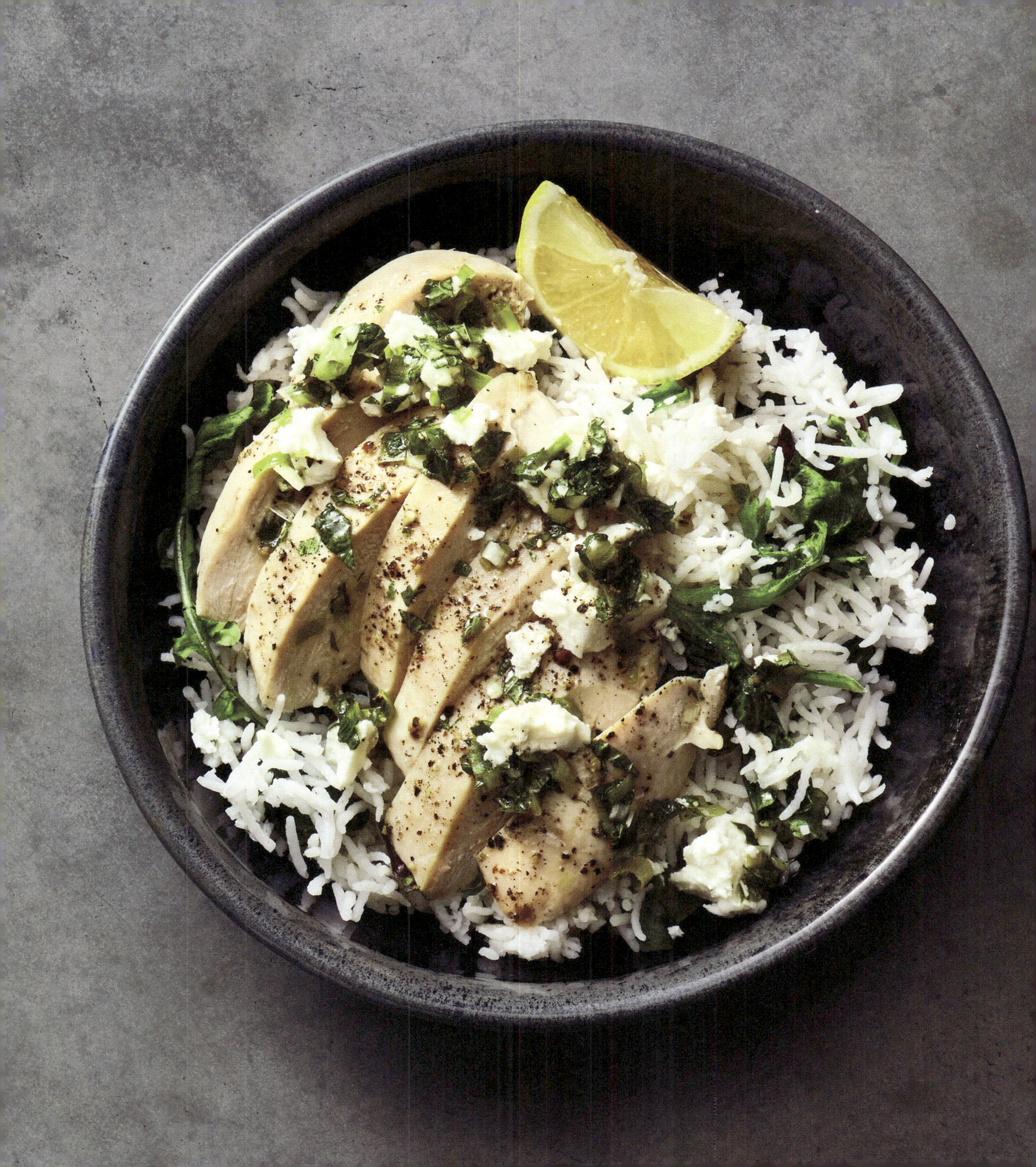

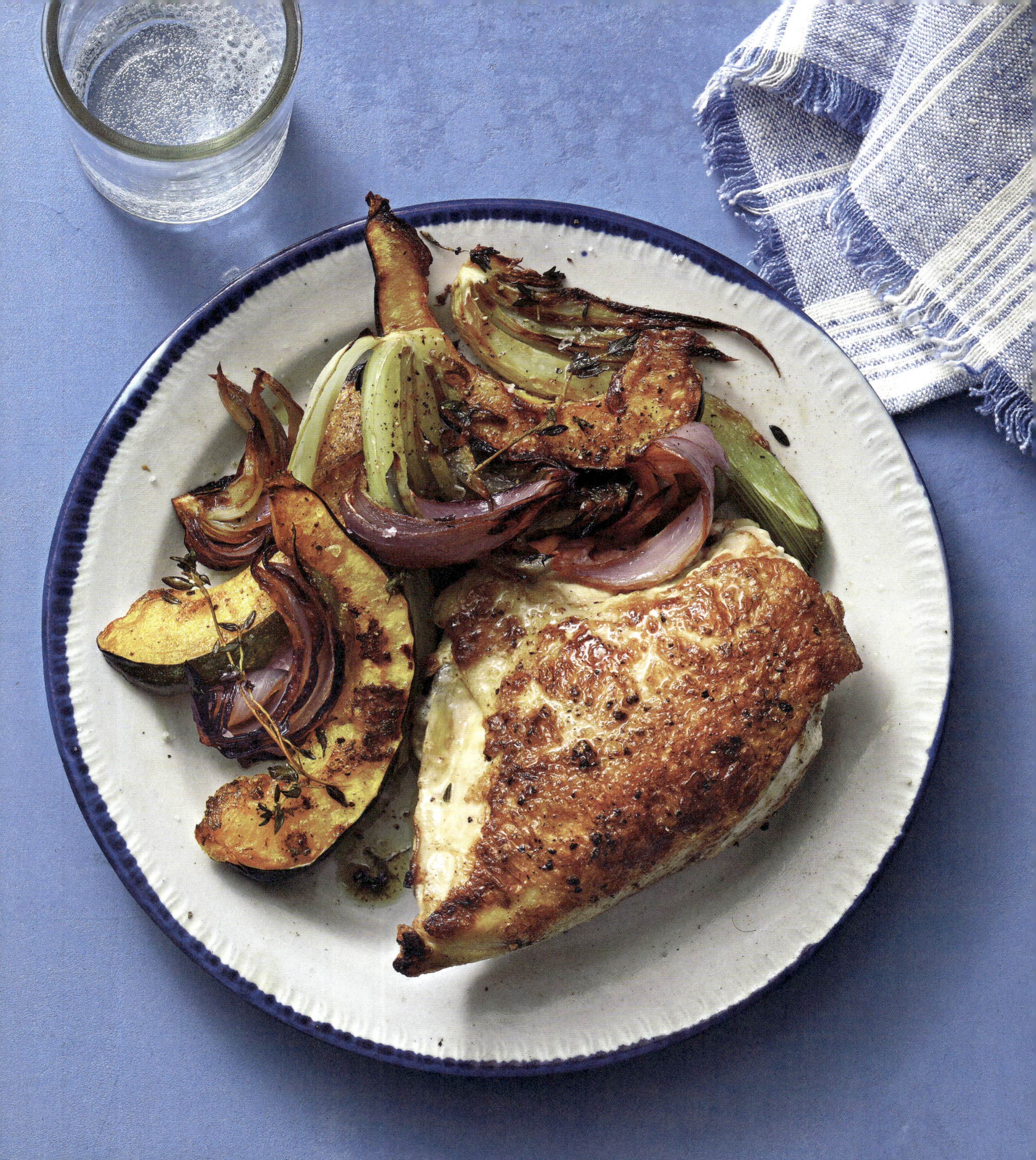

SHEET PAN ROASTED CHICKEN, ACORN SQUASH and FENNEL

ACTIVE 20 min. **TOTAL** 45 min. **SERVES** 4

- 4 small red onions, cut into ½-in.-thick wedges
- 2 small acorn squash (about 1 lb), cut into ¾-in.-thick wedges
- 2 bulb fennel, cut into ½-in-thick wedges
- 3 Tbsp olive oil, divided
- 8 sprigs thyme
- Kosher salt and pepper
- 4 small bone-in chicken breasts (about 1½ lb total)

1. Heat oven to 425°F. On a rimmed baking sheet, toss onions, squash, and fennel with 2 tablespoons oil, thyme, and ½ teaspoon each salt and pepper; transfer half to second sheet and roast 15 minutes.
2. Meanwhile, heat remaining tablespoon oil in large skillet over medium heat. Season chicken with ½ teaspoon each salt and pepper and cook, skin side down, until deep golden brown, 8 to 10 minutes. Flip and cook 3 minutes more.
3. Nestle 2 chicken breasts among veggies on each tray, rotate and swap positions of tray and roast until chicken is cooked through, 15 to 18 minutes. Transfer chicken to plates.
4. Return vegetables to oven and continue roasting until golden brown and tender, 5 minutes more.

PER SERVING *About 360 cal, 18 g fat (3.5 g sat), 83 mg chol, 614 mg sodium, 18 g carb, 5 g fiber, 8.5 g sugar (0 g added sugar), 32 g pro*

LOVE YOUR LEFTOVERS

Make a single-serve chicken and kale salad with any leftovers. In a large bowl, whisk together ½ tablespoon **olive oil**, 2 teaspoons **red wine vinegar**, ¼ teaspoon **Dijon mustard**, and a pinch each of **kosher salt and pepper**. Toss with 3 cups **baby kale**, then with a portion of **vegetables** and some sliced leftover **chicken**. Serve topped with crumbled **goat cheese**.

SMOKY CHICKEN THIGHS on BABY ROMAINE

ACTIVE 20 min. **TOTAL** 20 min. (plus marinating) **SERVES** 4

3 large cloves garlic, grated

⅓ cup fresh lemon juice

⅓ cup plus 2 tsp olive oil

1¾ tsp smoked paprika, divided

Kosher salt

4 5-oz boneless, skinless chicken thighs

3 slices sourdough bread

1 pt cherry or grape tomatoes, halved

2 jarred pepperoncini peppers, sliced

¼ cup flat-leaf parsley, chopped

4 heads baby romaine or little gem lettuce, halved or quartered if large

1 avocado, diced

1. In a medium bowl, whisk together garlic, lemon juice, ⅓ cup oil, 1½ teaspoons smoked paprika, and ½ teaspoon salt. Transfer ¼ cup dressing to a resealable bag, add chicken, and marinate at least 20 minutes, up to 2 hours; reserve remaining dressing.
2. Meanwhile, toast bread until golden brown, then tear into pieces and set aside.
3. Heat remaining 2 teaspoons oil in a large skillet over medium heat. Remove chicken from marinade, season with ¼ teaspoon salt, and cook until golden brown, 4 to 5 minutes per side. Transfer to a cutting board, sprinkle with remaining ¼ teaspoon smoked paprika, then slice.
4. To reserved dressing, add tomatoes, pepperoncini, and parsley and toss to combine.
5. Arrange lettuce on plates, top with torn sourdough, and top with tomato mixture, avocado, and sliced chicken.

PER SERVING *About 555 cal, 33 g fat (6 g sat), 130 mg chol, 808 mg sodium, 34 g carb, 7 g fiber, 5 g sugar (0 g added sugar), 32 g pro*

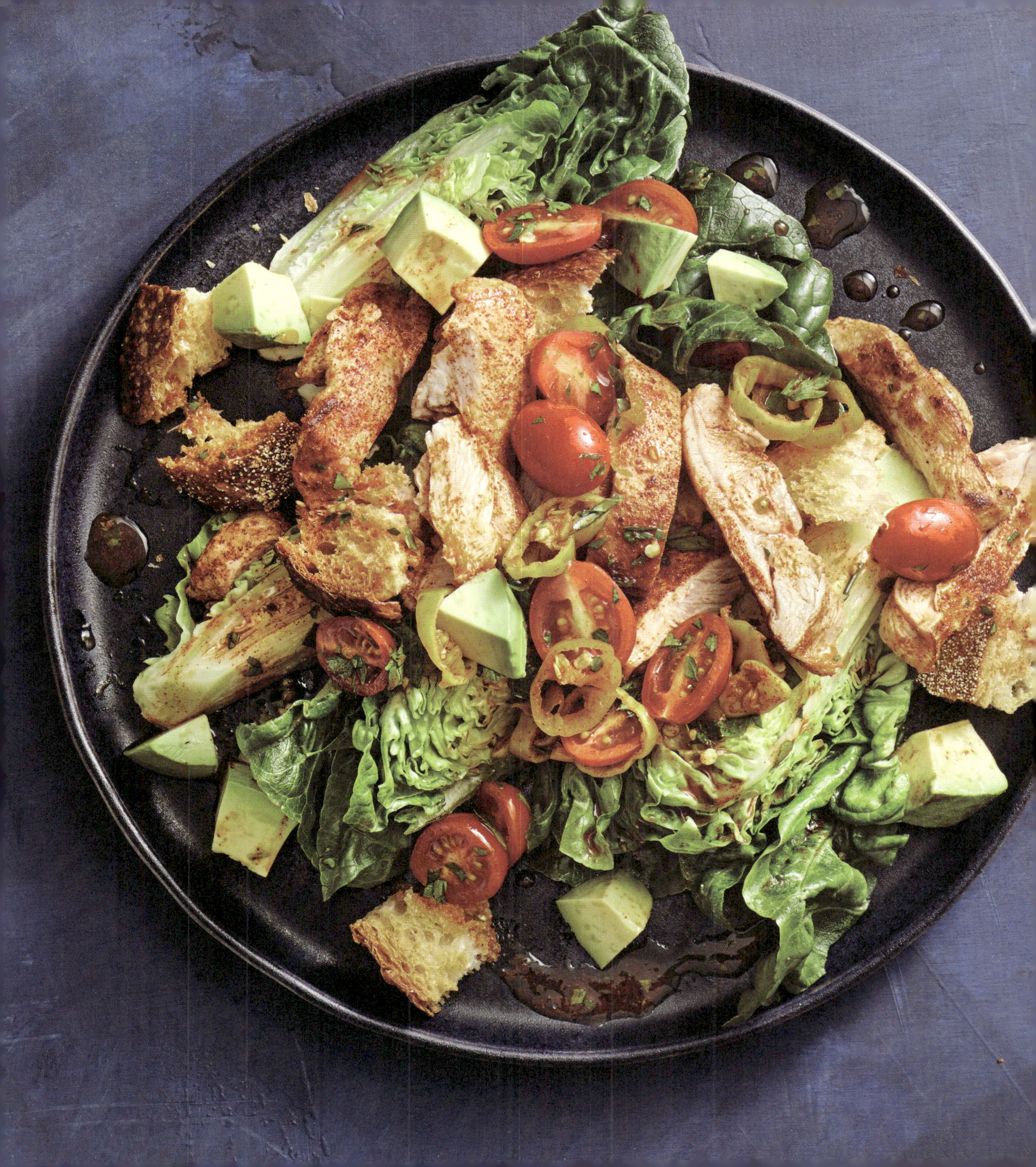

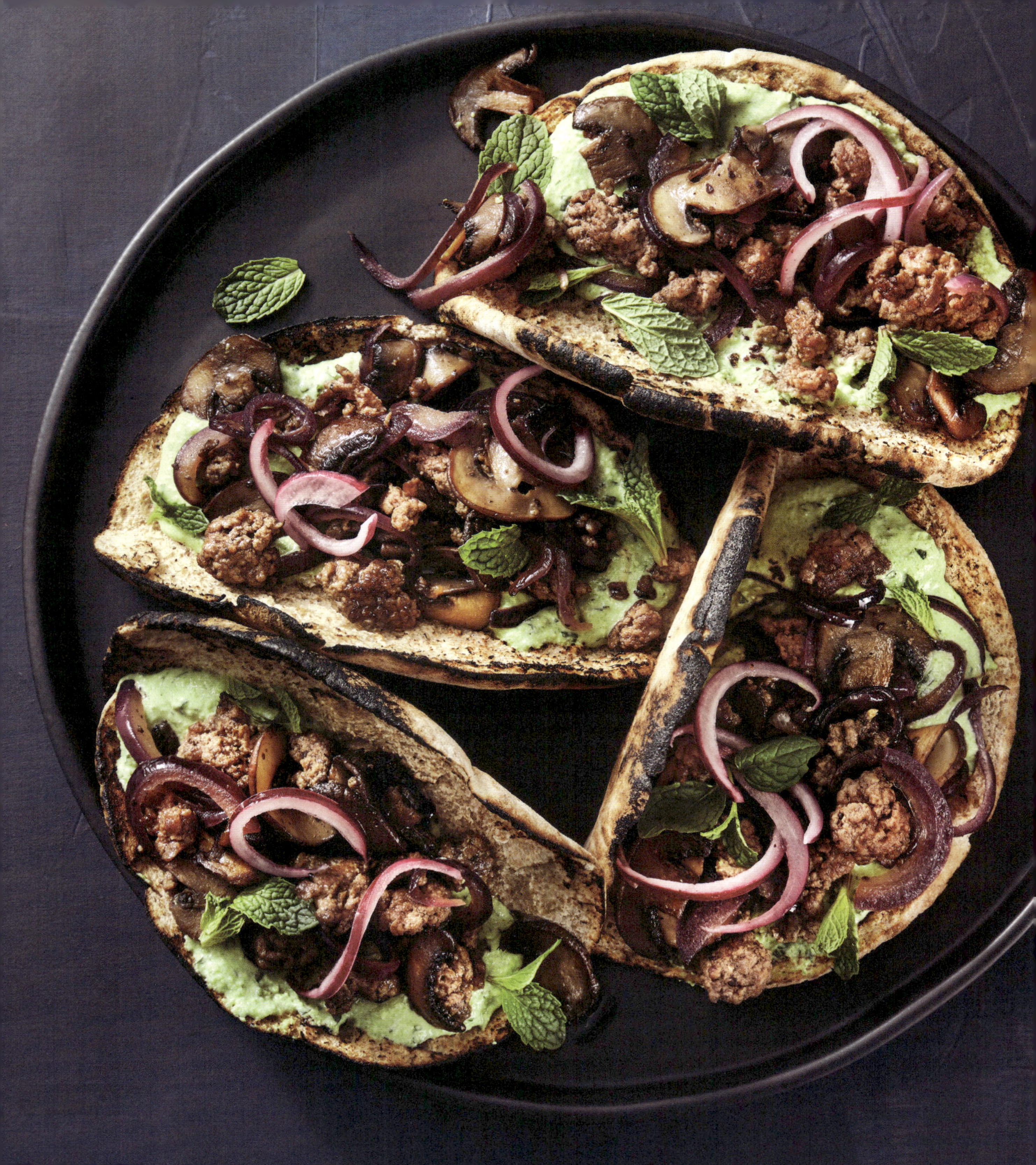

MINTY PEA & SPICED BEEF PITAS

ACTIVE 30 min. **TOTAL** 30 min. **SERVES** 4

2 Tbsp white wine vinegar, divided

¼ tsp sugar

Kosher salt

1 medium red onion, thinly sliced and divided

1½ cups frozen peas, thawed

⅓ cup low-fat cottage cheese

¼ cup mint leaves, plus more for topping

2 Tbsp olive oil

6 oz cremini mushrooms, very thinly sliced

12 oz lean ground beef (at least 90% lean), broken into pieces

¼ tsp sumac

2 whole-wheat pitas, split into 2 rounds and toasted

1. In a small bowl, whisk together 1 tablespoon vinegar, sugar, and ⅛ teaspoon salt. Toss in ¼ sliced onion and let sit until ready to use.
2. In a food processor, process peas, cottage cheese, and ⅛ teaspoon salt, scraping sides as necessary, until smooth. Pulse in mint until chopped.
3. Heat oil in a large skillet over medium-high heat. Add mushrooms in even layer and cook, undisturbed, until starting to brown, 4 to 5 minutes. Reduce heat to medium and sprinkle remaining onion on top; cook, undisturbed, until mushrooms are deep golden brown, 1 to 2 minutes more. Stir onion and mushrooms and scatter beef on top; season with ½ teaspoon each salt and pepper and sumac. Cook, breaking up beef and stirring occasionally, until beef is cooked through and browned, 5 to 6 minutes more. Remove from heat and stir in remaining 1 tablespoon vinegar.
4. Spread pitas with mint peas and top with beef mixture, pickled onions, and additional mint leaves.

PER SERVING *About 354 cal, 14 g fat (3.5 g sat), 56 mg chol, 617 mg sodium, 31 g carb, 6 g fiber, 6 g sugar (0 g added sugar), 27 g pro*

FIBER FIX

Tiny but mighty, peas add both sweet flavor and a surprising fiber boost. Just one cup delivers around 8 grams to help support digestion and keep you full longer.

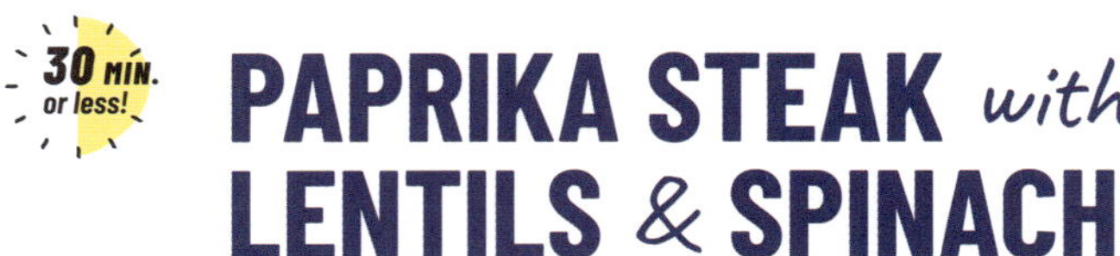

PAPRIKA STEAK *with* LENTILS & SPINACH

ACTIVE 30 min. **TOTAL** 30 min. **SERVES** 4

3 Tbsp olive oil, divided

1 clove garlic, finely chopped

1 cup dry lentils (we used black)

¼ cup dry white wine

3 cups low-sodium chicken broth

2 1-in.-thick strip steaks (about 1½ lb total)

1 Tbsp smoked paprika, plus more for serving

Kosher salt and pepper

5-oz pkg. baby spinach

Plain Greek yogurt and chopped flat-leaf parsley, for serving

1. In a medium saucepan, heat 1 tablespoon oil and garlic over medium heat until garlic is sizzling on the edges. Add lentils and toss to coat. Add wine and simmer 2 minutes. Add broth, partially cover, and bring to a boil, then reduce heat and simmer until tender, 20 to 22 minutes.
2. Meanwhile, pat steaks dry with a paper towel, then rub with paprika and ½ teaspoon each salt and pepper; shake off any excess. Heat 1 tablespoon oil in a large skillet over medium heat and cook to desired doneness, 4 to 5 minutes per side for medium-rare. Transfer to a cutting board and let rest at least 5 minutes before slicing.
3. Discard any excess liquid from lentils, then fold in spinach, remaining tablespoon oil, and ¼ teaspoon each salt and pepper.
4. Serve steak with lentils. Dollop with yogurt and sprinkle with paprika and parsley if desired.

PER SERVING *About 574 cal, 24.5 g fat (7.5 g sat), 102 mg chol, 518 mg sodium, 36 g carb, 11 g fiber, 1 g sugar (0 g added sugar), 54 g pro*

LOVE YOUR LEFTOVERS

Slice only the steak you plan on eating at this meal. Refrigerate the remaining steak and lentils in separate airtight containers for up to three days. For an easy lunch, spread yogurt in a pita pocket. Thinly slice steak and add to pita along with any leftover lentils and some mixed greens or arugula.

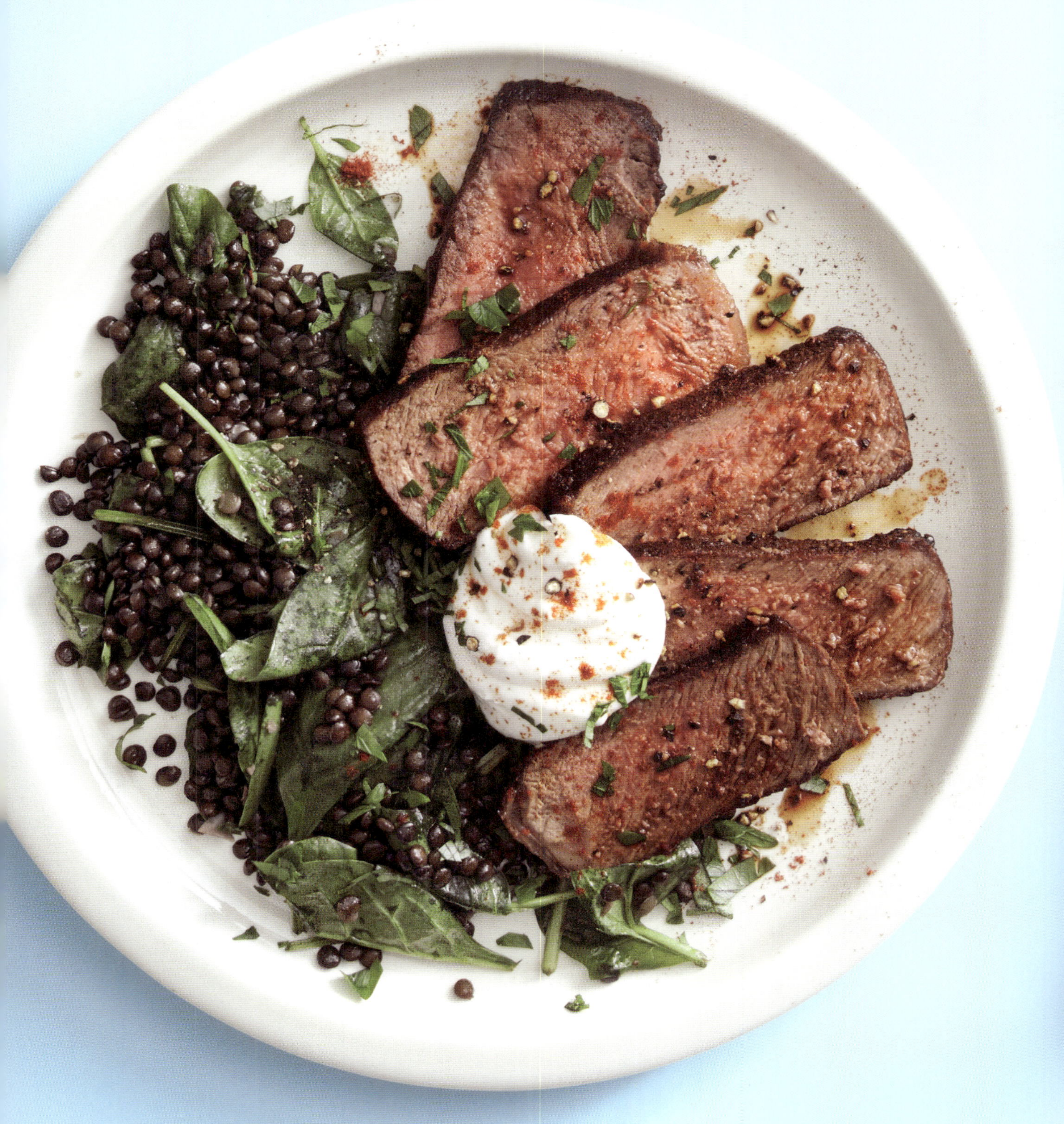

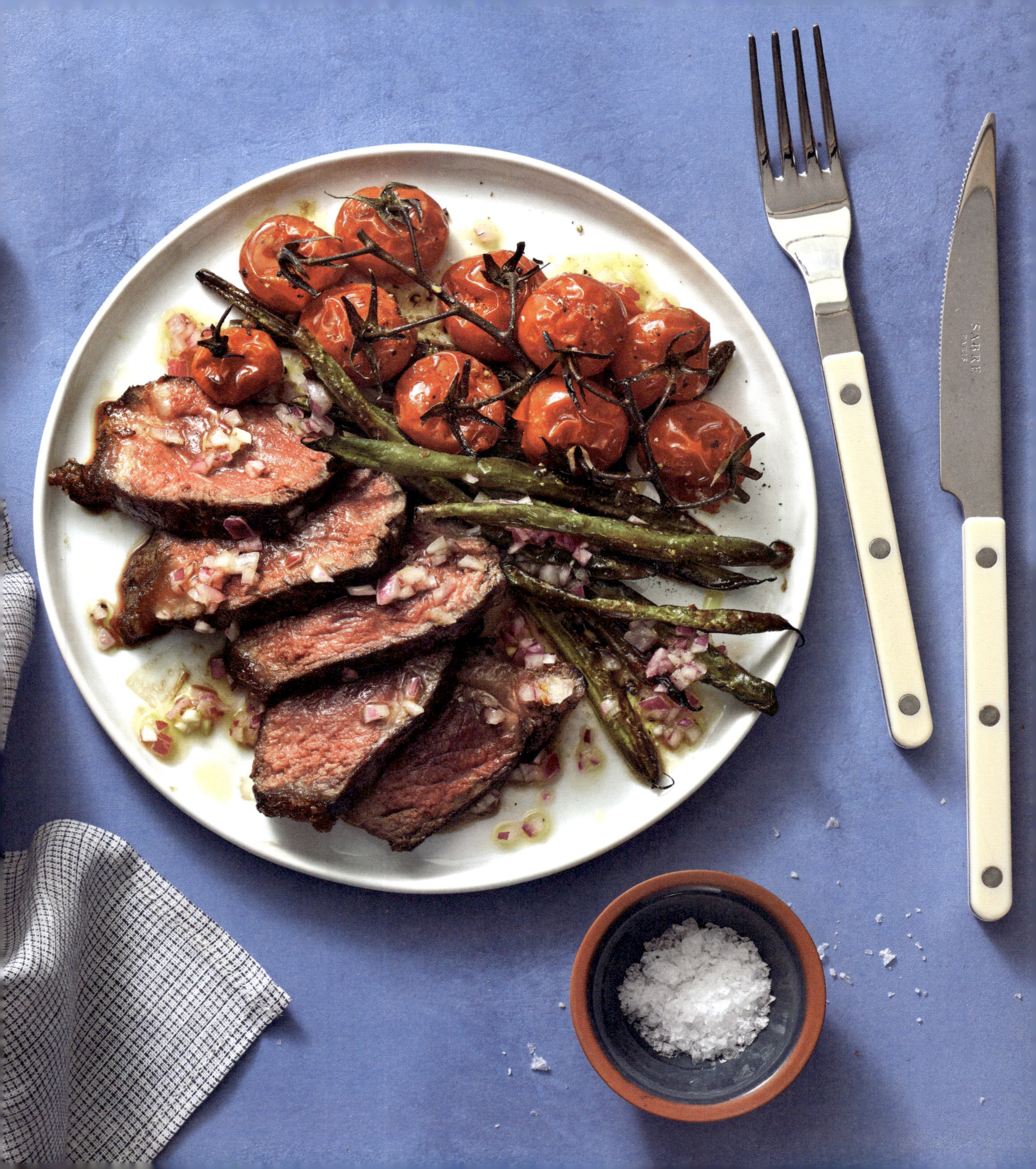
SABRE

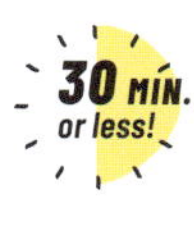

SEARED STEAK *with* BLISTERED TOMATOES & GREEN BEANS

ACTIVE 25 min. **TOTAL** 25 min. **SERVES** 4

1 lb green beans, trimmed

2 pints cherry or grape tomatoes on the vine

4 Tbsp plus 2 tsp olive oil, divided

Kosher salt and pepper

2 1½-in.-thick strip steaks (about 12 oz each)

2 Tbsp white wine vinegar

½ small red onion, finely chopped

1. Heat oven to 450°F. Toss green beans and tomatoes with 2 tablespoons oil and a pinch each salt and pepper on a large rimmed baking sheet. Roast until vegetables begin to brown, 10 to 12 minutes.
2. Meanwhile, heat 2 teaspoons oil in a large cast-iron skillet over medium heat. Season each steak with ¼ teaspoon each salt and pepper and cook until browned, 3 minutes per side. Transfer the skillet to oven and roast to desired doneness, 3 to 4 minutes for medium-rare. Transfer steaks to a cutting board and let rest at least 5 minutes before slicing.
3. In bowl, combine white wine vinegar, remaining 2 tablespoons oil, and ¼ teaspoon each salt and pepper; stir in onions. Serve sliced steak with vegetables and spoon vinegar-onion mixture on top.

PER SERVING *About 479 cal, 29.5 g fat (8 g sat), 104 mg chol, 479 mg sodium, 14 g carb, 5 g fiber, 7.5 g sugar (0 g added sugar), 40 g pro*

KITCHEN TIP

Make sure your skillet is nice and hot: If you add steak to a skillet that's warm but not hot, the outside will cook to a dull gray instead of developing a rich, golden-brown crust.

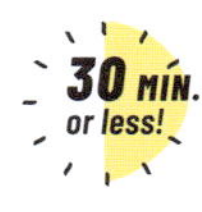

CUMIN AND CORIANDER RUBBED STEAK *with* CARROTS

ACTIVE 25 min. **TOTAL** 25 min. **SERVES** 4

- 1 cup packed cilantro
- 1 cup packed flat-leaf parsley, plus more for serving
- 1 tsp smoked paprika
- 1 large clove garlic
- ½ cup plus 1 Tbsp olive oil, divided
- 1 tsp lemon zest plus 2 Tbsp lemon juice
- Kosher salt and pepper
- 1 tsp ground cumin
- 1 tsp ground coriander
- ½ tsp ground cinnamon
- 1½ lb sirloin steak, cut into 4 pieces
- 1 lb small carrots, scrubbed, halved lengthwise if thick
- 1 oz feta, crumbled

1. Heat grill to medium. In a blender, puree cilantro, parsley, paprika, garlic, ½ cup oil, lemon zest and juice, and ¼ teaspoon each salt and pepper. Transfer to a small bowl.
2. In a separate small bowl, combine cumin, coriander, and cinnamon with ¼ teaspoon salt and ½ teaspoon pepper; rub all over steak. Rub carrots with remaining tablespoon oil and season with ¼ teaspoon each salt and pepper.
3. Grill steak and carrots, covered, until carrots are tender and steak is medium-rare, 3 to 5 minutes per side. Transfer steak to a cutting board and let rest 5 minutes before slicing.
4. Transfer carrots to a platter, drizzle with ¼ cup sauce and sprinkle with feta and parsley. Serve with steak and remaining sauce.

PER SERVING *About 635 cal, 46 g fat (11 g sat), 123 mg chol, 541 mg sodium, 14 g carb, 5 g fiber, 8.5 g sugar (0 g added sugar), 41 g pro*

MAKE IT AHEAD

This herby green sauce is inspired by chermoula, a North African sauce made with fresh herbs, garlic, lemon, oil, and spices. Prep it up to three days ahead and refrigerate in an airtight container with a thin layer of olive oil on top to keep it vibrant and green. Give it a quick stir before serving.

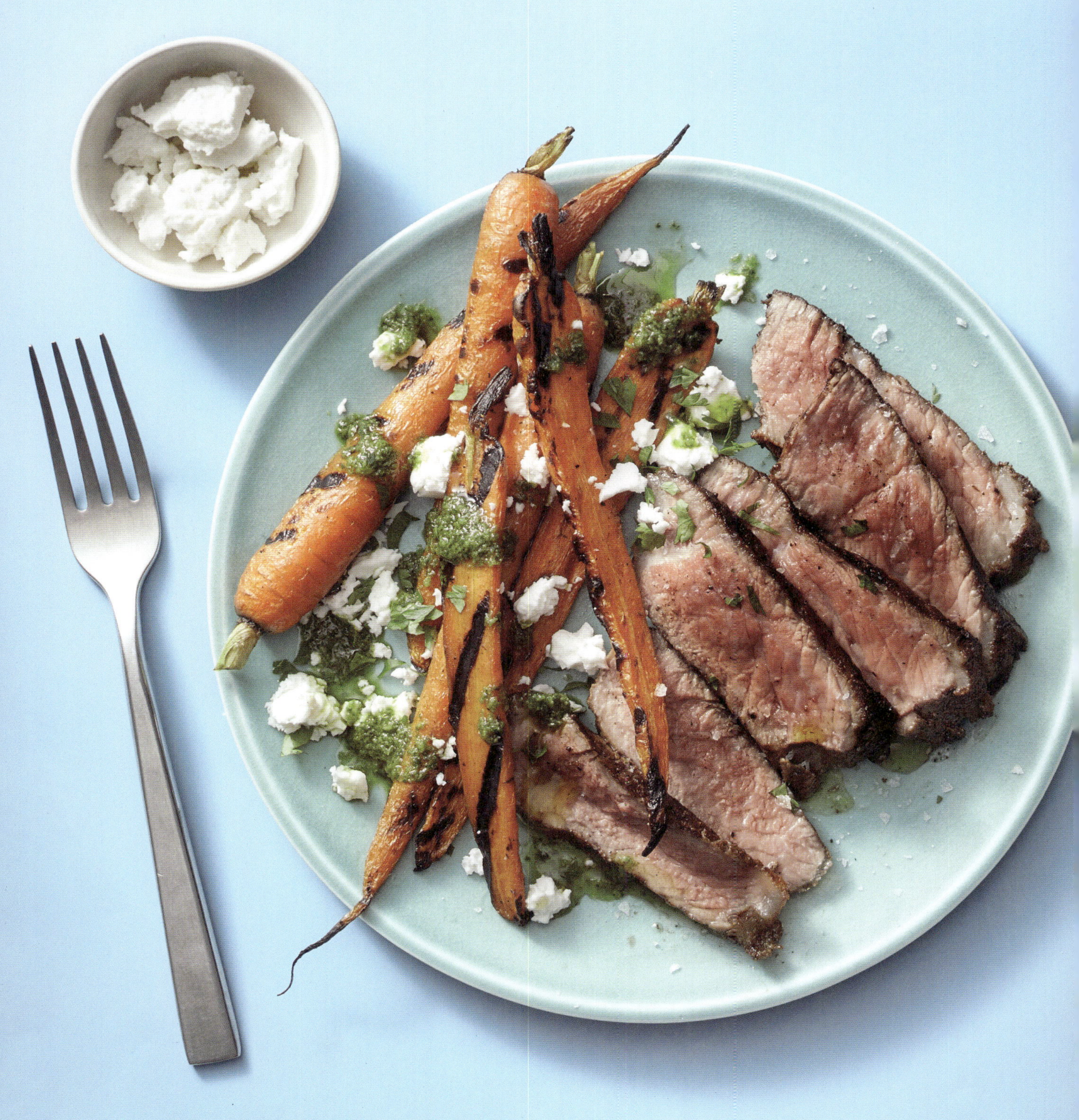

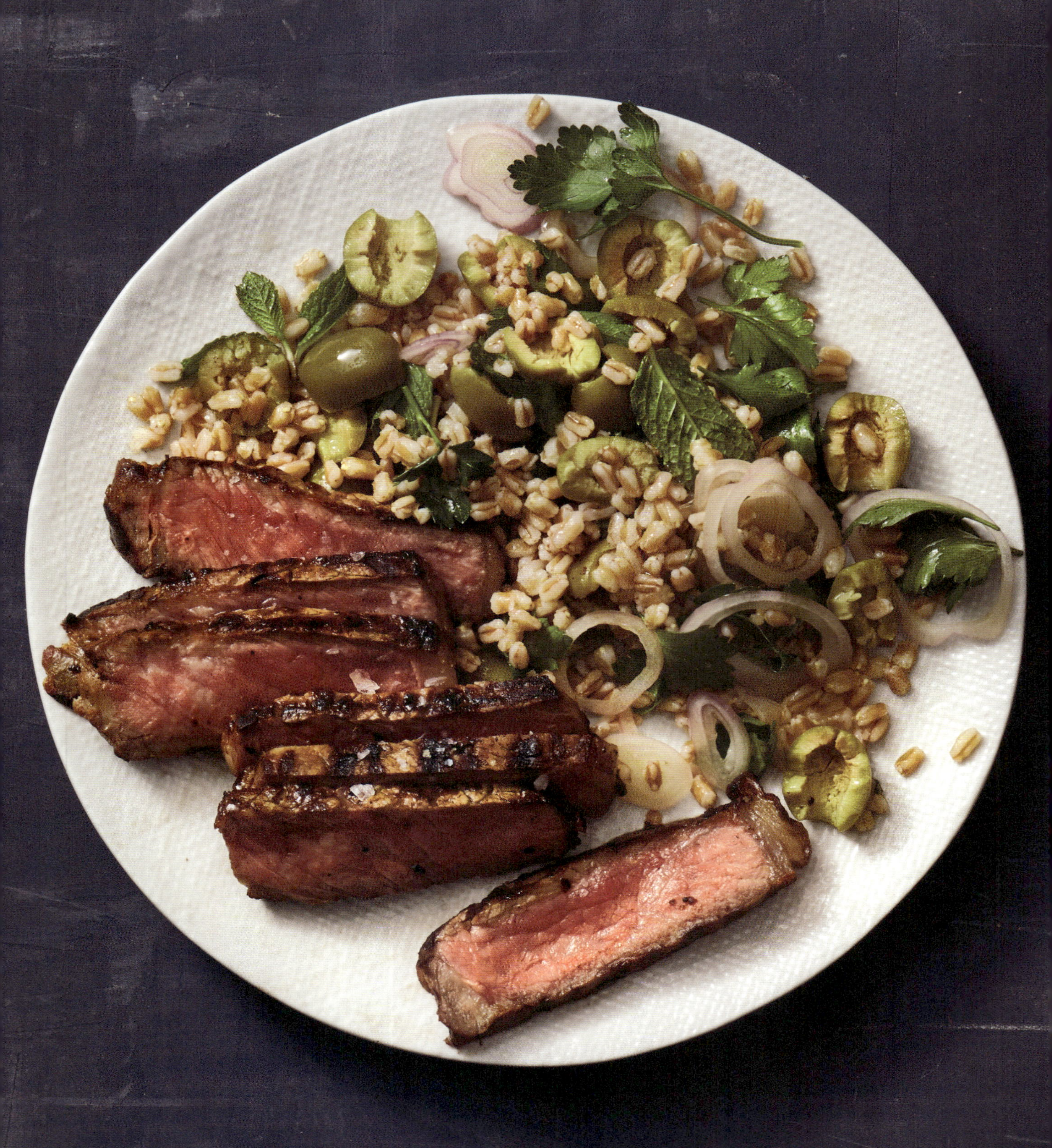

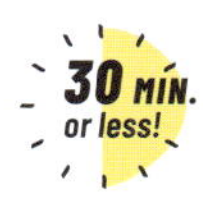

ALEPPO GRILLED STEAK *with* FARRO SALAD

ACTIVE 25 min. **TOTAL** 25 min. **SERVES** 4

- 1½ cups quick-cooking farro
- 2 12-oz strip steaks (each about 1½ in. thick)
- ¾ tsp Aleppo pepper
- Kosher salt and pepper
- 2 tsp grated lemon zest plus 3 Tbsp lemon juice
- 2 small shallots, thinly sliced
- 3 Tbsp olive oil
- ¾ cup pitted Castelvetrano olives, crushed and roughly chopped
- ¼ cup flat-leaf parsley, roughly chopped
- ¼ cup fresh mint torn or roughly chopped

1. Heat grill to medium. Cook farro per package directions.
2. Season steak with Aleppo pepper, ½ teaspoon salt, and ¼ teaspoon pepper and grill steak to desired doneness, 5 to 8 minutes per side for medium-rare. Transfer to a cutting board and let rest at least 5 minutes before slicing.
3. In a medium bowl, combine lemon zest and juice, shallots, and ½ teaspoon each salt and pepper and let sit 5 minutes. Stir in oil, then toss with farro. Fold in olives, parsley, and mint and serve with steak.

PER SERVING *About 698 cal, 31 g fat (10.5 g sat), 101 mg chol, 860 mg sodium, 57 g carb, 9.5 g fiber, 1 g sugar (0 g added sugar), 48 g pro*

MAKE IT AHEAD

Prep the farro salad without the herbs and refrigerate in an airtight container for up to two days. Fold in the herbs just before serving.

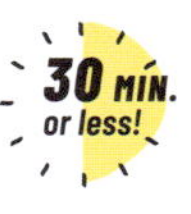

SEARED STEAK *with* CAULIFLOWER "TABBOULEH"

ACTIVE 25 min. **TOTAL** 25 min. **SERVES** 4

- 2 tsp olive oil
- 1 lb sirloin steak (1½-in. thick), cut into 2 pieces
- ½ tsp ground coriander
- Kosher salt and pepper
- 12 oz cauliflower florets
- 1¼ cups curly parsley (including stems), roughly chopped
- 1 cup mixed-color cherry tomatoes, halved
- 2 Persian cucumbers, sliced
- 3 Tbsp fresh lemon juice
- ½ small red onion, finely chopped
- ½ tsp ground cumin

1. Heat oil in a large cast-iron skillet over medium-high heat. Season steak with coriander and ½ teaspoon each salt and pepper and cook to desired doneness, 3 to 5 minutes per side for medium-rare. Transfer to a cutting board and let rest at least 5 minutes before slicing.
2. Meanwhile, in a food processor, pulse cauliflower until very finely chopped (you should have about 2½ cups). Transfer to a large bowl.
3. In the same food processor bowl, pulse parsley until very finely chopped. Add to bowl with cauliflower along with cherry tomatoes, cucumbers, lemon juice, onion, cumin, and ½ teaspoon each salt and pepper and toss to combine. Serve with steak.

PER SERVING *About 307 cal, 19 g fat (6.5 g sat), 75 mg chol, 573 mg sodium, 10 g carb, 3 g fiber, 3.5 g sugar (0 g added sugar), 25 g pro*

KITCHEN TIP
When making cauliflower tabbouleh or rice, don't over-pulse—stop when the pieces are the size of grains of rice. Over-processing can make it mushy instead of light and fluffy.

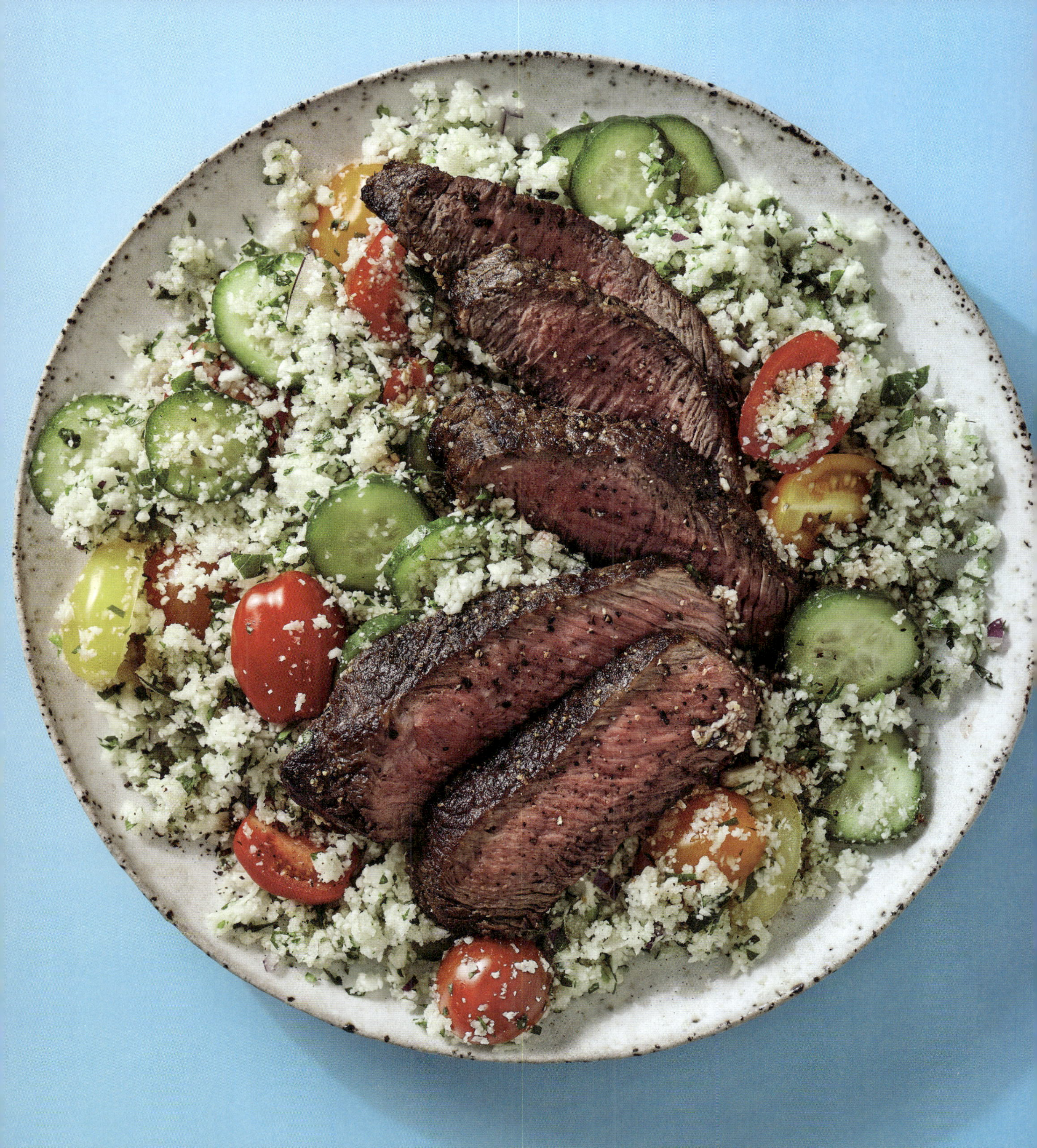

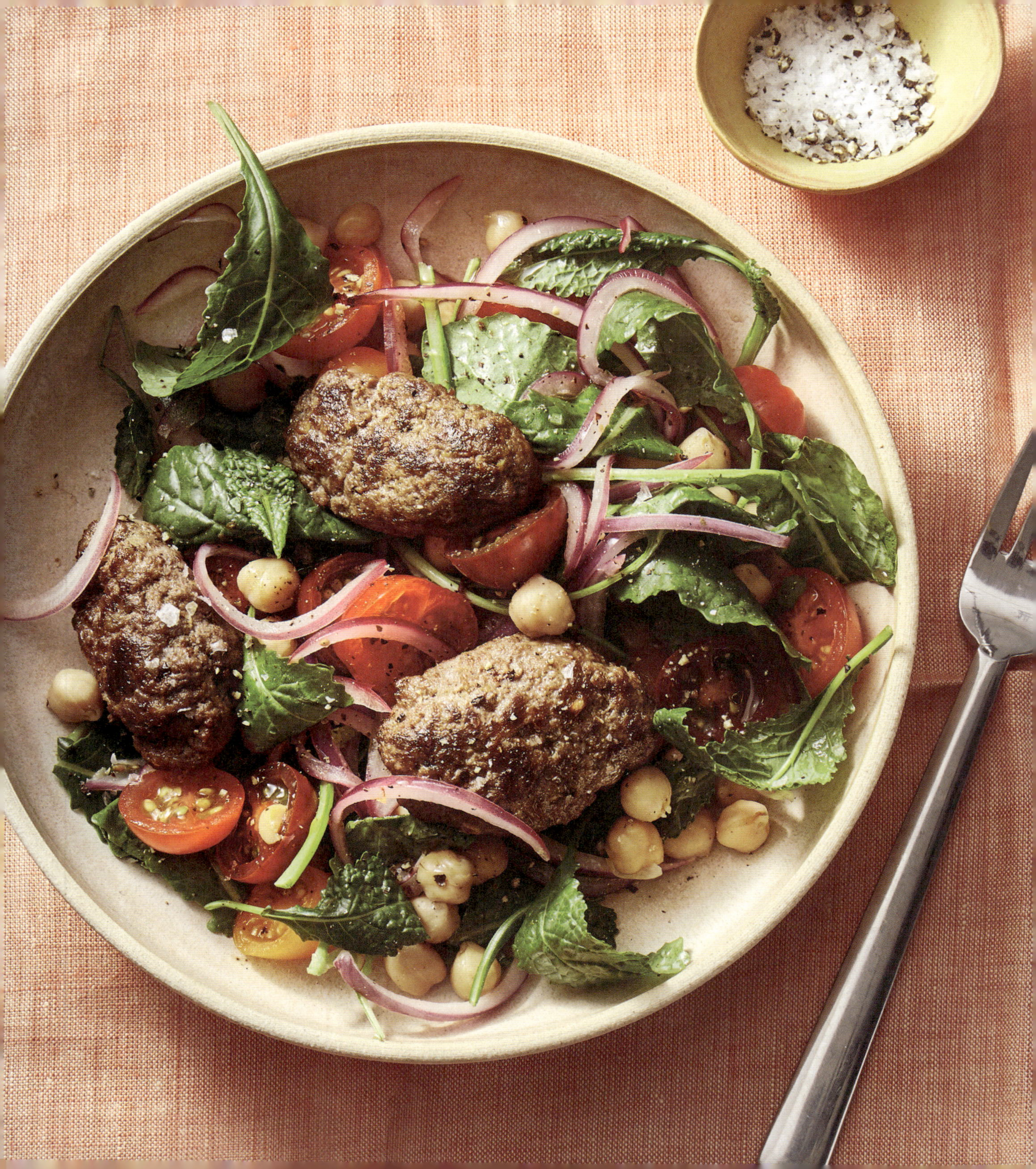

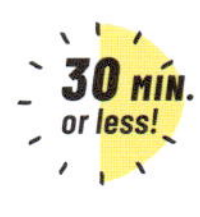

BEEF KOFTA *with* KALE *and* CHICKPEA SALAD

ACTIVE 20 min. **TOTAL** 20 min. **SERVES** 4

1 lemon

1 lb ground beef

2 cloves garlic, finely chopped

1½ tsp ground cumin

1½ tsp ground coriander

Kosher salt and pepper

3 Tbsp olive oil, divided

½ tsp dried oregano

1 small red onion, thinly sliced

15-oz can chickpeas, rinsed

4 cups baby kale

1 pint cherry tomatoes, halved if large

1. Finely grate zest of lemon and squeeze 3 tablespoons juice. In a large bowl, combine beef, garlic, cumin, coriander, lemon zest, 1 tablespoon lemon juice, and ½ teaspoon each salt and pepper. Form mixture into 12 flat ovals.
2. Heat 1 tablespoon oil in large skillet and cook kofta until browned and barely cooked through, 1½ to 2 minutes per side.
3. In another large bowl, whisk oregano with remaining 2 tablespoons oil and remaining 2 tablespoons lemon juice. Add onion and chickpeas and toss to combine. Let sit 5 minutes then toss with kale and tomatoes. Serve with kofta.

PER SERVING *About 386 cal, 20 g fat (5 g sat), 70 mg chol, 472 mg sodium, 23 g carb, 7 g fiber, 5.5 g sugar (0 g added sugar), 29 g pro*

MAKE IT AHEAD
Refrigerate cooked kofta in an airtight container for up to three days. Warm in a covered skillet over medium heat.

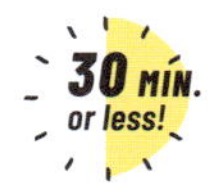

FRESH VEGGIE BEEF RAGU

ACTIVE 5 min. **TOTAL** 25 min. **SERVES** 4

12 oz linguine

1 lemon

2 Tbsp olive oil, divided

1 lb lean ground beef

2 cloves garlic

2 Tbsp tomato paste

½ cup dry white wine

1 pt cherry tomatoes

½ red onion

Parmesan and basil, if desired

1. Cook linguine according to package directions. Before draining, reserve 1 cup cooking liquid and set aside. Drain and return pasta to the pot. Grate the zest from the lemon directly into the pot. Then squeeze in the lemon juice. Add 1 tablespoon oil, and toss with pasta. Add reserved cooking liquid if the pasta seems dry.

2. While the pasta cooks, brown ground beef in a large skillet in 1 tablespoon oil, breaking it up into tiny pieces, 6 minutes. Finely chop garlic and stir into beef; cook 1 minute. Add tomato paste and cook, stirring, until beef starts to get crispy. Add wine and simmer until it evaporates, 3 minutes.

3. Thinly slice red onion. Cut cherry tomatoes in half. Toss the beef with pasta, cherry tomatoes, and red onion. Sprinkle with Parmesan and basil if desired.

PER SERVING *About 665 cal, 26 g fat (7.5 g sat), 77 mg chol, 328 mg sodium, 72 g carb, 5 g fiber, 5 g sugar (0 g added sugar), 34 g pro*

KITCHEN TIP
Choose at least 90% lean ground beef to cut down on saturated fat while still getting plenty of protein and flavor.

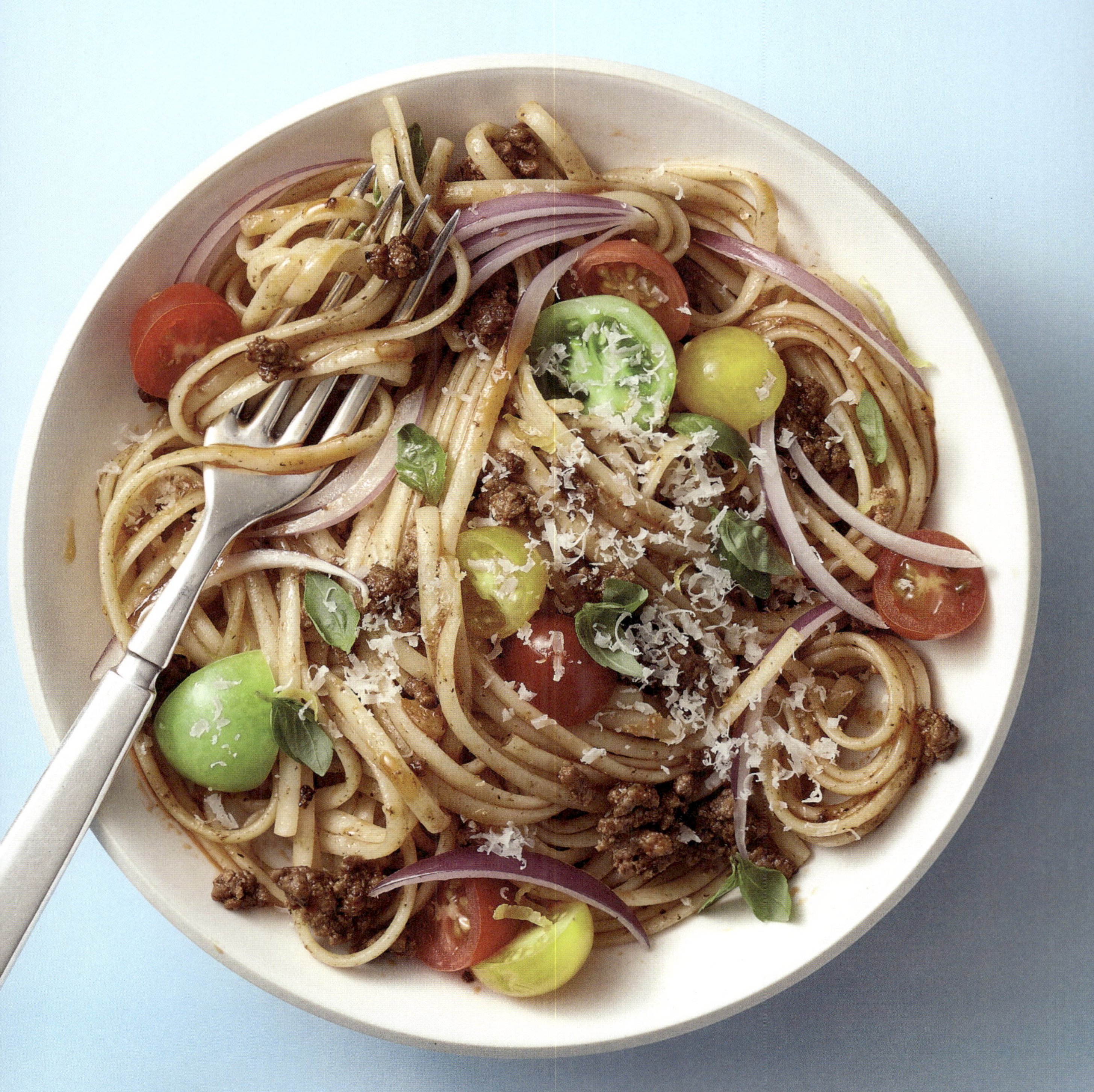

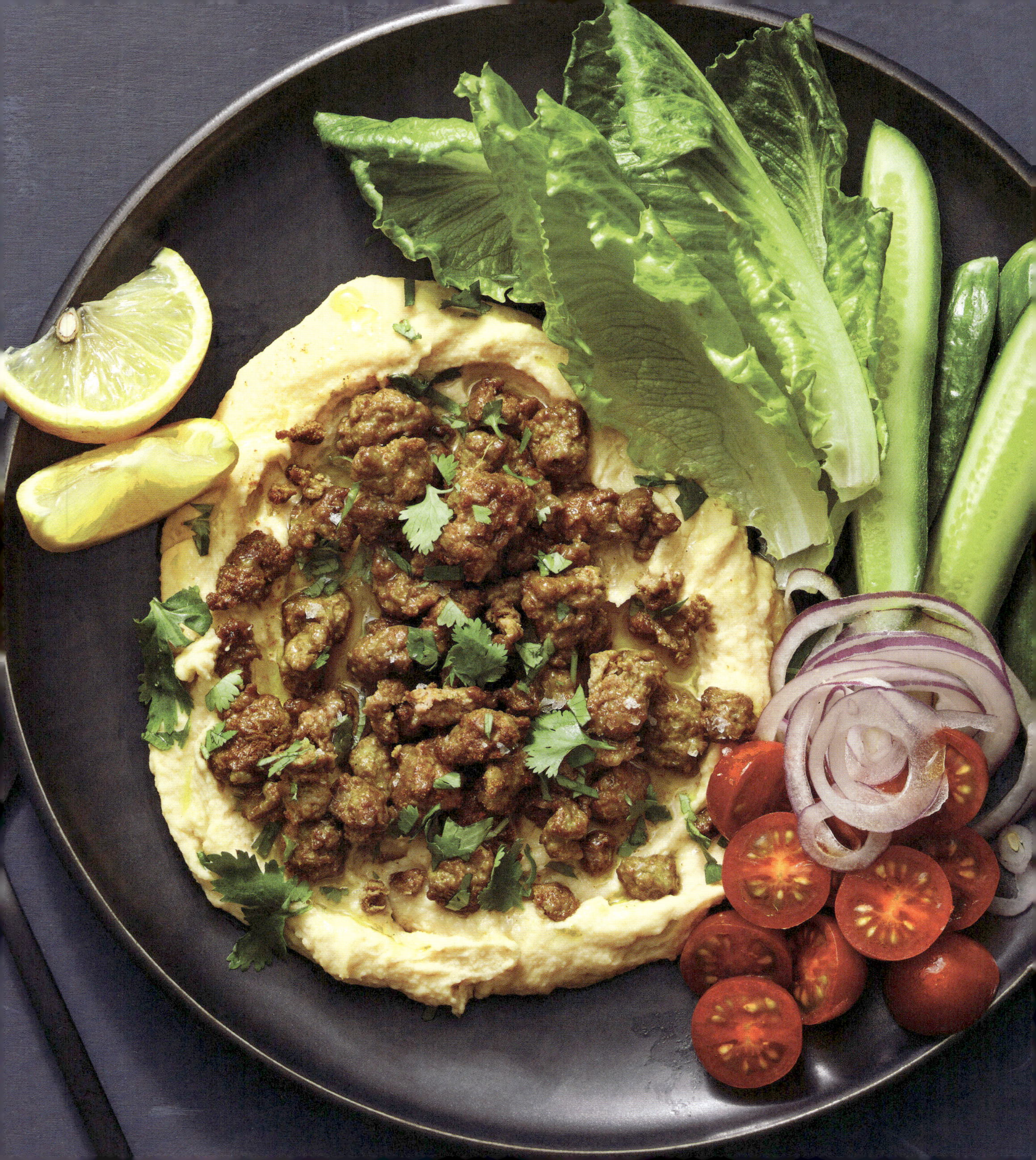

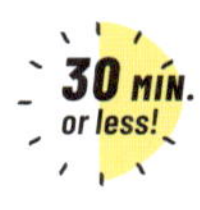

SPICED GROUND LAMB on WARM LENTIL HUMMUS

ACTIVE 30 min. **TOTAL** 30 min. **SERVES** 4

- ¾ cup split red lentils (masoor dal)
- 1 lb ground lamb (or dark meat ground turkey)
- 3 Tbsp shawarma seasoning
- 3 large cloves garlic, grated, divided
- Kosher salt
- 3½ Tbsp olive oil (4 Tbsp if using ground turkey), divided
- ½ tsp ground cumin
- ¼ cup plus 2 Tbsp fresh lemon juice, plus lemon wedges for serving
- ⅓ cup tahini
- Pinch of cayenne pepper
- ½ cup cilantro, chopped
- 2 heads Little Gem lettuce, leaves separated
- 4 small Persian cucumbers, quartered
- Halved cherry tomatoes and sliced red onion, for serving

1. In a small saucepan, combine lentils and 1¼ cups water; bring to a boil. Cover and simmer on very low until mostly tender and water is absorbed, 10 minutes. Remove from heat and let steam, covered, 5 minutes.

2. Meanwhile, in a bowl, combine ground lamb (or ground turkey) with shawarma seasoning, two-thirds of garlic, and ¾ teaspoon salt. Heat 1½ tablespoons oil (2 tablespoons for turkey) in large cast-iron skillet over medium-high heat. Cook lamb, breaking up a bit with wooden spoon, until turning brown and just cooked through, 5 to 6 minutes.

3. Transfer warm cooked lentils to a food processor with remaining garlic, cumin, and ¾ teaspoon salt and puree, scraping sides of bowl as necessary, until smooth, about 3 minutes. Pulse in lemon juice; add tahini and 1 tablespoon oil and puree until smooth, adding up to 2 more tablespoons lemon juice to taste.

4. Divide warm hummus among bowls and top with lamb. Sprinkle with remaining tablespoon oil, cayenne pepper, and cilantro. Serve with lettuce and cucumbers along with cherry tomatoes, red onion, and lemon wedges if desired.

PER SERVING *About 661 cal, 40.5 g fat (11.5 g sat), 61 mg chol, 829 mg sodium, 43 g carb, 9 g fiber, 4 g sugar (0 g added sugar), 35 g pro*

LOVE YOUR LEFTOVERS

Lentil hummus is a fun twist that adds extra protein and fiber while staying creamy. Make a double batch and refrigerate the extra in an airtight container for up to four days.

LAMB CHOPS & SNAP PEA SALAD

ACTIVE 25 min. **TOTAL** 35 min. **SERVES** 4

FOR LAMB CHOPS
½ red onion, finely chopped

2 Tbsp rice vinegar

Kosher salt and pepper

1 rack of lamb, trimmed

2 Tbsp olive oil, divided

2 tsp coriander, crushed

1 tsp ground sumac

¼ cup fresh mint, chopped

2 Tbsp flat-leaf parsley, chopped

FOR SALAD
1½ Tbsp fresh lemon juice

1 Tbsp olive oil

Pinch of sugar

Kosher salt and pepper

1 small fennel bulb very thinly sliced

¼ red onion, very thinly sliced

6 oz sugar snap peas, halved lengthwise

¼ cup flat-leaf parsley leaves

¼ cup small mint leaves

¼ cup small basil leaves

1. Heat oven to 425°F. In a small bowl, combine onion, vinegar, and ¼ teaspoon salt. Let sit until lamb is finished.
2. On a rimmed baking sheet, coat lamb with 1 tablespoon oil, then season with coriander, sumac, and ½ teaspoon each salt and pepper. Roast to desired doneness, 20 to 25 minutes for medium-rare. Let rest at least 10 minutes before slicing.
3. Meanwhile, in a medium bowl, whisk together lemon juice, oil, sugar, and ½ teaspoon each salt and pepper to dissolve. Add fennel and onion and let sit, tossing occasionally, 10 minutes then fold in snap peas and herbs.
4. While lamb is resting, stir remaining tablespoon oil into onion mixture, then fold in mint and parsley.
5. Cut lamb into chops and serve with salad and onion herb dressing.

PER SERVING *About 605 cal, 48.5 g fat (17.5 g sat), 124 mg chol, 782 mg sodium, 12 g carb, 5 g fiber, 4.5 g sugar (0 g added sugar), 30 g pro*

LOVE YOUR LEFTOVERS
Refrigerate any leftover lamb in an airtight container for up to three days. Reheat gently in a covered skillet over low heat with a splash of broth or water to keep them moist. Or wrap in foil and warm at 300°F for 10 to 15 minutes.

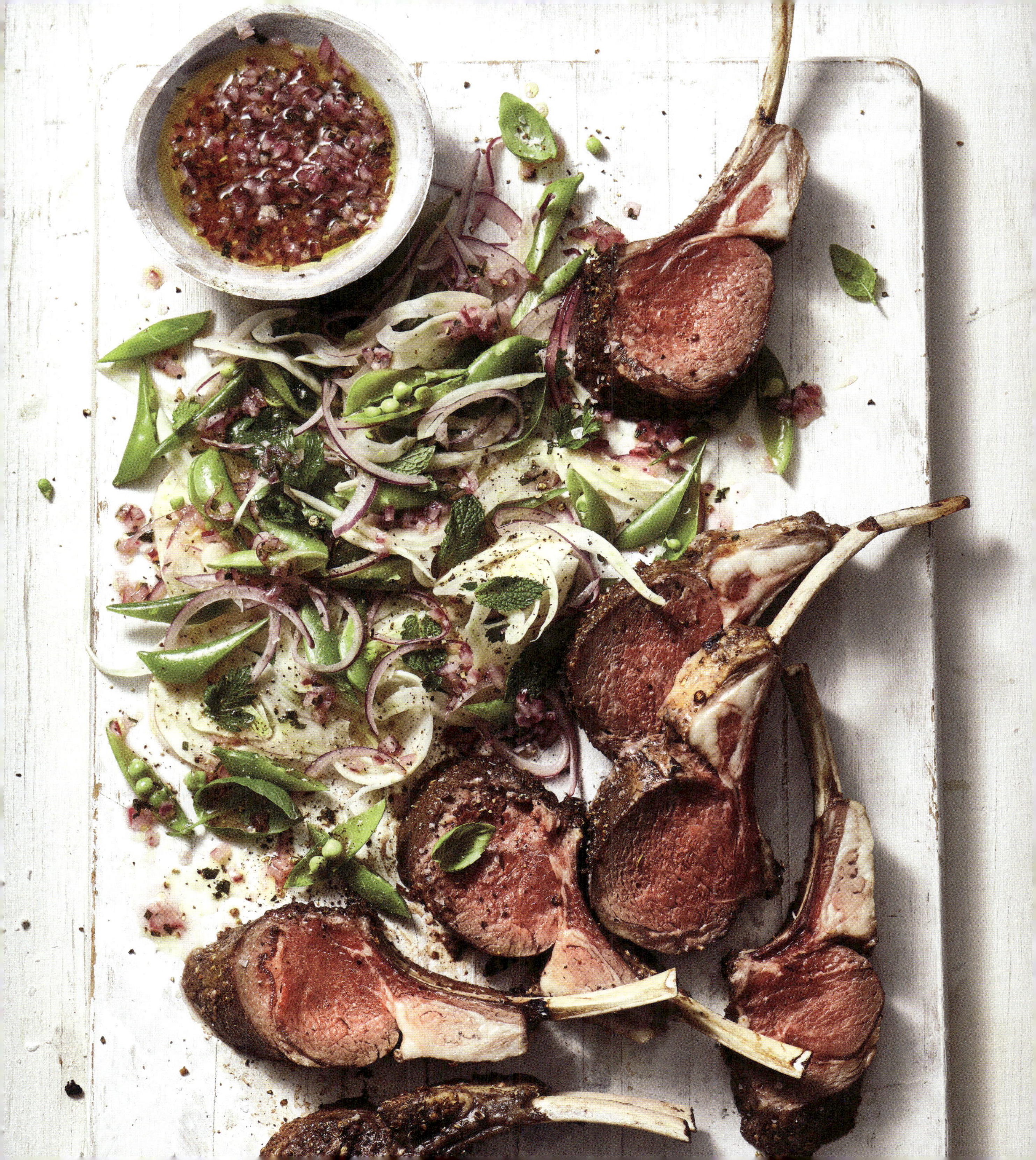

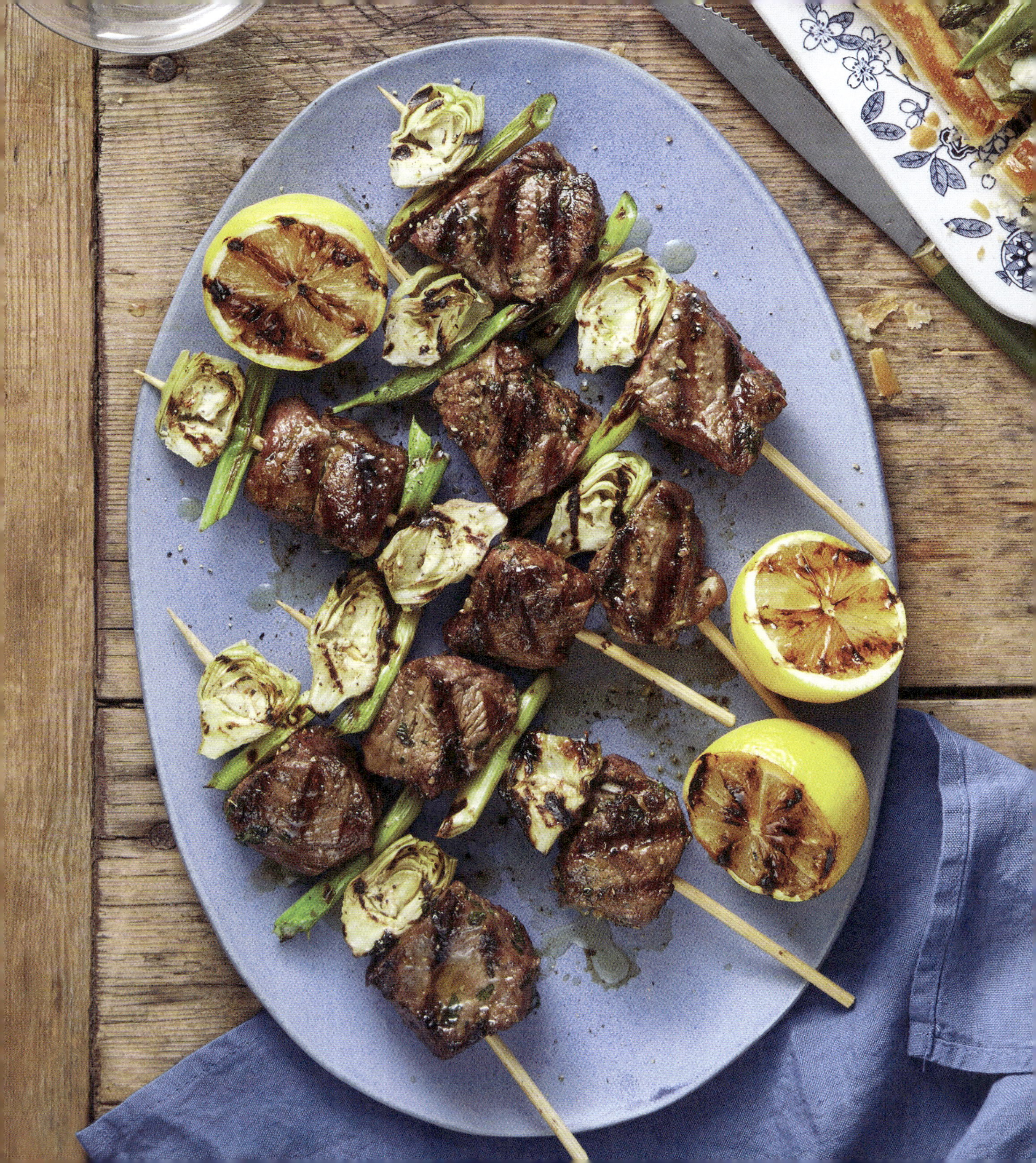

GRILLED LAMB & ARTICHOKE KEBABS

ACTIVE 25 min. **TOTAL** 1 hr. 30 min. **SERVES** 4

1½ lb boneless lamb leg, trimmed and cut into 1-in. chunks

3 Tbsp olive oil, divided

1 tsp ground coriander

1 tsp dried oregano

Kosher salt and pepper

3 lemons

2 cloves garlic, finely chopped

¼ cup flat-leaf parsley, chopped

¾ cup bulgur

1 bunch scallions

12 large marinated artichoke hearts

1. In a large bowl, toss lamb with 2 tablespoons oil, then coriander, oregano, and ½ teaspoon each salt and pepper. Finely grate zest of 2 lemons over lamb; add garlic and parsley and toss to combine. Let sit 1 hour or refrigerate overnight.
2. Meanwhile, In a medium saucepan, bring 1¼ cups water to a boil. Stir in bulgur and ½ teaspoon salt and simmer, covered, until nearly tender, 9 minutes. Remove from heat and let sit, covered, 3 minutes, then fluff with fork.
3. Thinly slice dark greens from 2 scallions and fold into bulgur along with remaining 1 tablespoon oil. Cut all lemons and artichokes in half and all remaining scallions crosswise into 2½-inch pieces.
4. Heat grill or a grill pan over medium-high heat. Thread artichokes, scallion pieces and lamb onto skewers.
5. Grill kebabs, turning occasionally, until lamb reaches desired doneness, 6 to 8 minutes for medium-rare. Grill lemons, cut sides down, until charred, 2 to 3 minutes. Squeeze over kebabs and serve with bulgur.

PER SERVING *About 507 cal, 27 g fat (5.5 g sat), 116 mg chol, 929 mg sodium, 31 g carb, 9 g fiber, 3 g sugar (0 g added sugar), 38 g pro*

FIBER FIX

While marinated artichoke hearts aren't as fiber-rich as their fresh, whole counterparts, artichokes are one of the best natural sources of inulin, a prebiotic fiber that feeds healthy gut bacteria and supports digestion.

HERB PORK with MUSHROOMS and KALE

ACTIVE 15 min. **TOTAL** 40 min. **SERVES** 4

- 3 Tbsp finely chopped mixed fresh herbs, such as parsley, mint, chives, rosemary, and thyme
- 1 small clove garlic, finely grated
- 1 tsp lemon zest
- ¼ tsp red pepper flakes
- 4½ Tbsp olive oil, divided
- 4 small shallots, peeled and halved
- Kosher salt and pepper
- 1 pork tenderloin (about 1¼ lb), halved crosswise
- 8 oz small cremini mushrooms, halved (or quartered if large)
- 1 large bunch green curly kale (about 1 lb), ribs removed, leaves torn into pieces

1. In a small bowl, combine herbs, garlic, lemon zest, red pepper flakes, and 1½ tablespoons oil.
2. Heat an air fryer to 400°F. In a large bowl, toss shallots with 1 tablespoon oil and ⅛ teaspoon each salt and pepper. Season pork with ¼ teaspoon salt. Transfer shallots and pork to the air fryer and cook 5 minutes.
3. Brush herb mixture over top and sides of pork, flip shallots, and continue cooking 5 minutes.
4. While pork and shallots cook, in the same large bowl, toss mushrooms with 1 tablespoon oil and a pinch each of salt and pepper. Add mushrooms to air fryer (with shallots and pork) and cook until pork registers 145°F on instant-read thermometer and mushrooms and shallots are golden brown and tender, 5 to 7 minutes more. Transfer pork to a cutting board and let rest at least 10 minutes before slicing. Transfer vegetables to a plate.
5. In the same large bowl, toss kale with remaining 1 tablespoon oil and a pinch each of salt and pepper, add to the air fryer basket and cook until kale has wilted and edges are slightly crisp, 3 to 5 minutes. Return mushrooms and shallots to the air fryer and toss to combine. Slice pork and serve with vegetables.

PER SERVING *About 307 cal, 19 g fat (6.5 g sat), 75 mg chol, 573 mg sodium, 10 g carb, 3 g fiber, 3.5 g sugar (0 g added sugar), 25 g pro*

KITCHEN TIP

To easily stem kale leaves, grab the stem by its bottom with one hand and strip the leave off by pulling them through your fingers on your other hand—like sliding off a zipper.

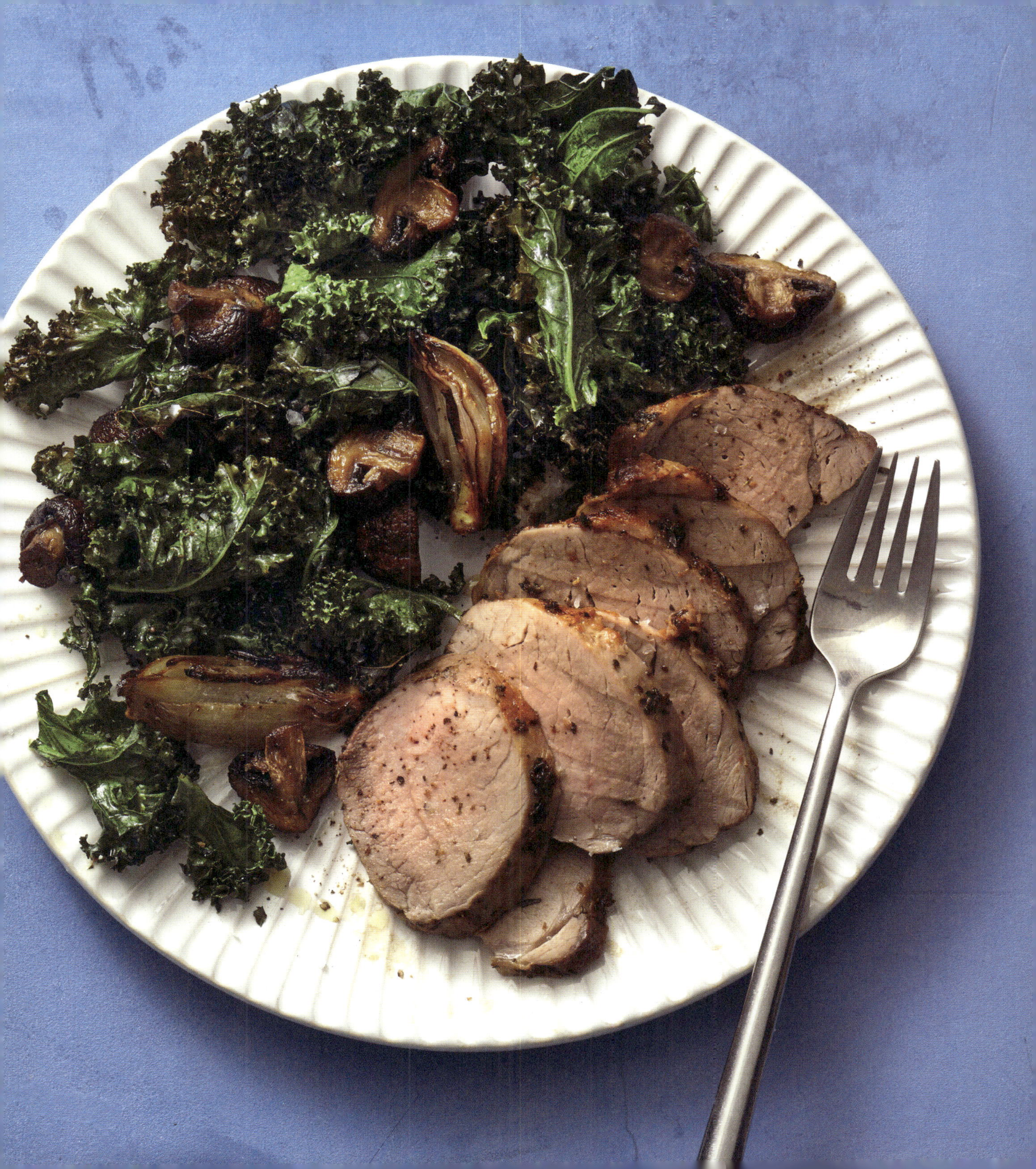

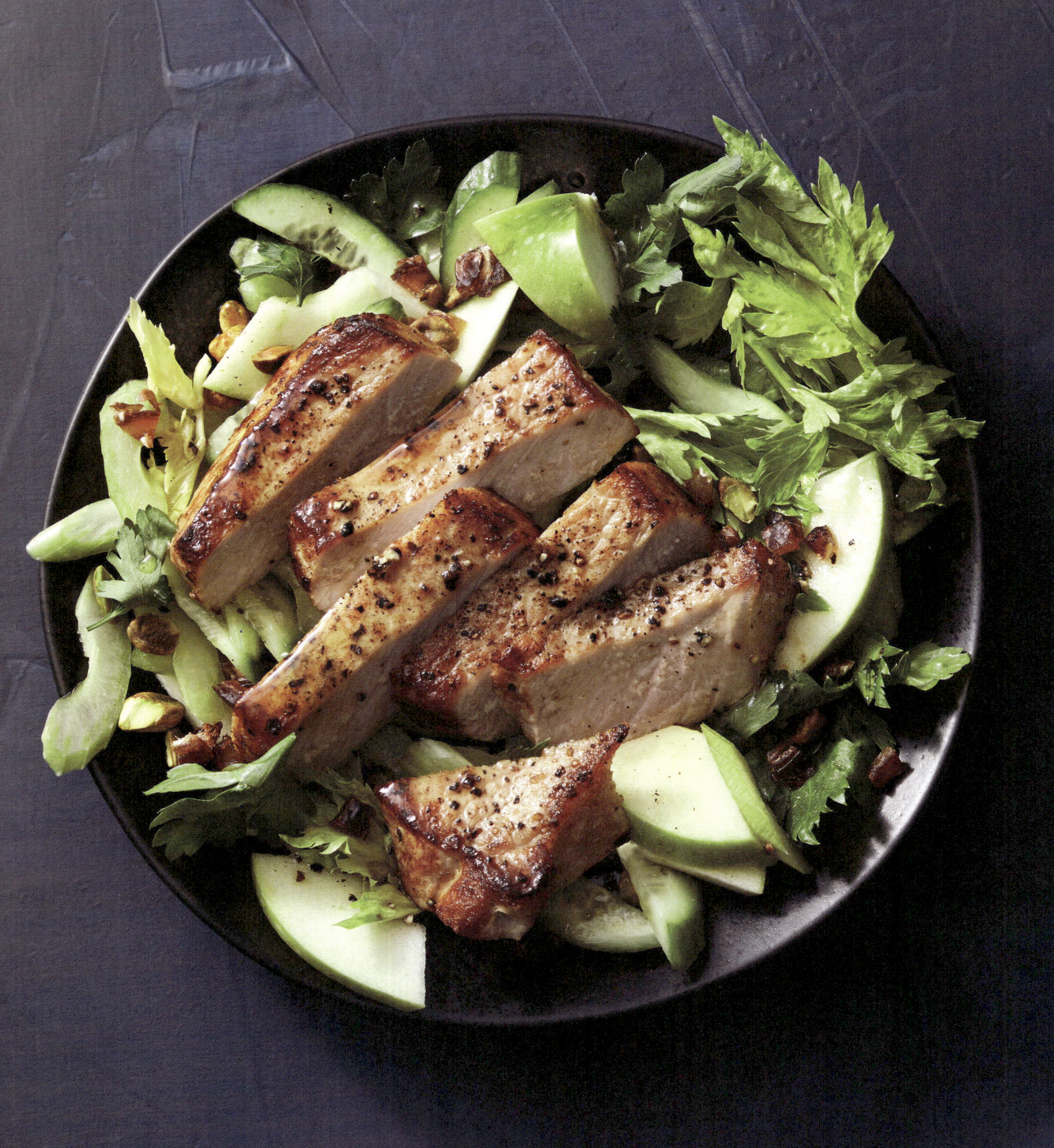

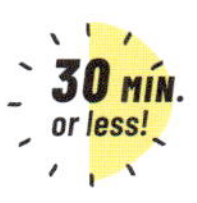

PORK CHOPS *with* CELERY *and* APPLE SALAD

ACTIVE 25 min. **TOTAL** 25 min. **SERVES** 4

- 3½ Tbsp olive oil, divided
- 4 6-ounce boneless pork chops (each about 1 inch thick)
- Kosher salt and pepper
- 1½ Tbsp fresh lemon juice
- 4 ribs celery, thinly sliced, plus ½ cup celery leaves
- 1 green apple, quartered, cored, and thinly sliced crosswise
- 2 Persian cucumbers, halved lengthwise, thinly sliced on bias
- 1 cup fresh flat-leaf parsley leaves
- 2 Medjool dates, pitted and chopped
- 3 Tbsp roasted salted pistachios, chopped and divided

1. Heat oven to 400°F. Heat 1 tablespoon oil in a large ovenproof skillet over medium heat. Season pork with ¼ teaspoon each salt and pepper. Cook until golden brown on one side, 4 to 5 minutes. Flip and cook 1 minute, then transfer a skillet to oven and roast until thermometer registers 145°F when inserted into thickest part, 2 to 4 minutes. Transfer to plates and let rest until ready to serve.

2. In a large bowl, whisk together lemon juice, ½ teaspoon salt, ¼ teaspoon pepper, and remaining 2½ tablespoon oil. Toss in celery and celery leaves, apple, cucumbers, parsley, dates, and half of pistachios.

3. Serve salad alongside pork sprinkled with remaining pistachios.

PER SERVING *About 501 cal, 31.5 g fat (8.5 g sat), 102 mg chol, 544 mg sodium, 17 g carb, 3 g fiber, 11.5 g sugar (0 g added sugar), 39 g pro*

FIBER FIX

Medjool dates are often mistaken for dried fruit, but they're actually fresh. Compared to regular dried dates, they're larger and softer in texture, sweeter and richer in flavor, and higher in fiber and potassium.

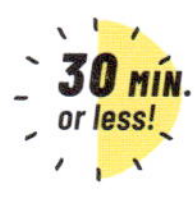

PORK *with* GRILLED SWEET POTATO FRIES

ACTIVE 30 min. **TOTAL** 30 min. **SERVES** 4

- ⅓ cup walnuts
- 1 small clove garlic
- 1 small jalapeño, cut up
- ½ cup mint leaves
- 1 Tbsp capers
- Kosher salt and pepper
- 1 Tbsp honey
- 1 Tbsp fresh lemon juice
- ⅓ cup plus 2 Tbsp olive oil, divided
- 3 large sweet potatoes, cut into 1-in. wedges
- 4 bone-in pork chops (about 1-in.-thick)

1. Heat grill over medium heat. Make salsa verde: In a food processor, finely chop walnuts, garlic, jalapeño, mint, capers, and a pinch of salt. Pulse in honey, lemon juice, and ⅓ cup oil.
2. Toss sweet potatoes with 1 tablespoon oil and ¼ teaspoon each salt and pepper. Brush pork chops with remaining tablespoon oil and season with ¼ teaspoon each salt and pepper.
3. Grill, covered, until potatoes are tender and the pork is just cooked through, 5 to 7 minutes per side. Serve with salsa verde.

PER SERVING *About 540 cal, 28.5 g fat (7 g sat), 132 mg chol, 442 mg sodium, 26 g carb, 5 g fiber, 10.5 g sugar (4.5 g added sugar), 44 g pro*

MAKE IT AHEAD

Classic Italian salsa verde leans on parsley, anchovies, and vinegar. This version puts a spicy-sweet spin on tradition with mint, jalapeño, and honey. Prep it up to three days ahead and refrigerate in an airtight container with a thin layer of olive oil on top to keep it vibrant and green. Give it a quick stir before serving.

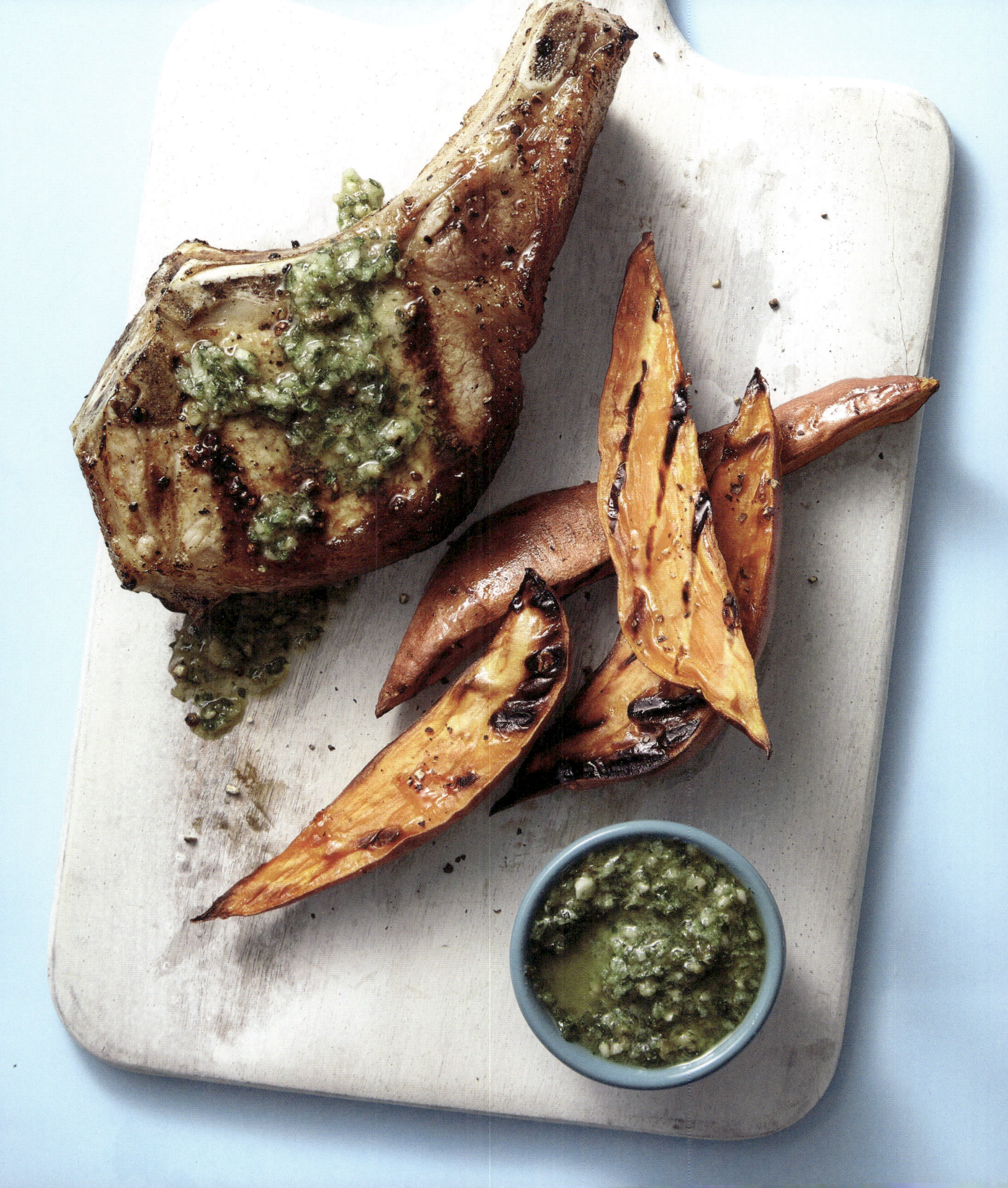

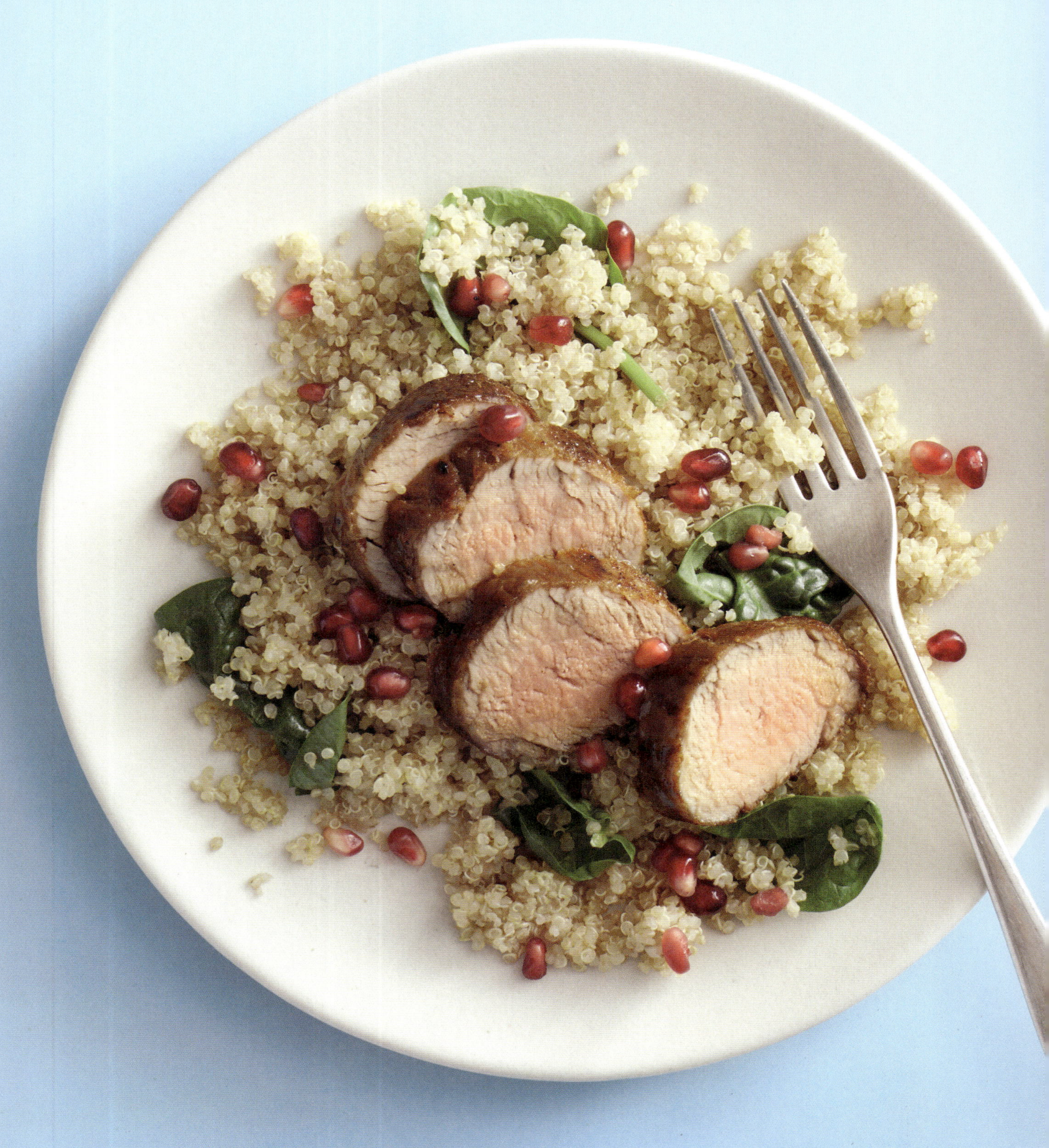

PORK TENDERLOIN *with* QUINOA PILAF

ACTIVE 25 min. **TOTAL** 35 min. **SERVES** 4

- 2 Tbsp olive oil, divided
- 1 clove garlic, thinly sliced
- 1½ cups quinoa
- 4 cups baby spinach (about 5 oz)
- 2 small pork tenderloins (about ¾ lb each), cut into 4 equal pieces
- Kosher salt and pepper
- 2 Tbsp white wine vinegar
- 2 Tbsp orange marmalade
- 2 tsp Dijon mustard
- ½ cup pomegranate seeds

1. Heat 1 tablespoon oil in a medium saucepan over medium heat. Add garlic and cook, stirring occasionally, until toasted, about 2 minutes. Add quinoa and cook per package directions. Fluff with a fork and fold in spinach.
2. While quinoa cooks, heat a skillet over medium heat. Add remaining tablespoon oil, season pork with ½ teaspoon each salt and pepper, and cook until browned on all sides and an instant-read thermometer registers 145°F, 12 to 14 minutes.
3. Meanwhile, in small bowl, whisk together vinegar, marmalade, and mustard. Transfer pork to a cutting board and let rest 5 minutes. Discard any oil left in the pan. Add mustard mixture to skillet and simmer until thickened, 2 to 3 minutes. Brush on pork.
4. Slice pork, serve over quinoa, and sprinkle with pomegranate seeds.

PER SERVING *About 544 cal, 16.5 g fat (3 g sat), 95 mg chol, 410 mg sodium, 54 g carb, 6 g fiber, 10.5 g sugar (0 g added sugar), 44 g pro*

LOVE YOUR LEFTOVERS

Slice only the pork you plan on eating at this meal. Store the remaining pork and quinoa in separate airtight containers for up to three days. You can slice and serve the pork cold in sandwiches, cube and toss into salads, or reheat, then slice and serve warm. Reheat quinoa in the microwave, covered, in 30-second intervals until heated through.

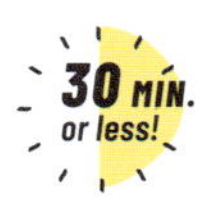

PORK TENDERLOIN SKEWERS *with* HERBED COUSCOUS

ACTIVE 30 min. **TOTAL** 30 min. **SERVES** 4

2 lemons

2 cloves garlic, pressed or finely grated

1 Tbsp olive oil

Kosher salt and pepper

1-lb pork tenderloin

5 scallions, each cut into four 2-in. pieces

1 cup couscous

1 cup fresh mint leaves, finely chopped

¾ cup flat-leaf parsley, finely chopped

½ seedless cucumber, cut into very small pieces

2 oz feta cheese, crumbled

1. Heat grill to medium-high. Finely grate the zest of 1 lemon into a medium bowl and squeeze in juice (you should get about 3 tablespoons). Add garlic, oil, and ½ teaspoon each salt and pepper and mix to combine. Thinly slice pork on a diagonal, add to the bowl along with scallions, and toss to coat.

2. Place couscous in a medium bowl. Finely grate the zest of the remaining lemon over the top; mix to combine. Add 1¼ cups boiling water, cover, and let sit until all the water has been absorbed, about 10 minutes.

3. Meanwhile, thread pork and scallions onto skewers and grill until just cooked through, 2 to 3 minutes per side. Squeeze juice of the zested lemon over the top; transfer to plates.

4. Fluff the couscous, then toss with mint, parsley, cucumber, and feta. Serve with pork skewers.

PER SERVING *About 412 cal, 12 g fat (4.5 g sat), 88 mg chol, 343 mg sodium, 41 g carb, 5 g fiber, 2.5 g sugar (0 g added sugar), 34 g pro*

KITCHEN TIP

Tenderloin typically has a strip of connective tissue, called silver skin, that's tough and chewy. To remove it before cooking, slip the tip of a sharp knife under one end of the silvery skin and carefully slice along its length, pulling it away with your other hand as you go.

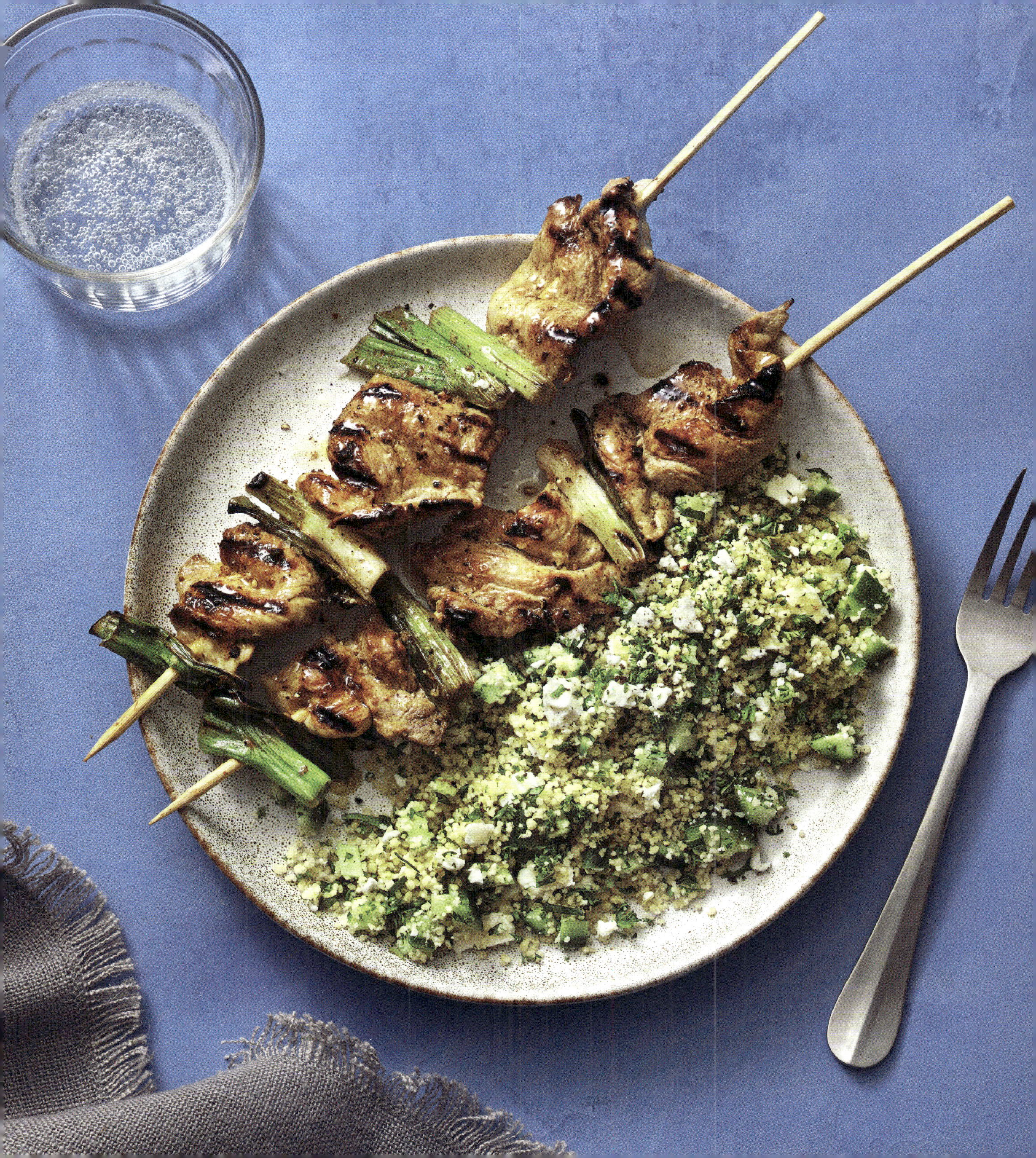

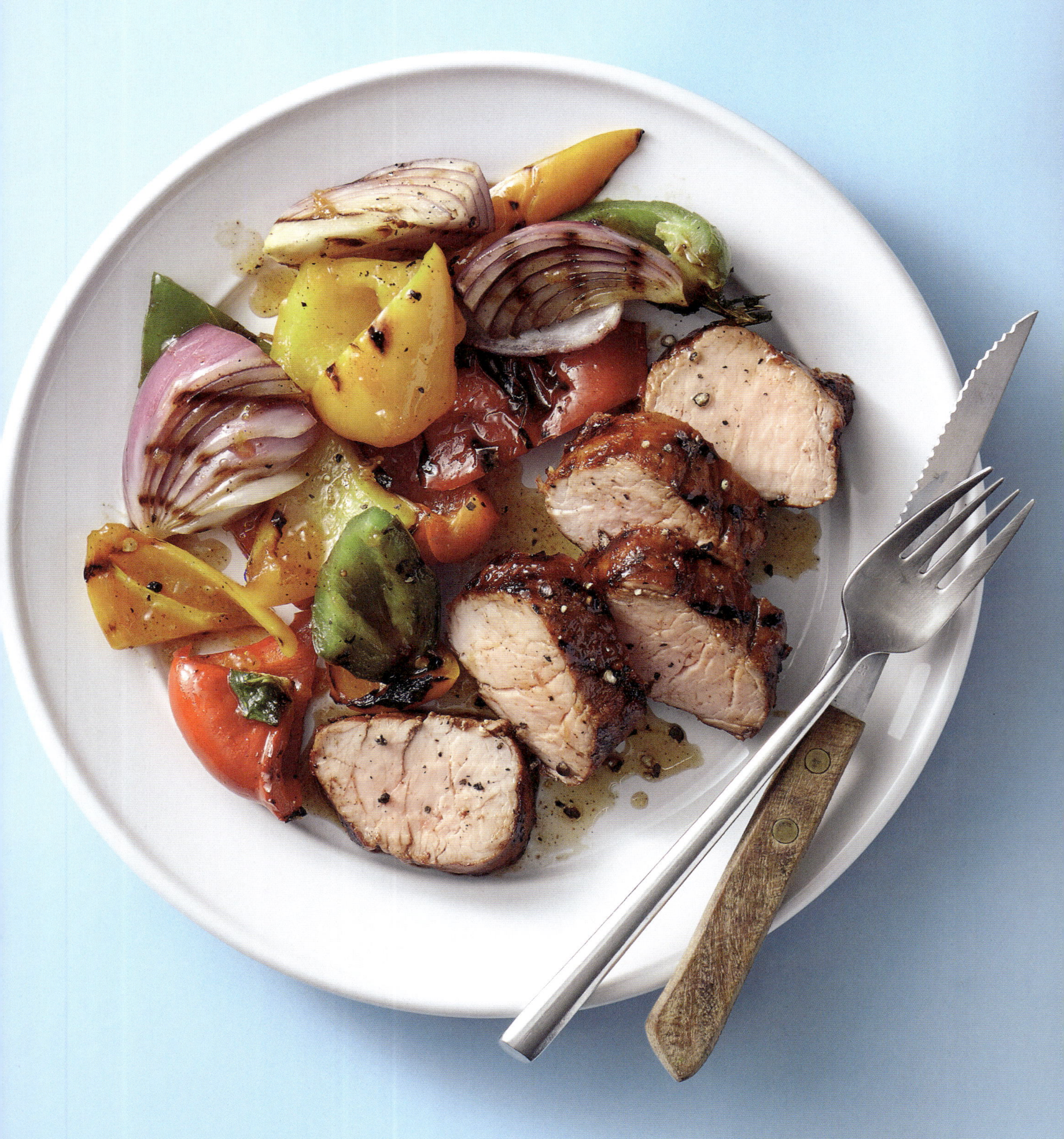

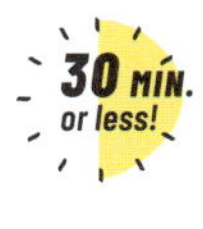

APRICOT GRILLED PORK TENDERLOIN & PEPPERS

ACTIVE 25 min. **TOTAL** 25 min. **SERVES** 4

- 4 peppers (red, yellow, or a combination), quartered
- 1 red onion, cut into ½-inch wedges
- 1 Tbsp olive oil
- 2 small pork tenderloins, about ¾ lb each
- Kosher salt and pepper
- ¼ cup apricot jam
- 2 Tbsp white wine vinegar

1. Heat grill over medium heat-high. Toss peppers and red onion with oil and season with salt and pepper.
2. Season pork tenderloins with ¼ teaspoon each salt and pepper. Grill vegetables and pork, covered, turning occasionally, until vegetables are tender, 8 to 10 minutes. Transfer vegetables to a cutting board.
3. Mix apricot jam and vinegar in a bowl. Continue grilling pork, basting with sauce until cooked through (145°F), 3 to 6 minutes. Let rest 5 minutes before slicing. Coarsely chop peppers and serve with onion, pork, and any remaining sauce.

PER SERVING *About 321 cal, 9 g fat (2.5 g sat), 95 mg chol, 333 mg sodium, 23 g carb, 3 g fiber, 14.5 g sugar (6 g added sugar), 36 g pro*

LOVE YOUR LEFTOVERS

Slice only the pork you plan on eating at this meal. Refrigerate the remaining pork and vegetables in separate containers for up to three days. You can slice and serve the pork cold in sandwiches alongside the peppers and onions or reheat all, then slice the pork.

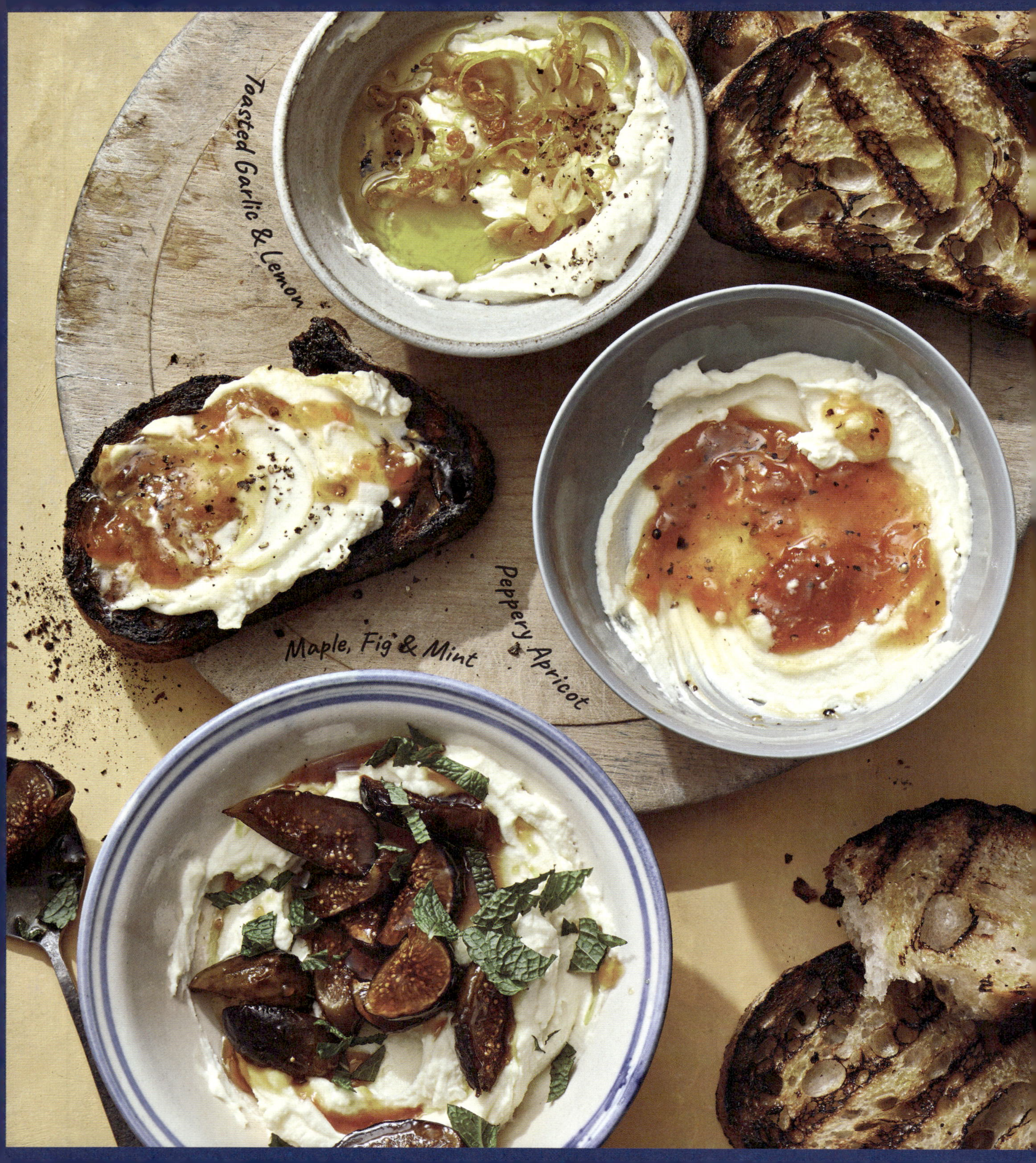
Toasted Garlic & Lemon
Maple, Fig & Mint
Peppery Apricot

Dip Dip Hooray!

Looking for a snack that's both tasty and satisfying? Scoop into these protein-packed dips with crunchy cucumber slices, sweet bell pepper strips, or warm whole-grain pita wedges.

WHIPPED RICOTTA THREE WAYS

ACTIVE 15 min. **TOTAL** 15 min. **SERVES** 8

1½ cups ricotta cheese

Milk, for thinning (if ricotta is low-moisture)

Kosher salt

Apricot, fig and lemon-garlic toppings

8 slices sourdough bread, grilled

Using electric mixer, beat ricotta on medium, adding milk if needed, until light and fluffy, 2 to 3 minutes. Taste and season with ⅛ teaspoon salt if needed. Transfer to bowl, top as desired, and serve with bread.

TOASTED GARLIC & LEMON

Heat 3 tablespoons **olive oil** in a small skillet on low. Add 2 cloves **garlic** (thinly sliced) and one 2-inch-long strip **lemon zest** (thinly sliced) and cook until garlic is golden brown, 4 to 6 minutes.

PER SERVING *About 269 cal, 12 g fat (4.5 g sat), 24 mg chol, 387 mg sodium, 29 g carb, 1.5 g fiber, 1.5 g sugar (0 g added sugar), 11 g pro*

PEPPERY APRICOT

In a small bowl, whisk together 3 tablespoons **apricot preserves**, 1 teaspoon **rice vinegar**, and coarsely cracked **black pepper**.

PER SERVING *About 241 cal, 7 g fat (4 g sat), 24 mg chol, 393 mg sodium, 34 g carb, 1.5 g fiber, 5 g sugar (0 g added sugar), 11 g pro*

MAPLE, FIG & MINT

Heat oven to 350°F. In an 8- by 8-inch glass baking dish, toss 8 oz **figs** (trimmed and quartered) with 1 tablespoon **olive oil** and ½ tablespoon **pure maple syrup**. Bake until juicy and caramelized, about 20 minutes. Top with ¼ cup **mint leaves** (chopped).

PER SERVING *263 cal, 8.5 g fat (4.5 g sat), 24 mg chol, 388 mg sodium, 35 g carb, 2.5 g fiber, 7 g sugar (0.5 g added sugar), 11 g pro*

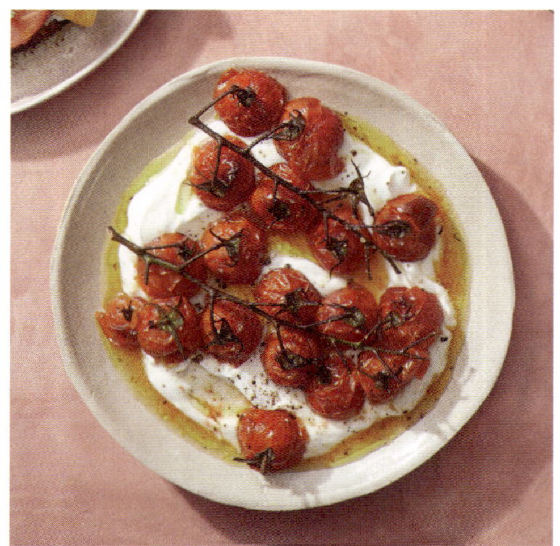

WHIPPED COTTAGE CHEESE *with* ROASTED TOMATOES

ACTIVE 5 min. **TOTAL** 15 min. **SERVES** 4

On a small rimmed baking sheet, toss 1 pound **cherry tomatoes** with 2 tablespoons **olive oil** and ¼ teaspoon each **kosher salt** and **pepper**; roast at 425°F until some start to burst, 8 to 10 minutes. In a mini food processor, puree 1 cup **cottage cheese** until smooth. Spoon cottage cheese onto a plate and top with tomatoes and any juices in pan. Top with cracked **pepper** if desired.

PER SERVING *About 135 cal, 9.5 g fat (2.5 g sat), 13 mg chol, 296 mg sodium, 8 g carb, 1.5 g fiber, 5.5 g sugar (0 g added sugar), 7 g pro*

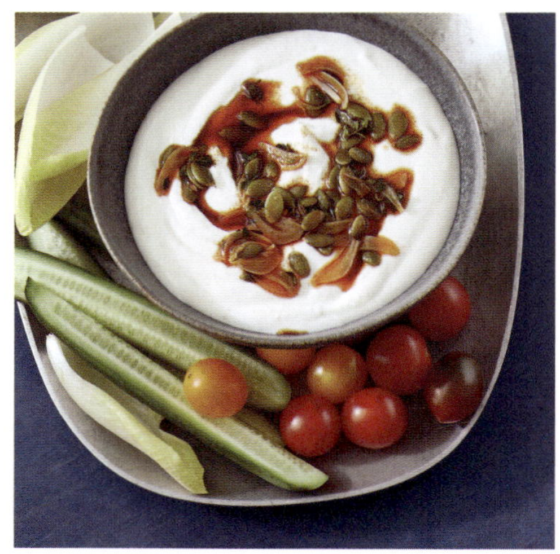

WHIPPED COTTAGE CHEESE *with* SMOKY GARLIC OIL

ACTIVE 15 min. **TOTAL** 15 min. **SERVES** 4

In a mini food processor, puree 1½ cups **cottage cheese** until smooth; transfer to serving bowl. In a small skillet, cook 2 cloves **garlic** (thinly sliced) in 2 tablespoons **olive oil** on medium, stirring until garlic begins to brown lightly around edges, 2 minutes. Add 2 tablespoons **pepitas**, 1 teaspoon fresh **thyme**, ¼ teaspoon **smoked paprika**, and a pinch of **kosher salt** and cook 1 minute more; transfer to bowl and let cool 5 minutes. Spoon over whipped cheese and serve with vegetables and bread.

PER SERVING *About 162 cal, 12 g fat (2.5 g sat), 13 mg chol, 316 mg sodium, 4 g carb, 0.5 g fiber, 2 g sugar (0 g added sugar), 10 g pro*

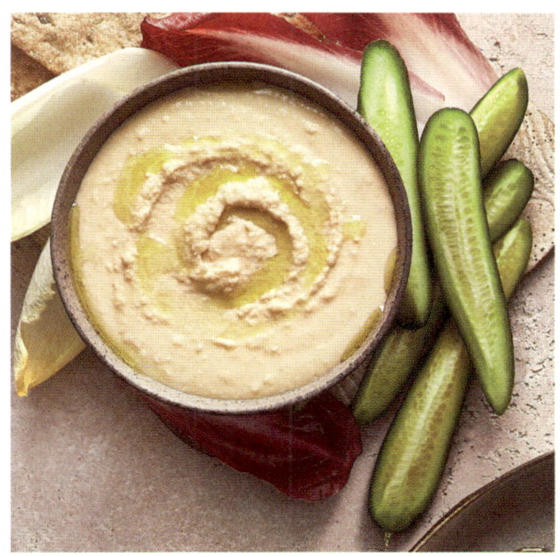

RED LENTIL HUMMUS

ACTIVE 5 min. **TOTAL** 20 min. **SERVES** 8

Cook 1 cup **red lentils** per package directions; reserve ½ cup cooking liquid and transfer lentils to a food processor. Add 1 large clove **garlic** (grated), ¼ cup **tahini**, 2 teaspoons grated **lemon zest** plus 3 tablespoons **lemon juice**, and ½ teaspoon each **ground cumin**, **ground coriander**, **kosher salt**, and **pepper**, then puree until smooth, adding some of reserved liquid if hummus seems too thick. Serve with fresh vegetables for dipping.

PER ¼-CUP PER SERVING *About 134 cal, 4.5 g fat (0.5 g sat), 0 mg chol, 131 mg sodium, 18 g carb, 3.5 g fiber, 0.5 g sugar (0 g added sugar), 7 g pro*

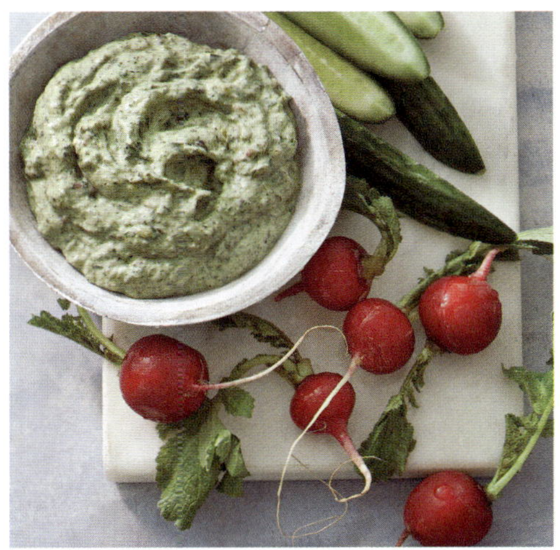

CREAMY CHARRED SCALLION DIP

ACTIVE 15 min **TOTAL** 15 min. **SERVES** 4

Toss 1 bunch **scallions** (trimmed) with 2 teaspoons **olive oil** and a pinch each of **kosher salt** and **pepper**. Grill on medium-high, turning often, until tender and lightly charred, about 2 minutes. Cut into pieces and transfer to a blender along with ⅔ cup plain **Greek yogurt**, ½ ripe **avocado**, ½ cup each **mint** and **flat-leaf parsley**, ¼ cup fresh **lemon juice**, 2 tablespoons **water**, and ¼ teaspoon salt; blend until smooth. Serve with vegetables or tortilla chips for dipping.

PER ¼-CUP PER SERVING *About 127 cal, 8.5 g fat (2 g sat), 6 mg chol, 199 mg sodium, 9 g carb, 3.5 g fiber, 3 g sugar (0 g added sugar), 6 g pro*

SPINACH *and* YOGURT DIP

ACTIVE 25 min. **TOTAL** 25 min. **SERVES** 8

- 3 Tbsp olive oil, divided
- 1 small onion, finely chopped
- 1 large clove garlic, finely chopped
- 8 oz frozen leaf spinach, thawed and squeezed dry
- 2 cups plain Greek yogurt
- 1 Tbsp fresh lemon juice
- Kosher salt and pepper
- ¼ cup fresh mint leaves, chopped

1. Heat 1 tablespoon olive oil in a large skillet on medium. Cook onion, stirring occasionally, until tender, 5 to 6 minutes. Stir in garlic and cook 2 minutes; transfer to bowl.

2. Chop spinach and toss with onion mixture. Fold in yogurt, lemon juice, and ½ teaspoon each salt and pepper.

3. Heat remaining 2 tablespoons oil in a skillet until shimmering. Add mint and cook until sizzling and fragrant, 1 minute. Let cool slightly, then spoon over yogurt dip. Makes 2⅔ cups.

PER SERVING *About 121 cal, 8.5 g fat (2.5 g sat), 8 mg chol, 165 mg sodium, 5 g carb, 1.5 g fiber, 3 g sugar (0 g added sugar), 7 g pro*

GREEK YELLOW SPLIT PEA DIP

ACTIVE 10 min. **TOTAL** 1 hr. 10 min. **SERVES** 8

- 1 cup yellow split peas
- 1 small onion, finely chopped
- 1 large clove garlic, pressed
- 1 bay leaf
- ½ tsp ground turmeric
- Kosher salt
- 2 Tbsp olive oil, plus more for serving
- 1 Tbsp fresh lemon juice
- Finely chopped red onion, finely chopped parsley, and paprika, for serving

1. In a small saucepan, combine split peas with 2½ cups water and bring to a boil, skimming foam that rises to surface. Lower heat and add onion, garlic, bay leaf, turmeric, and ½ teaspoon salt and simmer until split peas are very tender, 50 to 60 minutes.

2. Discard bay leaf and transfer to a food processor with any remaining liquid. Add olive oil and lemon juice and puree until smooth.

3. Transfer to a serving bowl, drizzle with additional olive oil, and top with red onion, parsley, and sprinkle of paprika if desired. Makes 2¼ cups.

PER SERVING *About 133 cal, 4.5 g fat (0.5 g sat), 0 mg chol, 121 mg sodium, 17.5 g carb, 6.5 g fiber, 1 g sugar (0 g added sugar), 6 g pro*

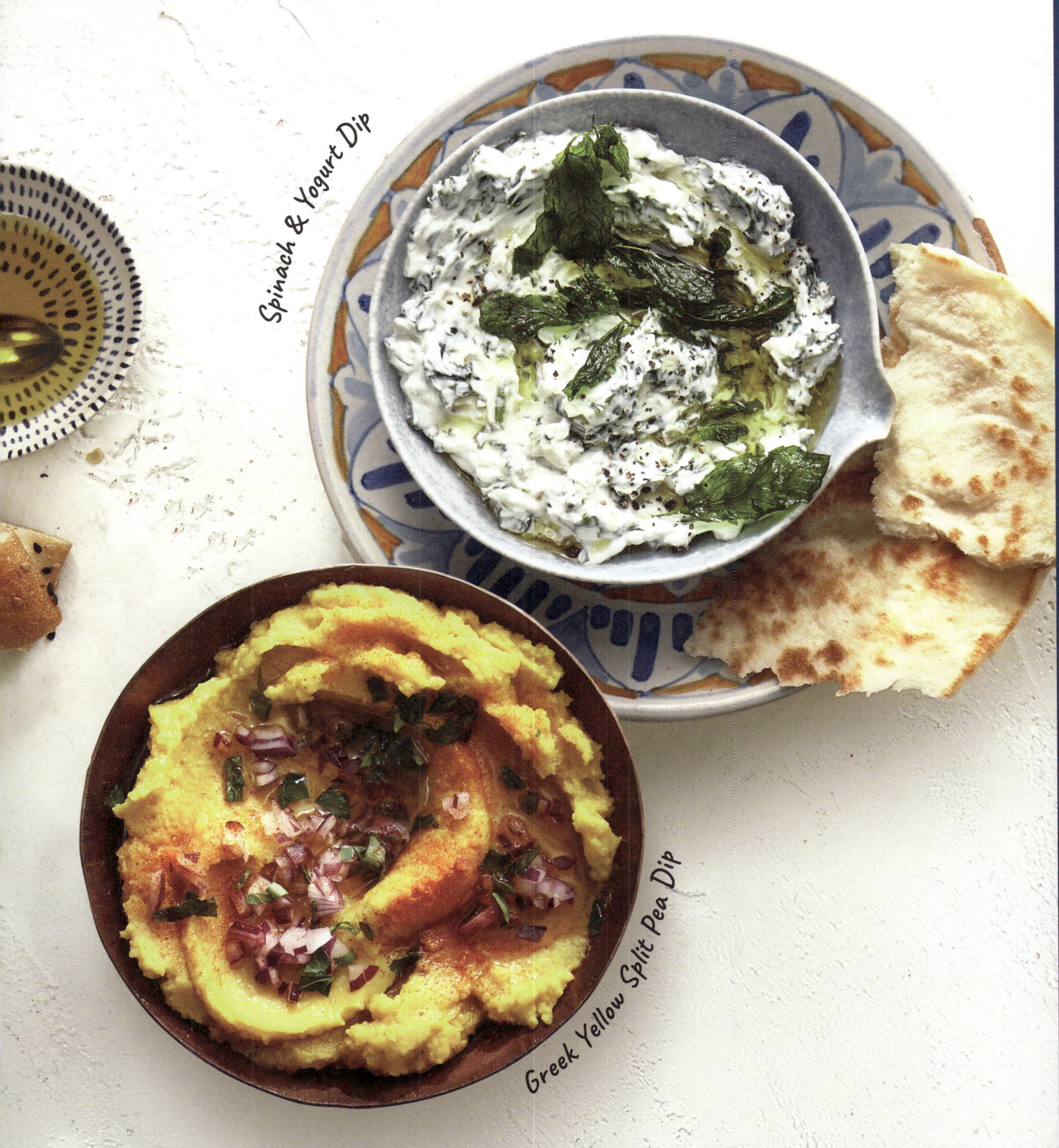
Spinach & Yogurt Dip
Greek Yellow Split Pea Dip

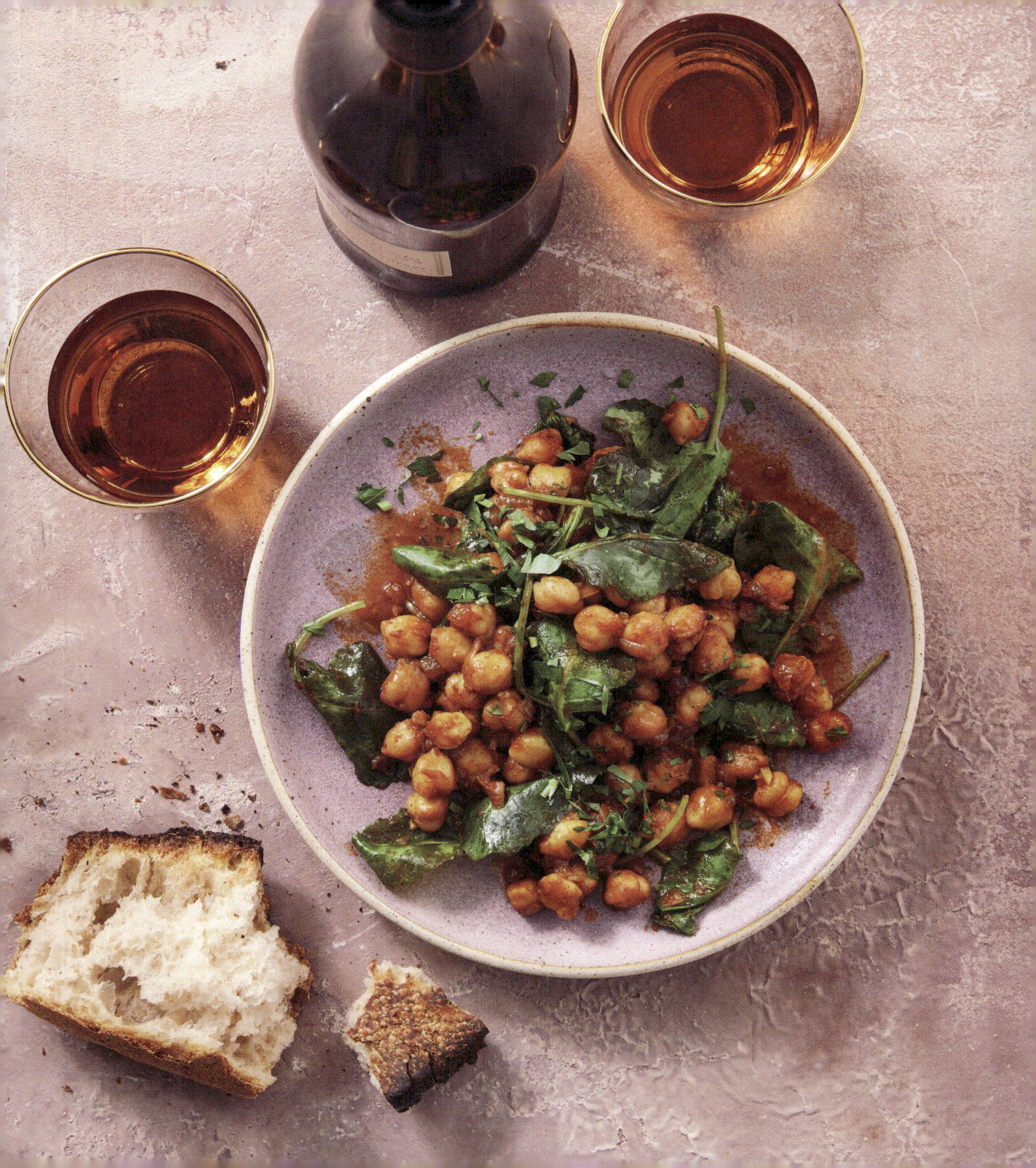

SMOKY GLAZED CHICKPEAS & GREENS

ACTIVE 20 min. **TOTAL** 20 min. **SERVES** 4

- 2 Tbsp olive oil
- 1 medium onion, finely chopped
- 2 cloves garlic, finely chopped
- 1 tsp ground cumin
- 1 tsp paprika
- ½ tsp smoked paprika
- ½ tsp dried oregano
- Kosher salt and pepper
- 2 Tbsp tomato paste
- ½ cup dry sherry, such as Manzanilla
- 2 15-oz cans chickpeas, rinsed
- ½ cup low-sodium vegetable broth
- 5-oz pkg. baby kale
- Chopped parsley and crusty bread, for serving

1. Heat oil in a large skillet on medium. Add onion and cook, stirring occasionally, until tender and beginning to brown, 6 to 8 minutes.
2. Stir in garlic, cumin, paprika, smoked paprika, oregano, and ¼ teaspoon each salt and pepper; cook, stirring, 2 minutes. Add tomato paste and cook, stirring, until dark red, 3 minutes. Add sherry and cook, scraping up any browned bits, until sherry has mostly evaporated, about 2 minutes.
3. Add chickpeas and vegetable broth and cook, tossing occasionally, until heated through, 3 minutes.
4. Add kale and ½ teaspoon salt and cook, tossing, until just beginning to wilt, about 1 minute. Sprinkle with chopped parsley and serve with crusty bread if desired.

PER SERVING *About 286 cal, 10.5 g fat (1.5 g sat), 0 mg chol, 688 mg sodium, 38 g carb, 11 g fiber, 8 g sugar (0 g added sugar), 12 g pro*

FIBER FIX

Beans like chickpeas are high in soluble fiber, which helps slow digestion, stabilize blood sugar and support heart health. They also contain insoluble fiber, which aids digestion and keeps things moving smoothly.

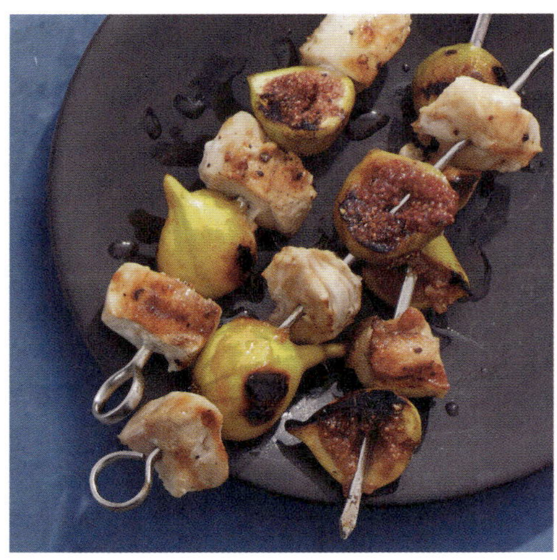

FIG & CHICKEN KEBABS

ACTIVE 10 min. **TOTAL** 20 min. **SERVES** 4

Thread 1¼ pounds boneless, skinless **chicken breasts** (cut into chunks) and 8 fresh **figs** (halved) onto skewers. Brush with 1 tablespoon **olive oil** and season with ½ teaspoon each **salt** and **pepper**. Grill on medium, turning occasionally, until chicken is cooked through, 5 to 7 minutes. Mix 2 tablespoons **orange marmalade** with 1 tablespoon **balsamic vinegar** and brush over skewers.

PER SERVING *About 286 cal, 7 g fat (1.5 g sat), 78 mg chol, 316 mg sodium, 27 g carb, 3 g fiber, 23 g sugar (6 g added sugar), 29 g pro*

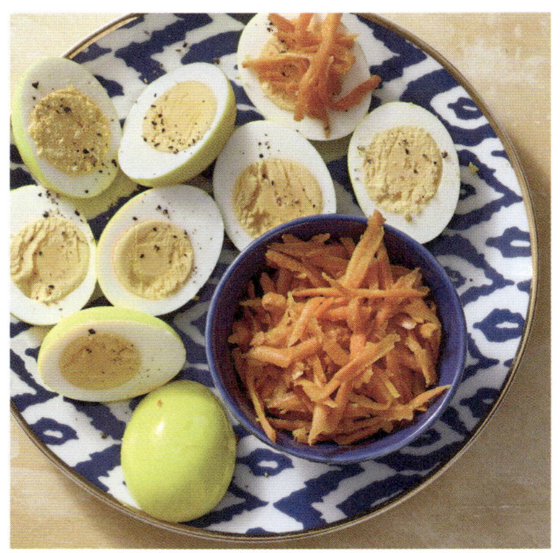

GOLDEN TURMERIC PICKLED EGGS

ACTIVE 10 min.
TOTAL 10 min. (plus 4 hr. chilling)
SERVES 4

Place 4 medium **carrots** (10 ounces scrubbed and coarsely grated) in a heatproof quart jar. In a small saucepan, bring 1 cup **water**, ½ cup **distilled white vinegar**, 2 teaspoons **sugar**, one 1-inch piece each fresh **turmeric** and fresh **ginger** (both peeled and finely grated), and 1½ teaspoons **kosher salt** to a boil. Pour over carrots. Let cool 15 minutes. Add 4 large **hard-boiled eggs** (peeled). Cover and refrigerate at least 4 hours, up to 5 days. Serve sprinkled with cracked black **pepper**.

PER SERVING *About 111 cal, 5.5 g fat (1.5 g sat), 187 mg chol, 346 mg sodium, 8 g carb, 2 g fiber, 4 g sugar (0.5 g added sugar), 7 g pro*

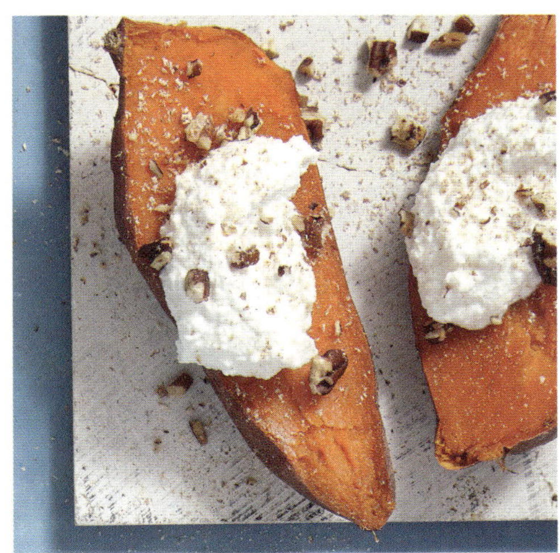

SWEET POTATO *with* SPICED RICOTTA *and* PECANS

ACTIVE 5 min. **TOTAL** 10 min. **SERVES** 4

Cook one 7-ounces **sweet potato** (pricked all over) until soft and beginning to ooze (50 to 60 minutes in 375°F oven or 6 to 7 minutes in microwave on High). Combine ½ cup **ricotta** and ½ teaspoon freshly grated **nutmeg**. Halve sweet potato, transfer to plates, and top each half with ricotta, then sprinkle with 2 tablespoons **pecans** (toasted and chopped).

PER SERVING *About 209 cal, 13 g fat (5.5 g sat), 32 mg chol, 74 mg sodium, 16 g carb, 3 g fiber, 4.5 g sugar (0 g added sugar), 9 g pro*

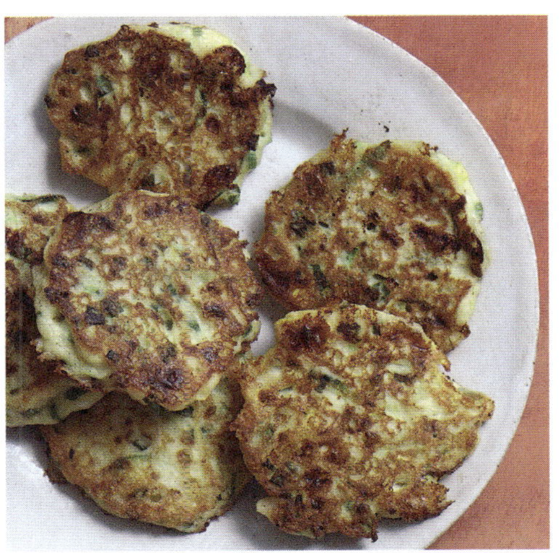

SUMMER SQUASH PANCAKES

ACTIVE 1 hr. **TOTAL** 1 hr. **SERVES** 4 to 6

In a medium bowl, whisk 3 large **eggs** and stir in 1 cup **low-fat cottage cheese** (drained if needed), 1 **zucchini**, and 1 **yellow squash** (6 ounces each; coarsely grated—3 cups total), and ½ cup each finely grated **Parmesan cheese** and chopped **chives**. In second bowl, whisk ⅔ cup **almond flour**, ¼ cup **cassava flour**, and ¼ teaspoon **pepper**; fold into squash mixture. Heat 1½ teaspoons **olive oil** in large nonstick pan on medium. Working in batches, spoon in 3-tablespoon mounds to make 2½-inch cakes. Cook, lowering heat and adding 1 teaspoon oil for next batch as needed, until deep golden and mostly set, 4 to 5 minutes. Flip and repeat cooking on other side, 3 to 4 minutes.

PER SERVING *About 245 cal, 15 g fat (3.5 g sat), 124 mg chol, 349 mg sodium, 15 g carb, 3 g fiber, 4 g sugar (0.5 g added sugar), 15 g pro*

STONE FRUIT *with* TAHINI YOGURT

ACTIVE 15 min. **TOTAL** 30 min. (plus chilling) **SERVES** 4

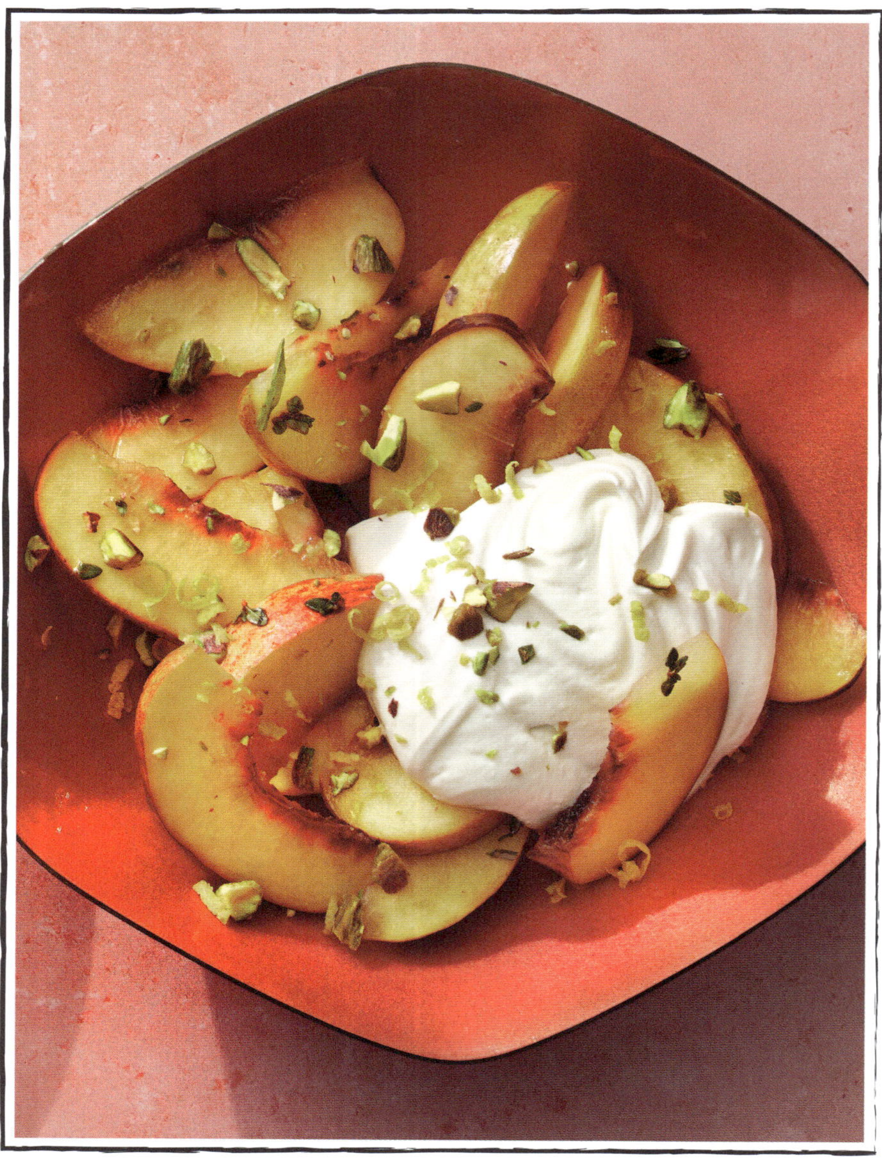

1. In a large bowl, whisk together 2 tablespoons fresh **lemon juice**, 1 teaspoon **honey**, ½ teaspoon **thyme** leaves, chopped. Add **nectarines** (4 nectarines or small peaches (1 pound, 2 ounce), pitted and cut into ¼-inch-thick wedges) and toss to coat. Refrigerate, tossing every 10 minutes, for 30 minutes total.

2. Meanwhile, in a small bowl, stir together 1 cup plain whole-milk **Greek yogurt**, 2 tablespoons **tahini**, and 2 teaspoons **honey**. Refrigerate until ready to serve.

3. Divide nectarines among bowls. Top with tahini yogurt, ¼ cup lightly salted shelled **pistachios**, roughly chopped, and **lemon zest**.

PER SERVING *About 219 cal, 11 g fat (2.5 g sat), 8 mg chol, 70 mg sodium, 24 g carb, 3 g fiber, 17 g sugar (4.5 g added sugar), 10 g pro*

SAVORY YOGURT PARFAIT

ACTIVE 20 min. **TOTAL** 20 min. **SERVES** 4

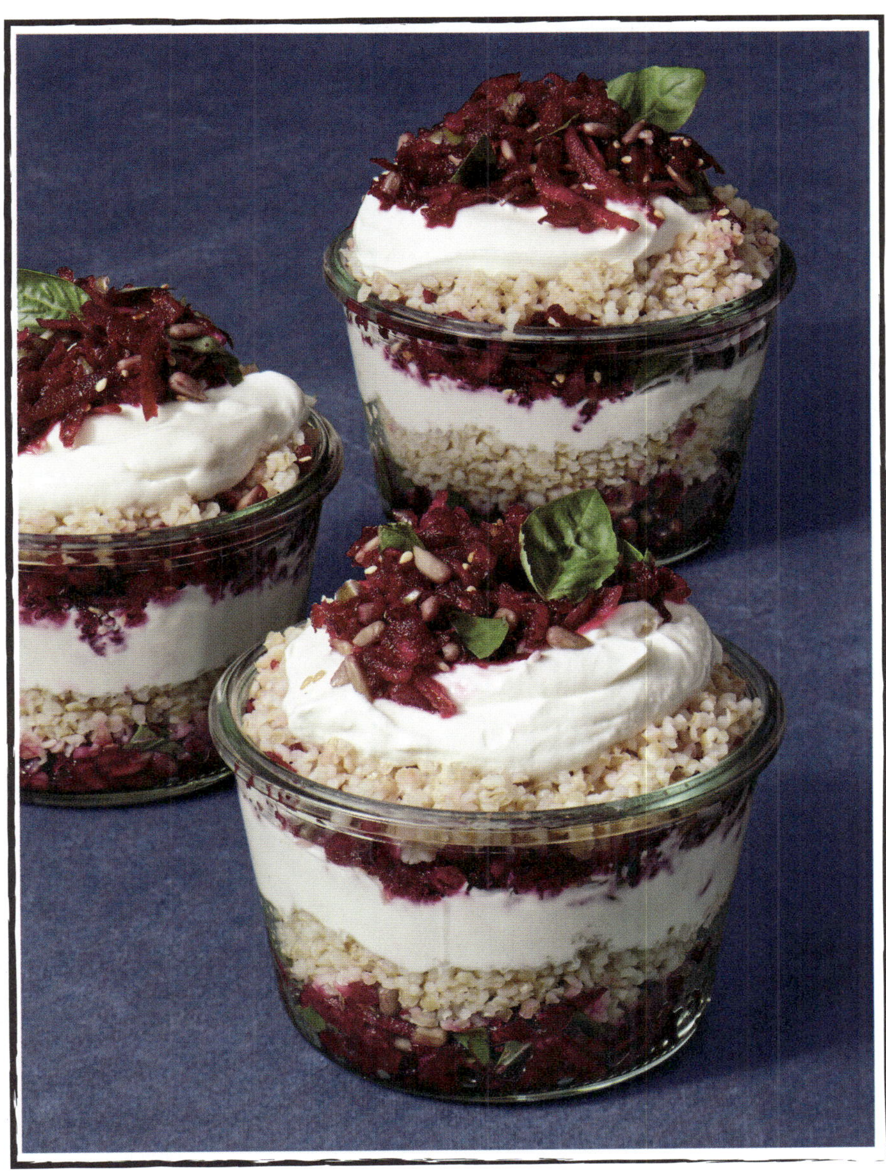

1. In a medium saucepan, bring ¾ cup water to a boil. Stir in ⅓ cup **bulgur**, reduce heat, and simmer, covered, until nearly tender, 8 to 10 minutes. Remove from heat; let sit, covered, 3 minutes, then fluff with fork.

2. Meanwhile, in a medium bowl, toss together 2 medium **Granny Smith apples** (about 7 ounces each; unpeeled and coarsely grated) and 2 small **beets** (about 3 ounces each; peeled and coarsely grated), 1 tablespoon **honey**, ½ teaspoon **cumin** seeds (toasted), and ¼ teaspoon each **kosher salt** and **pepper**, then toss with ¼ cup **roasted salted sunflower seeds**, ⅓ cup fresh **basil leaves** (chopped), and 1 tablespoon **toasted sesame seeds**.

3. In four 12-ounce jars, layer ¼ cup apple-beet mixture, 2 tablespoons cooked bulgur, and ⅓ cup plain **Greek yogurt**. Repeat layering process once more for each jar, then divide any remaining apple-beet mixture on top.

PER SERVING *About 345 cal, 14 g fat (4.5 g sat), 22 mg chol, 261 mg sodium, 36 g carb, 6 g fiber, 21.5 g sugar (4.5 g added sugar), 20 g pro*

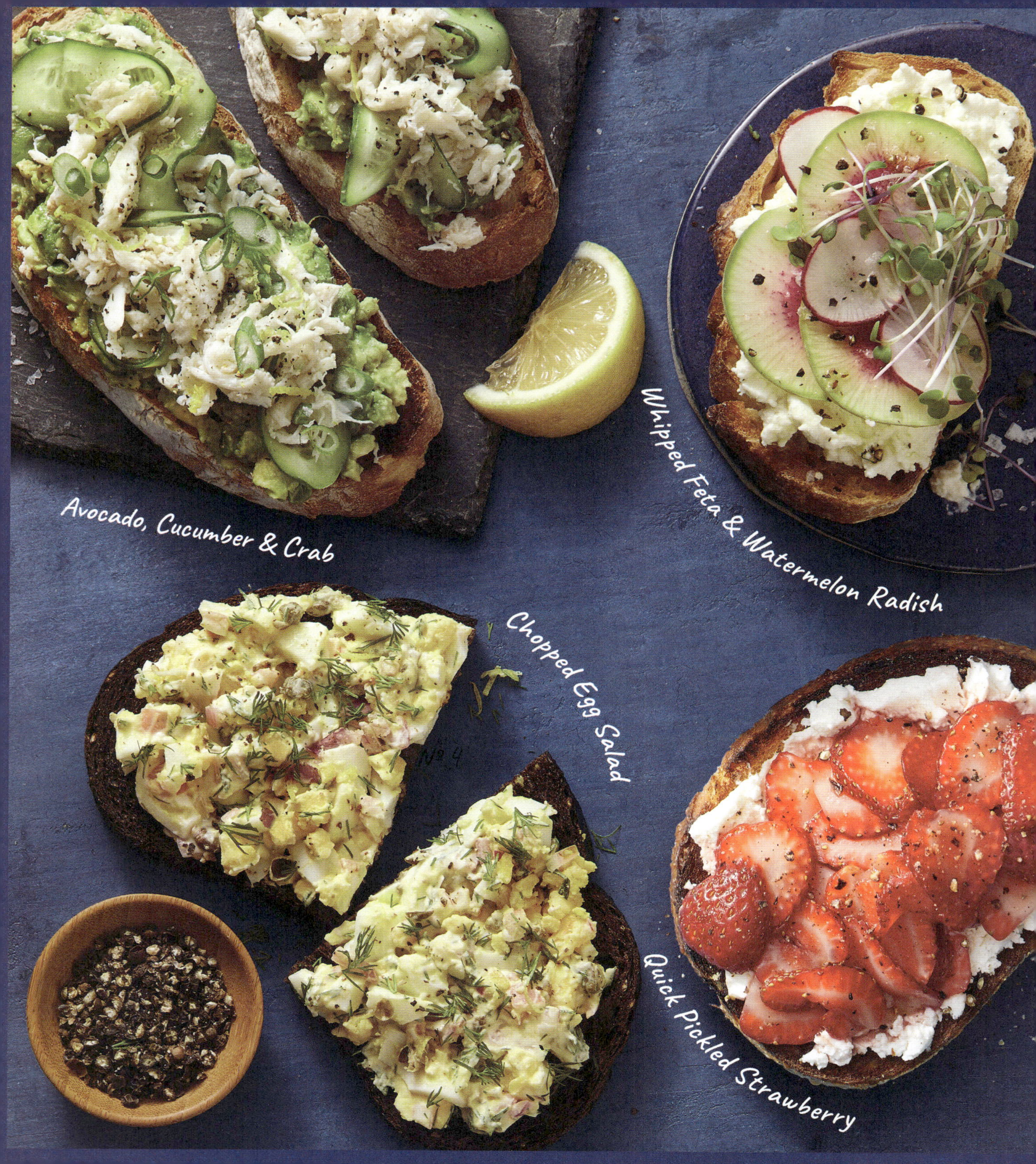

Avocado, Cucumber & Crab
Whipped Feta & Watermelon Radish
Chopped Egg Salad
Quick Pickled Strawberry

A Special Toast

Pile on the protein with these tasty toast creations. Each one starts with crispy bread to deliver big flavor and a well-balanced boost of nutrition.

AVOCADO, CUCUMBER, & CRAB TOAST

ACTIVE 10 min.
TOTAL 10 min.
SERVES 4

Divide 1 ripe **avocado** among 4 slices toast, season with a pinch each of **salt** and **pepper** and mash with fork. Using vegetable peeler, thinly slice 2 **Persian cucumbers** lengthwise and arrange on top. Top with 8 ounce **lump crabmeat** and 1 **scallion** (thinly sliced on bias). Grate **lemon zest** on top, then squeeze on a touch of **lemon juice** and season with a pinch each of **salt** and **pepper**.

PER SERVING *About 234 cal, 9.5 g fat (1.5 g sat), 55 mg chol, 424 mg sodium, 25 g carb, 4.5 g fiber, 3 g sugar (1.5 g added sugar), 14 g pro*

WHIPPED FETA & WATERMELON RADISH TOAST

ACTIVE 10 min.
TOTAL 10 min.
SERVES 4

In a mini food processor, puree 3 ounces **feta cheese** (broken into pieces) and 2 tablespoons **milk** until smooth, adding more milk as necessary; spread on 4 thick slices sourdough toast. Top with 1 medium **watermelon radish** and 2 **red radishes** (all very thinly sliced) and ½ cup **radish** or **broccoli sprouts**. Drizzle with **olive oil** and sprinkle with **salt** and **pepper**.

PER SERVING *About 278 cal, 9.5 g fat (4 g sat), 20 mg chol, 676 mg sodium, 37 g carb, 2 g fiber, 3.5 g sugar (0 g added sugar), 11 g pro*

QUICK PICKLED STRAWBERRY TOAST

ACTIVE 10 min.
TOTAL 10 min.
SERVES 4

Whisk together 2 teaspoons each **honey** and **red wine vinegar** and ¼ teaspoon each **kosher salt** and coarsely ground **pepper**. Fold in 8 ounces **strawberries** (hulled and sliced) and let sit, tossing occasionally, 5 minutes. Spread 3 ounces **goat cheese** on 4 pieces toasted rustic bread and spoon strawberries on top. Sprinkle with additional pepper if desired.

PER SERVING *About 185 cal, 5.5 g fat (3 g sat), 10 mg chol, 398 mg sodium, 25 g carb, 2 g fiber, 6.5 g sugar (3.5 g added sugar), 7 g pro*

CHOPPED EGG SALAD TOAST

ACTIVE 10 min.
TOTAL 10 min.
SERVES 4

In a bowl, whisk together 3 tablespoons plain **Greek yogurt**, ½ teaspoon grated **lemon zest** plus 1 tablespoon **lemon juice**, and ¼ teaspoon each **salt** and **pepper**. Gently mix in 4 large **hard-boiled eggs** (peeled and roughly chopped). Fold in ¼ small **red onion** (finely chopped), 1 heaping tablespoon **capers** (chopped), and 1 tablespoon chopped **dill**. Divide among 4 pieces pumpernickel toast and sprinkle with additional dill and cracked pepper.

PER SERVING *About 173 cal, 6.9 g fat (2.1 g sat), 188 mg chol, 427 mg sodium, 17 g carb, 2.5 g fiber, 1.5 g sugar (0 g added sugar), 10 g pro*

TOASTS WITH MINT YOGURT & SUMAC VINAIGRETTE

ACTIVE 10 min.
TOTAL 10 min.
SERVES 4

In a bowl, combine ½ cup plain **Greek yogurt**, 1 **scallion** (finely chopped), ¼ cup **mint** (chopped), and 2 teaspoons grated **lemon zest**. In a second bowl, whisk together 2 tablespoons **olive oil**, 1 teaspoon **lemon juice**, and ¼ teaspoon each **cumin seed**, **ground sumac**, coarsely cracked **pepper**, and **kosher salt**. Spread yogurt on 4 pieces toasted bread, top with 3 medium **heirloom tomatoes** (sliced), and spoon vinaigrette on top. Sprinkle with additional chopped scallion if desired.

PER SERVING *About 182 cal, 9.8 g fat (2 g sat), 4 mg chol, 243 mg sodium, 17 g carb, 4 g fiber, 5.5 g sugar (0 g added sugar), 7.5 g pro*

LEMONY WHIPPED GOAT CHEESE CROSTINI

ACTIVE 5 min.
TOTAL 5 min.
SERVES 4

In a mini food processor, pulse 4 ounces slightly softened **goat cheese** with 1½ teaspoons grated **lemon zest** for 30 seconds. Spread on 12 pieces of crostini, drizzle with 2 teaspoons **honey**, and top with 2 **scallions** (thinly sliced), 2 tablespoons **pomegranate seeds**, and freshly ground **black pepper**.

PER SERVING *About 160 cal, 6.5 g fat (4.5 g sat), 13 mg chol, 281 mg sodium, 17.5 g carb, 1 g fiber, 5 g sugar (3.5 g added sugar), 8 g pro*

SARDINE TOAST WITH QUICK-PICKLED SPICY SHALLOTS

ACTIVE 15 min.
TOTAL 15 min.
SERVES 4

In a bowl, toss 1 **shallot** and 1 small **red chile** (both thinly sliced) with 1 tablespoon **lemon juice** and ¼ teaspoon **kosher salt**; let sit 8 minutes. In mini food processor, puree one 15-ounce can **low-sodium white beans**, 2 tablespoons **olive oil**, and ¼ teaspoon each **salt** and **pepper** until smooth. Spread about 3 tablespoons each on 4 slices toast (save the rest for another use). Divide two 3.75-ounce cans **smoked sardines** (drained) among toast slices. Toss shallot mixture with½ tablespoon oil and spoon over top of sardine toast.

PER SERVING *About 283 cal, 12.5 g fat (2.5 g sat), 18 mg chol, 503 mg sodium, 26 g carb, 5.5 g fiber, 3.5 g sugar (0 g added sugar), 17 g pro*

CHERRY, GOAT CHEESE & CRESS TOASTS

ACTIVE 20 min.
TOTAL 20 min.
SERVES 4

Heat grill to high. Grill four ½-inch-thick slices **sourdough bread** until lightly toasted, 30 to 45 seconds per side; rub 1 clove **garlic** on 1 side of each slice. Toss 8 ounces **cherries** (halved and pitted) with 1½ teaspoons **red wine vinegar**, 2 teaspoons **olive oil**, 1 large **scallion** (thinly sliced), and ⅛ teaspoon **kosher salt**. Spread bread with 4 ounces fresh **goat cheese** and top with ½ cup **watercress**. Spoon cherry mixture on top and sprinkle with freshly cracked **pepper**.

PER SERVING *About 266 cal, 9.5 g fat (4.5 g sat), 13 mg chol, 499 mg sodium, 35 g carb, 2.5 g fiber, 8.5 g sugar (0 g added sugar), 12 g pro*

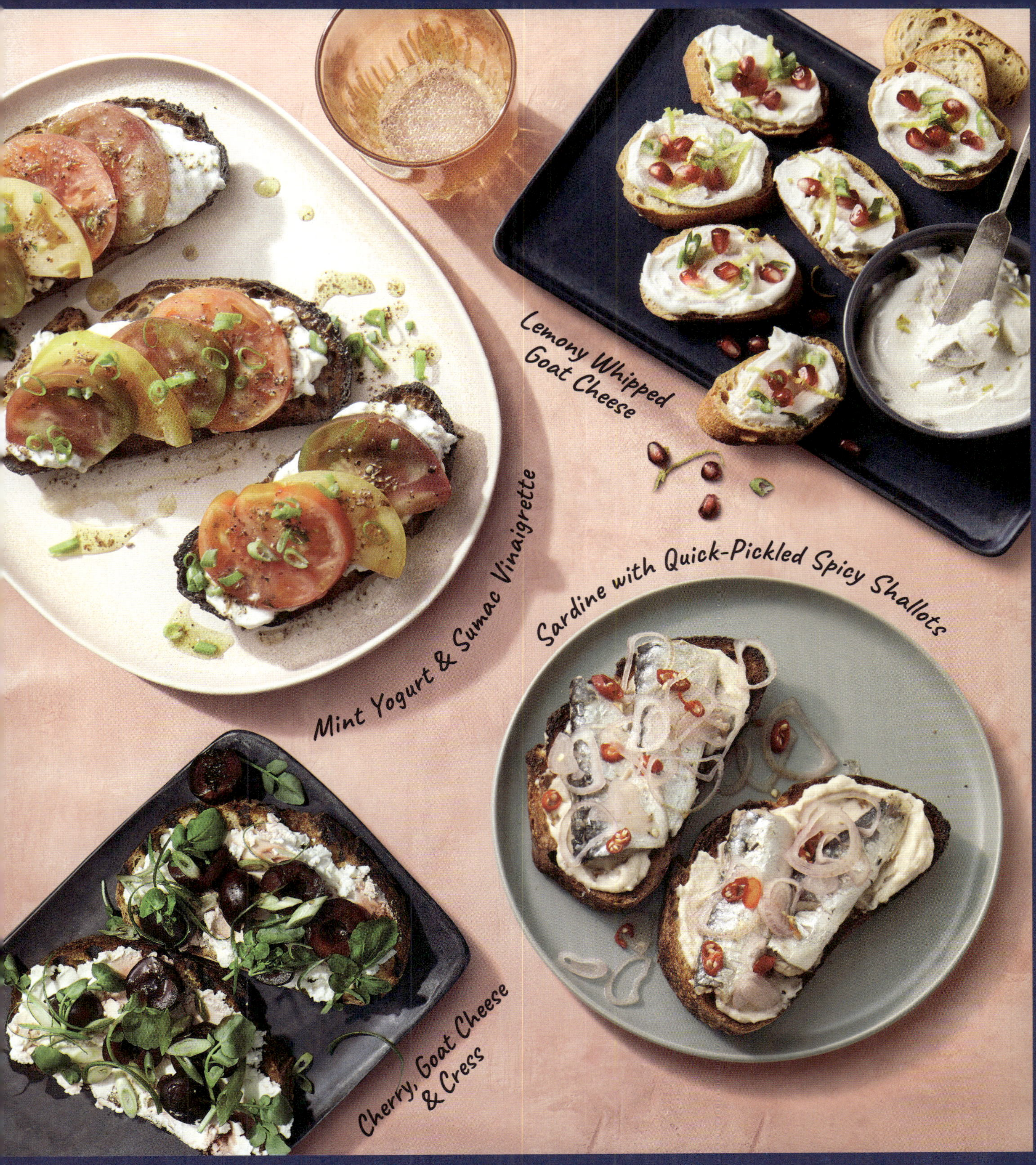
Lemony Whipped Goat Cheese
Mint Yogurt & Sumac Vinaigrette
Sardine with Quick-Pickled Spicy Shallots
Cherry, Goat Cheese & Cress

PART 3

7-DAY JUMPSTART

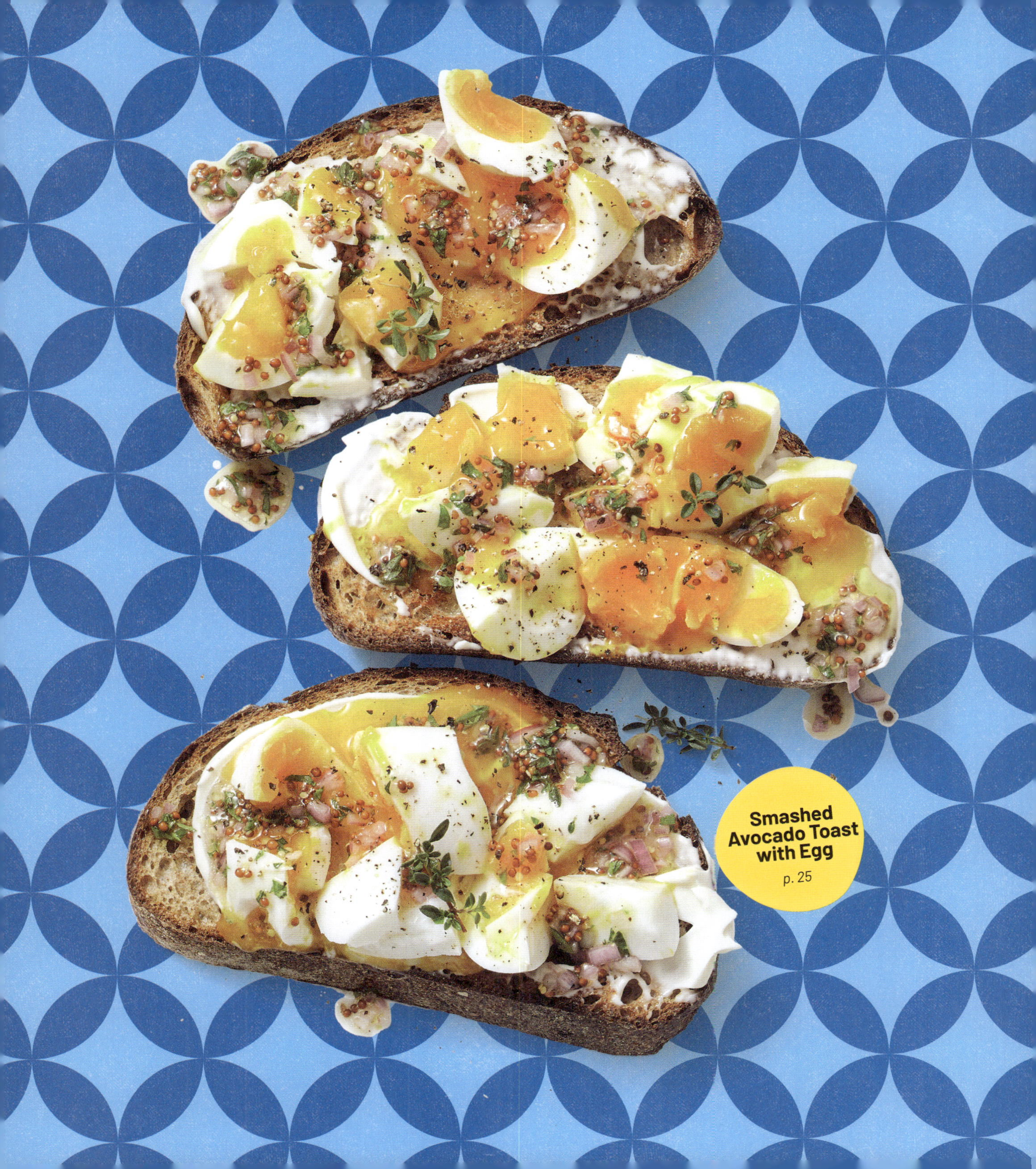
Smashed Avocado Toast with Egg
p. 25

Welcome to Your 7-Day High-Protein Mediterranean Meal Plan

This isn't your average meal plan—it's a flexible, flavorful, and protein-packed way to nourish your body, support your muscles, balance your blood sugar, and keep you feeling full and energized, plus lose a little weight too.

Our food and nutrition experts have designed a full week of easy-to-make recipes with a mix of meal prep and creative twists on leftovers to help you hit your protein goals without counting every gram.

Each day includes three balanced meals and optional snacks, built around whole, nutrient-dense ingredients like lean proteins, colorful fruits and vegetables, healthy fats, and fiber-rich grains and legumes.

Many of the meals make 4 servings, perfect for sharing or saving. If you're cooking solo, freeze leftovers for the future or halve recipes if needed. Unless noted, enjoy one serving.

This meal plan starts on a Saturday, so that your weekend features make-ahead meals to set yourself up for success in the week ahead. The rest of the recipes take under 30 minutes (some as little as 5), making them perfect for weeknight cooking (because we all know the temptation for takeout is strong midweek).

Each day is perfectly portioned with:

- Around 1,500–1,600 calories, a good target for most people aiming to lose weight safely. For weight maintenance, feel free to add in an extra snack or dessert. If you're not sure what the appropriate amount of calories is for you, consult with your physician or a registered dietitian.
- At least 90 grams of protein, as many researchers recommended getting between 0.55 to 0.68 grams of protein per pound of body weight daily.
- Between 25 and 40 grams of fiber, to align with the Dietary Guidelines for Americans' recommended intake of 25 grams per day for women and 30–38 grams per day for men.
- Mindful amounts of added sugars, in line with the guidelines from the American Heart Association.

Let's get cooking!

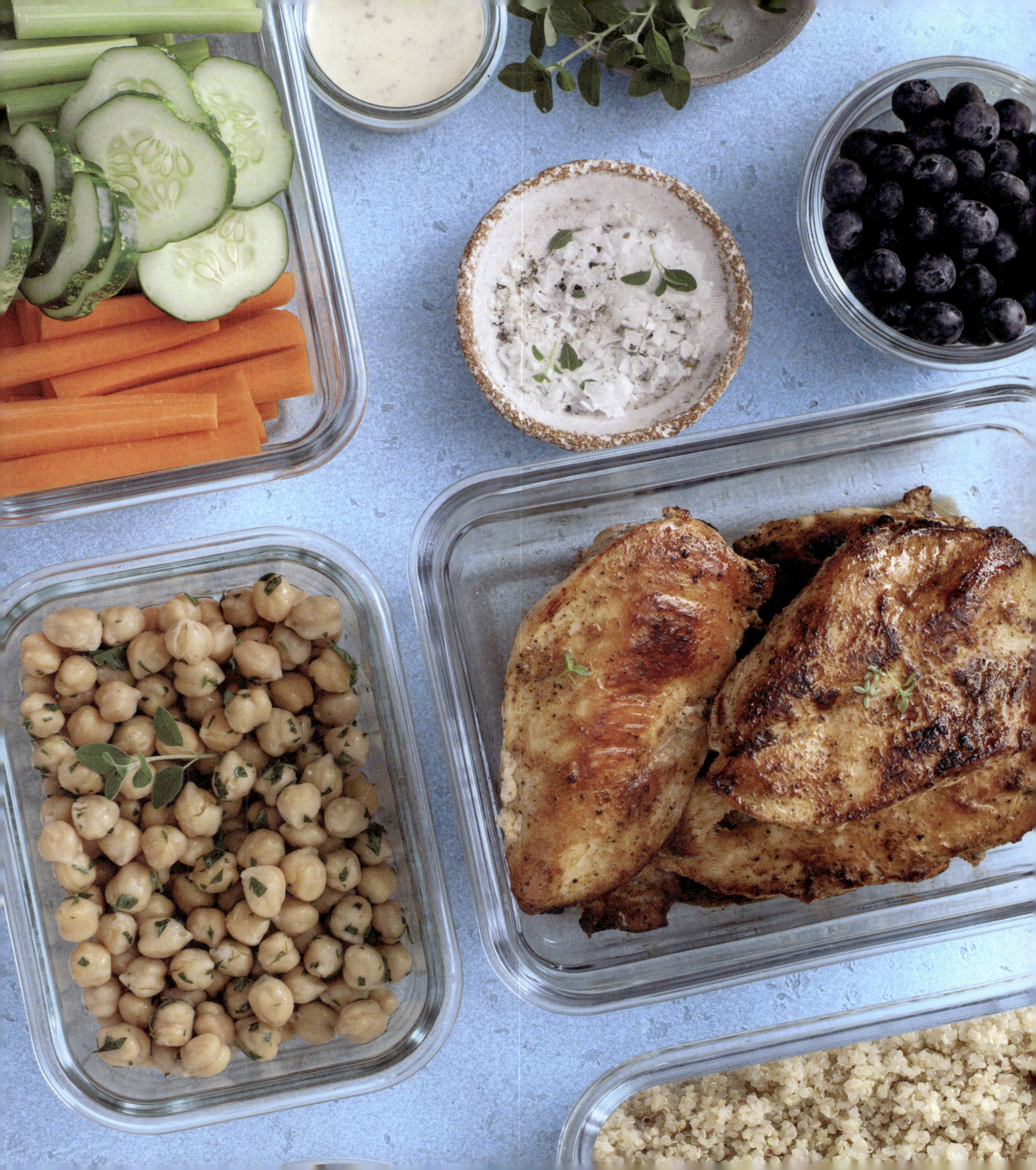

MEAL PLANNING 101: 6 TIPS TO SAVE YOURSELF TIME AND ENERGY

Our 7-Day Jumpstart is the perfect way to kick off a high-protein Mediterranean lifestyle, combining fast and flavorful meals that help you hit your protein targets. To keep the momentum going, here are some meal-plan tips for long-term success.

1

BUILD IN BATCH PREP

Meal prep can feel like a lot if you try to do it all in one day. Spread it out throughout the week. Making quinoa for dinner? Cook a double batch and save the rest for salads. Assembling chia pudding? Triple the recipe so breakfast is covered for days. Small, intentional steps make healthy eating feel effortless.

2

SIMPLIFY DINNER DECISIONS

Streamline meal planning with a simple weekly formula: Assign each day of the week its own category, like Meatless Mondays, Taco Tuesdays, Pasta Wednesdays, and so on. Or, cut down on decision fatigue by building out a weekly rotation of tried-and-true recipes the whole family loves.

3

BUILD FLAVOR EFFORTLESSLY

Adopt simple swaps to boost flavor (and nutrients) to your big-batch base ingredients (like grains) without any extra work. For example, cook rice, quinoa, or farro in low-sodium bone broth instead of water for a savory taste and a bonus boost of protein. Or, stir in some flavor upgrades to the cooking water, such as herbs like thyme sprigs or rosemary (remove before serving), lemon or orange zest, a splash of soy sauce, or a Parmesan rind.

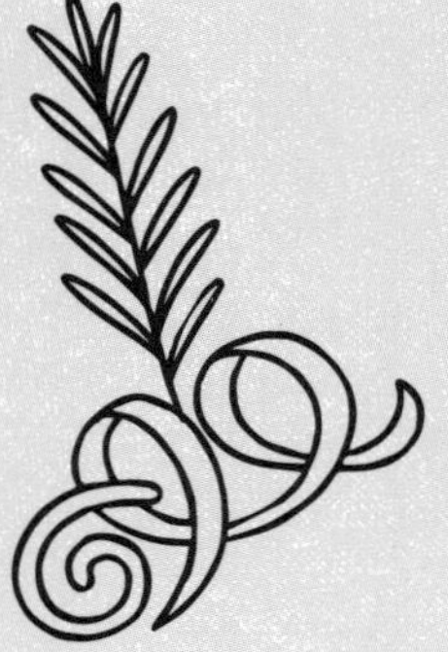

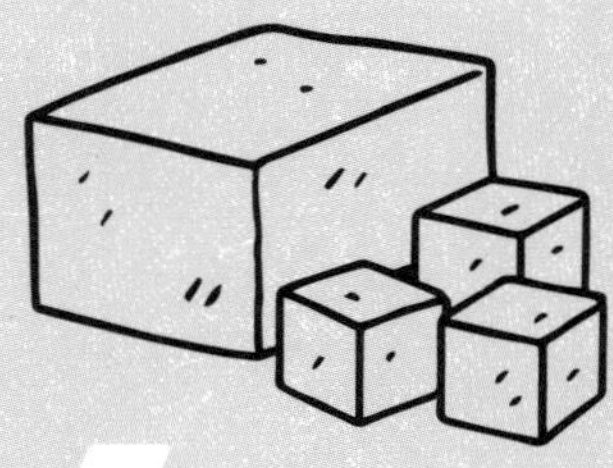

4

SWITCH IT UP

Make any recipe your own by swapping out ingredients based on your personal preferences or dietary needs. Most grains can be replaced with gluten-free alternatives, such as brown rice and quinoa. Even breads can easily be swapped out for gluten-free versions—just aim for minimally processed versions when possible. If you're vegetarian or plant-based, use vegan protein sources like tofu, tempeh, beans and lentils, or even a dairy-free yogurt in place of Greek yogurt. It's all about making it work for you.

5

REINVENT LEFTOVERS

Eating the same leftovers day after day can get boring fast and leave you wanting something different. But cooking every single meal from scratch is time-consuming and exhausting. The solution? Keep flavors fresh with simple and creative ways to upgrade your leftovers. For example, transform last night's grilled chicken and chickpeas into today's toppings for a grain bowl paired with a drizzle of tahini or tzatziki. Or repurpose roasted potatoes and peppers into a protein-packed breakfast hash topped with a quick fried egg.

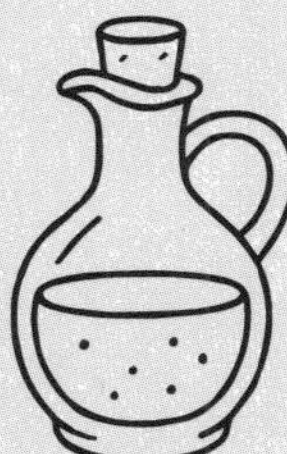

6

STORE FOOD PROPERLY

Most leftovers can be refrigerated in airtight containers for two to five days.

Store separately: Meats and vegetables reheat at different rates. Storing them apart gives you meal prep flexibility to use them in different dishes.

Keep it whole: Leave cooked meats unsliced until you're ready to reheat to prevent drying out.

Add toppings later: Store dressings, herbs, or nuts separately and add them just before serving so nothing wilts or softens if it sits too long.

Meal Plan FAQs

Does it matter what brand of food I buy?
Buy what you prefer. A few tips:

- The fewer ingredients that are listed, the better.
- Check to see if the first ingredient is a whole real food, as the ingredients are listed by weight.
- Keep an eye out for added sugar. For packaged goods like Greek yogurt or bread, aim to keep added sugars at a minimum—less than 8 grams per serving.

Should I eat my meals at a certain time?
The best times to eat are dictated by your body. Practice listening and becoming more familiar with your hunger cues. A good rule of thumb is to eat three meals (including a protein-rich breakfast) and two snacks (if needed) throughout the day. Constant snacking can lead to elevated insulin levels, which makes it harder for your body to lose weight in the long run. On the other hand, going too long without food can make you feel ravenous and reach for a quick fix. Tune in to your body, including your mood and energy levels, to make sure you are adequately nourished.

What should I do if I miss a day?
Don't sweat it, you're only human! Get right back on track with the plan and resume the next day. There is no need to resort to detox methods or extreme restriction. Just get back to the plan and recommit as best you can.

WELLNESS BASICS

A Mediterranean lifestyle isn't just a way of eating--it's a well-rounded approach to living well.

Hydration

Staying hydrated does more than quench your thirst. Water carries nutrients and oxygen to cells, lubricates joints, and helps your liver and kidneys flush out waste. Since our brains can sometimes mistake thirst for hunger, it's helpful to know how much your body needs. Instead of the old "eight cups a day" goal, aim to drink half your body weight in ounces. (For a 160 lb person, shoot for 80 oz, or 10 cups.) Water is best, including sparkling and fruit-infused waters. Don't sleep on hydrating foods too, like cucumbers, tomatoes, and watermelon (all that fiber will help fill you up too!)

Movement

There are a million reasons to get moving: Exercise helps strengthen your heart, muscles, and bones, and can also reduce your risk of cancer or diabetes, lower your stress levels, and boost your mood and energy. Luckily, exercise doesn't have to mean burpees or 5Ks. Day-to-day activities like walking your dog, raking leaves, or dancing in the kitchen count too. The American Heart Association recommends 150 minutes of moderate exercise a week. To make it more manageable, break it into 20 to 30 minutes a day.

Sleep

Quality shut-eye is about more than rest—it's your body's nightly reset button. Getting regular, consistent sleep can help your mind stay sharp, your mood stay bright, and your energy stay high. When you're tired, you're also more likely to cave to cravings. For better sleep, start with good habits—and stick to them. Keeping a consistent bedtime and wake-up time trains your body's internal clock to work like clockwork, making it easier to fall asleep, stay asleep, and wake up feeling refreshed.

Emotional Health

Less-than-perfect days are part of life, but how you handle stress is key for overall wellness. Research has shown that ongoing stress can take a toll on your heart, metabolism, mood, muscles, sleep, and immune system. To help feel more calm and in control, try some simple mindfulness tricks to manage stress, like deep breathing or gentle movement like yoga or walking.

Connection

Eating together isn't just about food—it's about community. Sharing meals with others can boost mood, reduce stress, and help us slow down and truly enjoy what we eat. Connecting over food with good conversation (phones down!) is a simple, powerful way to nourish both your body and soul.

Your 7-Day Meal Plan

Fuel your week with quick, tasty meals that bring together Mediterranean-inspired eating and the power of protein.

Day	Breakfast	Snack	Lunch	Dinner	Snack/Dessert
1 Saturday	Almond-Buckwheat Granola with Yogurt & Berries, p. 45	½ c shelled unsalted pistachios	Chickpea Salad Sandwich, p. 82	Chicken with Stewed Peppers and Tomatoes, p. 189	1 square (1 oz) dark chocolate (at least 70%)
2 Sunday	Open-Face Frittata Sandwiches, p. 28		Chicken with Stewed Peppers and Tomatoes + ½ c cooked brown rice + 1 c mixed greens + crispy chickpeas + a drizzle of red wine vinegar, p. 189 or leftover from Saturday	Skillet Shrimp with Tomato-Feta Orzo, p. 147	1 large apple + 2 Tbsp unsalted peanut butter
3 Monday	Smoked Salmon Omelet, p. 36	1 c air-popped popcorn	Chickpea Salad Sandwich, p. 82 or leftover from Saturday	Butternut Squash White Bean Soup, p. 68	½ c whole-milk Greek yogurt + ¼ c shelled unsalted pistachios
4 Tuesday	Five-Spice Apple Cottage Cheese Bowl, p. 55	Cucumber slices + 2 Tbsp hummus	Open-Face Chicken & White Bean Salad Sandwiches, p. 177	Paprika Steak with Lentils & Spinach, p. 210	1 square (1 oz) dark chocolate (at least 70%) + ½ c raspberries
5 Wednesday	Almond-Buckwheat Granola with Yogurt & Berries, p. 45 or leftover from Saturday	¼ c crispy chickpeas	Open-Face Chicken & White Bean Salad Sandwiches, p. 177 or leftover from Tuesday	Tomato-Roasted Cod with Spiced Almonds, p. 119	1 large apple + 2 Tbsp unsalted peanut butter
6 Thursday	Open-Face Frittata Sandwiches, p. 28 or leftover from Sunday	Cucumber slices + 2 Tbsp hummus	Butternut Squash White Bean Soup, p. 68 or leftover from Monday	Roasted Salmon with Charred Lemon Vinaigrette, p. 159	½ c whole-milk Greek yogurt + ½ c raspberries
7 Friday	Smashed Avocado Toast with Egg, p. 25		Roasted Salmon with Charred Lemon Vinaigrette + ¼ c green beans + 1 hard-boiled egg + 2 boiled golden new potatoes, p. 159 or leftover from Thursday	Sardine Pasta with Burst Tomatoes, p. 151	1 square (1 oz) dark chocolate (at least 70%) + 1 large apple

INDEX

C

F

G

H

I

J

K

L

M

N

O

T

V

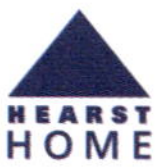

PROJECT EDITOR Drew Salvatore
COVER AND BOOK DESIGN Erynn Hassinger
GROUP EXECUTIVE DIRECTOR, CREATIVE Melissa Geurts
DEPUTY ART DIRECTOR Laura Formisano
PHOTO RESEARCH Roni Martin-Chase, Bruce Perez
COPY EDITOR Lauren Spencer

Library of Congress Cataloging-in-Publication Data Available on Request

10 9 8 7 6 5 4 3 2 1

Published by Hearst Home, an imprint of
Hearst Books/Hearst Magazine Media, Inc.
300 W 57th Street
New York, NY 10019

For information about custom editions, special sales, premium and corporate purchases: hearst.com/magazines/hearst-books

Printed in China
978-1-958395-54-7

photo credits **Alex Lau** 41; **Allison Gootee** 250 (kebabs); **Armando Rafael** 245 (hummus); **Chelsea Kyle** 10, 35, 37, 82, 133; **Con Poulos** 157; **Chris Court** 149; **Danielle Daly** 69, 77, 84, 99, 136, 137, 161, 185, 192, 211, 215, 223, 235, 236, 240, 244, 257; **David Malosh** 111; **Erik Bernstein** 114, 248; **Getty Images** 13, 14, 261; **Joe Lingeman** 29, 50, 53, 54, 61, 81, 162, 177; **Julia Gartland** 74; **Laura Murray** 49; **Lucy Schaeffer** 34, 46, 95, 121, 251; **Linda Xiao** 130, 176; **Mike Garten** Cover, 2, 4, 5, 7, 21, 23, 24, 25, 26, 30, 31, 32, 34, 38, 42, 44, 47, 57, 58, 62, 65, 66, 70, 73, 78, 83, 87, 88, 91, 92, 94, 96, 100, 102-108, 115, 117, 118, 122, 125, 129, 138-146, 150, 158, 165-174, 178, 181, 182, 186-191, 195-208, 212, 216, 220, 224-232, 239, 242, 244, 245 (scallion), 247, 249, 250 (eggs), 252, 253, 254, 257 (crostini, sardine toast), 259; **Nico Schinco** 154, 219; **Paola & Murray** 126; **Rocky Luten** 134, 153; **Ryan Dausch** 165; **Sam Kaplan** 43; **Stocksy** 9